DIARRHEA AND MALNUTRITION
Interactions, Mechanisms, and Interventions

W0235246

DIARRHEA AND MALNUTRITION

Interactions, Mechanisms, and Interventions

Edited by

Lincoln C. Chen

Ford Foundation
New Delhi, India

and

Nevin S. Scrimshaw

Institute Professor, Massachusetts Institute of Technology
Director, MIT/Harvard International Food and Nutrition Program
Senior Adviser, World Hunger Program, United Nations University

Sponsored by the United Nations University, Tokyo, Japan

PLENUM PRESS • NEW YORK AND LONDON

Library of Congress Cataloging in Publication Data

Main entry under title:

Diarrhea and malnutrition.

  Bibliography: p.
  Includes index.
  1. Diarrhea in children—Complications and sequelae. 2. Malnutrition in children. I.
Chen, Lincoln C. II. Scrimshaw, Nevin S. III. United Nations University.
RJ456.D5D5 1982   618.92'3427   82-18894
ISBN-13: 978-1-4615-9286-0   e-ISBN-13: 978-1-4615-9284-6
DOI: 10.1007/978-1-4615-9284-6

ᶜ 1983 The United Nations University
Softcover reprint of the hardcover 1st edition 1983
Plenum Press is
a Division of Plenum Publishing Corporation
233 Spring Street, New York, N.Y. 10013

Contributors

MARÍA A. ALLEN • Instituto de Investigaciones en Salud, Universidad de Costa Rica, San Pedro, Costa Rica.

*ROBERT E. BLACK • University of Maryland School of Medicine, Center for Vaccine Development, Baltimore, Maryland 21201.

KENNETH H. BROWN • Division of Geographical Medicine, School of Medicine, Johns Hopkins University, Baltimore, Maryland 21205.

*OSCAR BRUNSER • Laboratorio de Investigaciones Pediatricas, Casilla 5370, Santiago, Chile.

*RICHARD A. CASH • Harvard Institute for International Development, Cambridge, Massachusetts 02115.

*RANJIT K. CHANDRA • Memorial University of Newfoundland, St. John's, Newfoundland.

*LINCOLN C. CHEN • Ford Foundation, New Delhi Field Office, c/o 320 East 43 Street, New York, New York 10017.

MARIA E. GARCÍA • Instituto de Investigaciones en Salud, Universidad de Costa Rica, San Pedro, Costa Rica.

*WILLIAM B. GREENOUGH • International Centre for Diarrhoeal Disease Research—Bangladesh, Dacca-2, Bangladesh.

*RICHARD L. GUERRANT • Division of Geographic Medicine, University of Virginia School of Medicine, Charlottesville, Virginia 22908.

*OSCAR HARKAVY • Population Office, The Ford Foundation, 320 East 43 Street, New York, New York 10017.

PATRICIA JIMÉNEZ • Instituto de Investigaciones en Salud, Universidad de Costa Rica, San Pedro, Costa Rica.

Asterisk (*) precedes names of participants at the conference upon which this volume is based

*GERALD T. KEUSCH • Division of Geographic Medicine, Tufts University School of Medicine–New England Medical Center Hospital, 136 Harrison Avenue, Boston, Massachusetts 02111.

M. KHATOON • International Centre for Diarrhoeal Disease Research—Bangladesh, Dacca-2, Bangladesh.

*DILIP MAHALANABIS • Kothari Centre of Research in Gastroenterology, Calcutta, India.

*REYNALDO MARTORELL • Food Research Institute, Stanford University, Stanford, California 94305.

*LEONARDO J. MATA • Instituto de Investigaciones en Salud, Universidad de Costa Rica, San Pedro, Costa Rica.

MICHAEL H. MERSON • International Centre for Diarrhoeal Disease Research—Bangladesh, Dacca-2, Bangladesh.

*A. MAJID MOLLA • International Centre for Diarrhoeal Disease Research—Bangladesh, Dacca-2, Bangladesh.

*AYESHA MOLLA • International Centre for Diarrhoeal Disease Research—Bangladesh, Dacca-2, Bangladesh.

ELIZABETH D. MOYER • Research Division, Cutter Laboratories, Berkeley, California.

*IMRAN OZALP • Hacettepe University, Faculty of Medicine, Department of Biochemistry, Hacettepe, Ankara, Turkey.

MICHAEL C. POWANDA • Department of the Army, Division of Cutaneous Hazards, Letterman Army Institute of Research, Presidio of San Francisco, California 94129.

*M. MUJIBUR RAHAMAN • International Centre for Diarrhoeal Disease Research—Bangladesh, Dacca-2, Bangladesh.

MARÍA E. RODRÍGUEZ • Instituto de Investigaciones en Salud, Universidad de Costa Rica, San Pedro, Costa Rica.

*JON E. ROHDE • c/o Management Sciences for Health, P.O. Box 2560, Port-au-Prince, Haiti.

*M. G. M. ROWLAND • MRC Laboratories Fajara, P.O. Box 273, Banjul, The Gambia, West Africa.

S. SAHNI • Janeway Child Health Center, St. John's, Newfoundland.

S. A. SARKER • International Centre for Diarrhoeal Disease Research—Bangladesh, Dacca-2, Bangladesh.

*NEVIN S. SCRIMSHAW • The United Nations University World Hunger Programme, Massachusetts Institute of Technology, Cambridge, Massachusetts 01239.

*BENJAMIN TORÚN • Institute of Nutrition of Central America and Panama, Division of Physiology and Clinical Nutrition, Guatemala City, Guatemala, Central America.

CARLOS VALERIN • Instituto de Investigaciones en Salud, Universidad de Costa Rica, San Pedro, Costa Rica.

*AREE VALYASEVI • Mahidol University Research Center, Ramathibodi Hospital, Bangkok 4, Thailand.

WILLIAM VARGAS • Instituto de Investigaciones en Salud, Universidad de Costa Rica, San Pedro, Costa Rica.

M. A. WAHED • International Centre for Diarrhoeal Disease Research —Bangladesh, Dacca-2, Bangladesh.

*KENNETH S. WARREN • The Rockefeller Foundation, 1133 Avenue of the Americas, New York, New York 10009.

CHARLES YARBROUGH • Computers for Marketing Corporation, San Francisco, California.

*CHENG-CHIEN WU • Chinese Academy of Medical Sciences, Beijing, People's Republic of China.

Preface

There are several reasons why a consolidation of recent advances in our understanding of the interaction of diarrhea and malnutrition is indicated and timely. It is now widely recognized that diarrhea is a major cause of morbidity and mortality among children of poor countries. Due to recent advances in laboratory and field diagnostic techniques, many of the previously unrecognized etiologic agents responsible for diarrhea have been identified, thereby providing new scientific knowledge for rational control strategies. Increasingly these advances suggest that the morbidity burden of diarrhea may be of equal, if not greater, public health consequence than mortality. Diarrhea only rarely causes disease severe enough to require institutionalized medical care. The vast majority of diseases are of mild or moderate severity, and because of high prevalence, diarrhea imposes an enormous morbidity burden and exerts a significant negative impact on child growth and development. Moreover, the effects of successive episodes of diarrhea are likely to be cumulative. In contrast to several other childhood infections, the treatment of the diarrheal diseases is feasible because it uses simple, effective, and low-cost medical technologies.

Within the context of these developments, there has been a major resurgence of international interest in, and commitment to, the control of the diarrheal diseases. The World Health Organization recently has launched a global program for the control of diarrhea, and simultaneously, an independent international research center on diarrhea has been established in Bangladesh. The promise of effective treatment has stimulated many governments and nongovernmental organizations to implement large-scale oral rehydration programs, usually integrated into community-based health services. There has also been demand for the incorporation of new knowledge in the design and evaluation of water and environmental sanitation programs and in the formulation of international standards for protein and energy requirements by FAO/WHO/ UN University.

The purpose of this volume is to contribute to these international initiatives. The overarching theme and purpose of this book is to consolidate new knowledge to enhance the capacity of people to improve their own health and nutrition through the prevention and treatment of diarrheal diseases. More specifically, the objectives are to (1) consolidate the current state of knowledge of the epidemiology and pathogenesis of the major diarrheal diseases of childhood; (2) clarify and quantify the mechanisms through which the diarrheal diseases cause, precipitate, or worsen protein-calorie malnutrition; (3) derive policy implications, including high-priority research needs, improved strategies for disease prevention, improved therapeutic interventions, and sound international guidelines for protein and energy requirements.

The editors began the planning of this volume in May 1980. Over the ensuing months, scientists who were actively pursuing relevant advanced research on diarrhea and malnutrition were commissioned to produce background papers for an international workshop. A major objective in the selection of participants was not only relevance and quality of research productivity but also the desire to promote the interchange of concepts, knowledge, and methodologies between scientists studying diarrhea and nutritionists, representing disciplines that have not commonly interacted either in person or through the highly compartmentalized published literature. Drafts of the commissioned papers were produced in early 1981, and the workshop, involving most of the contributors to this volume, was conducted at the Bellagio Conference Center in Bellagio, Italy, May 10 to 15, 1981. The chapters in this book represent revised versions of the commissioned background papers, supplemented by four concluding chapters produced by working groups comprised of workshop participants.

The book is divided into five parts. Part I attempts to provide an overview of the book's contents. The five chapters in Part II provide updated information on the basic pathophysiology and epidemiology of the diarrheal diseases, and on the interaction of nutritional status and host defenses against infection. Part III summarizes past evidence and presents new findings on the mechanisms by which diarrhea causes malnutrition. Interventions against the diarrheal diseases, integrating the concept of diarrhea-and malnutrition prevention and treatment, are presented in Part IV. The final Part V provides a summary of the deliberations of four working groups in an attempt to synthesize information of relevance for policy, planning, and implementation.

This volume should not be viewed as comprehensive. Rather, like most topics dominated by the medical profession, it is biased toward the biological sciences. It is recognized by the editors that the diarrhea–malnutrition problem has important socioeconomic, political, and cultural dimensions. Although diarrhea–malnutrition at the individual level is primarily a biological problem, its genesis and the basis for its ultimate control probably lie beyond the biological sciences. Today, in rich and poor countries alike, the prevalence of poverty shows few signs of abating. New patterns and densities of human settlement in periurban slums and rural villages are generating unprecedented conditions for disease transmission.

The alarming decline in breast-feeding in many communities—exacerbated by commercial interests, stressful economic and time demands on mothers, and other forces of "modernization"—are compromising natural host defense mechanisms and precipitating high diarrhea attack rates. Although new and promising technologies have been and are being developed (such as oral rehydration and a potential vaccine against rotavirus) their delivery places demands on nonexistent or underdeveloped health care systems.

It is within this social context that this volume has been produced. Our hopes are that the information consolidated here is useful.

We are grateful to the sponsoring organizations for their support of the Bellagio workshop: The United Nations University World Hunger Programme, the Rockefeller Foundation, the Ford Foundation, and the International Centre for Diarrhoeal Disease Research, Bangladesh. Special thanks are also given to Miss Jane Dittrich, who provided invaluable editorial assistance during the workshop and in the production of this volume, and to Ms. Patricia Jayson for administrative assistance.

Lincoln C. Chen
Nevin S. Scrimshaw

Contents

PART III—Mechanisms of Diarrhea and Malnutrition

PART IV—Interventions against Diarrhea and Malnutrition

PART V—Policy, Planning, and Implementation

I

Overview

Interactions of Diarrhea and Malnutrition

Mechanisms and Interventions

LINCOLN C. CHEN

SIGNIFICANCE OF DIARRHEA

The diarrheal diseases are a major cause of death in all poor societies. Typically, these populations have a youthful age structure, with nearly half under 15 years of age and one-sixth under age 5.[1] Yet over half of all deaths occur in children under 5 years, the age group at highest risk for diarrhea and malnutrition.[2,3] In Latin America, for example, diarrhea was found to be by far the major infectious cause of death in children below age 5, and malnutrition was noted to be a direct or underlying cause of most deaths.[3] In-depth longitudinal surveillance in rural Bangladesh has shown diarrhea to be responsible for 28.6% of all deaths in children under 5. Diarrhea accounted for 13.7% of all infant deaths, while among children 1 to 4 years of age, diarrhea was responsible for 44%.[2]

These mortality statistics reflect much heavier burdens of morbidity. Investigations worldwide have found diarrhea incidence peaking between the ages of 6 months to 3 years, with an annual rate ranging from 2 to 12 episodes, averaging about 4 per year in most poor communities.[4–7] The point prevalence of diarrhea ranges from 5 to 15%, averaging about 10%. The global implications of these findings are crudely estimated in Table I. World population in 1980 was estimated at 4.4 billion.[1] Of 559 million children under age 5, 474 million reside in less

LINCOLN C. CHEN • The Ford Foundation, New Delhi Field Office, 55 Lodi Estate, New Delhi, India.

Table I.   Global and Regional Population in 1980 and Estimated Number
(Millions) and Distribution of the Diarrheal Diseases

Region	Population	Children < 5 years		Children diarrhea episodes	
		N	%	N	%
Global	4415	559	100.0	1507	100.0
More developed countries	1131	85	15.2	85	5.6
Less developed countries	3284	474	84.8	1422	94.4
Africa	469	86	15.4	258	17.1
Asia	2447	331	59.2	993	65.9
Latin America	368	57	10.2	171	11.3

developed countries. Assuming an average of one and three episodes per child per year in more and less developed countries, respectively, there would be over 1.5 billion episodes of diarrhea annually.[6,8] Of these, 1.4 billion (94.4%) would be in developing countries, with 1.0 billion (65.9%) in Asia.

Another way of interpreting these global statistics is to focus on the community level. A village health worker is commonly responsible for delivering health care to a target population of about 5000. Typically, therefore, a village health worker can expect to be confronted with nearly 3000 diarrhea cases annually among 750 preschool children. This averages out to about 8 new cases daily. On any given day, roughly 75 children will be experiencing diarrhea (old and new cases). Of perhaps 50 childhood deaths annually, 10 to 20 will be caused by diarrhea. Furthermore, much of the growth retardation of the surviving children in this community can be attributed directly to previous bouts of diarrhea.

Diarrhea rarely operates alone. The classic work by Scrimshaw, Taylor, and Gordon postulated that malnutrition and infections, including diarrhea, operate in a synergistic manner.[9] A bidirectional causal relationship is hypothesized wherein malnutrition predisposes the host to diarrhea, and conversely, diarrhea exerts a negative impact on nutritional status. While recognizing the interactive, synergistic relation between these two processes, it is the latter diarrhea–malnutrition interaction that is the central focus of this volume.

Epidemiologic studies in Guatemala, Bangladesh, and The Gambia[4,10–13] have demonstrated a marked negative relationship between diarrhea and child physical growth and development. Longitudinal follow-up of a cohort of Guatemalan children by Mata has confirmed the importance of childhood infections in causing retardation of physical growth.[4] Similar findings in Guatemala of growth retardation in association with child diarrhea were also reported by Martorell.[11] Regressing infectious disease prevalence by monthly body length and weight gain in Gambian children, Rowland and Whitehead estimated that monthly diarrhea prevalence was associated with − 4.2 mm and − 746 grams in linear growth and weight gain, respectively.[13] Although malaria exerted a larger effect than diarrhea, its overall impact was less because of lower prevalence. In contrast, the nutritional impact of respiratory infection was insignificant statistically. Measles was excluded because the population had been previously immunized, and the possible nutritional effects of whooping cough were obscured because pertussis was not distinguished from other respiratory infections. Seasonally standardized regressions of the diarrhea and growth data, moreover, suggested that, had gastroenteritis been eliminated completely, Gambian children would have achieved growth rates of 200 to 400 grams per month in 10 months of the year, a velocity similar to that of well-nourished reference populations in industrialized countries.

EPIDEMIOLOGY AND PATHOPHYSIOLOGY

Table II summarizes evidence of the epidemiology and transmission of the major etiologic agents responsible for childhood diarrhea in rural Bangladesh.[14,15] Regional differences may be anticipated, but the Bangladesh studies provide insights on diarrheal patterns in one intensively studied community. Eighty-six percent of children presenting to a rural diarrhea treatment center in Bangladesh had an identifiable enteropathogen isolated. The most common was rotavirus (45%), followed by *Escherichia coli* (28%). A lower identification rate of 48% was achieved in field surveillance. The major agents associated with diarrheas among children surveyed were *E. coli* (20%), *Shigella* (15%), and rotavirus (11%). These

Table II. Epidemiology and Transmission of Diarrheal Diseases

Etiologic agent	Percent (< 2 years)		Seasonality	Asymptomatic infections	Transmission		
	Hospital	Field			Water	Food	Person-person
V. cholerae	8	1	Fall	+	+	0	0
E. coli	28	20	Spring-summer	+	+	+	0
Rotavirus	45	11	Winter	+	?	?	+
Shigella	5	15	All year	+	+	±	+
	(86)	(47)					

three agents accounted for 46% of diarrheas found in the field survey. Each of these agents displayed a characteristic but largely unexplained seasonal pattern, and all possessed a pyramidal structure of disease severity, ranging from severe, clinical disease to mild to moderate illness and to large numbers of asymptomatic infections.[16-18]

Other bacterial *(Salmonella, Yersinia)*, viral (Norwalk agent), and parasitic agents *(Giardia* and *Entamoeba histolytica)* have also been documented to cause acute diarrhea. It seems likely, however, given the evidence from available epidemiologic studies, that their significance is of lower order than *E. coli*, rotavirus, and *Shigella*.

These major infectious agents responsible for childhood diarrhea are transmitted via a fecal-oral route. Cholera is primarily a waterborne disease. Enterotoxigenic *E. coli* are commonly found in food, particularly weaning food contaminated by impure water, unclean utensils, and unhygienic food-handling. Rotavirus and *Shigella* are infectious in relatively small doses, and thus person-to-person transmission is important. Although all of these pathogens are fecal-orally transmitted, the multiplicity of transmission pathways is an important characteristic, compromising the impact of unidimensional interventions, such as water or sanitation.

Of the various diarrheas, the pathogenesis of *Vibrio cholerae* is best understood.[6,19,20] The organism is introduced through the ingestion of contaminated water, and very large numbers of the bacteria are necessary to survive passage through the gastric acid barrier. In the small intestine, *Vibrio cholerae* multiply, adhere to epithelial cells, and elaborate a protein enterotoxin. The integrity of the gut epithelium is maintained, and neither bacterium nor toxin invades the systemic circulation. The beta subunit of cholera toxin binds in a specific manner to cell receptors consisting of gangliosides, and the alpha subunit of the toxin stimulates the adenyl cyclase enzyme system. The consequent elevation of intracellular cyclic AMP leads to the reduction of sodium absorption in villus tip cells and the enhancement of chloride secretion in crypt cells, resulting in loss of fluids and electrolytes.[19,21] All of the clinical signs and symptoms of cholera can be traced back to this basic sequence of events.

Table III contrasts the mechanisms of disease pathogenesis between cholera and the three major agents responsible for childhood diarrhea. *E. coli*, presumably because, like cholera, it is acid-sensitive, also requires large infective doses to cause clinical disease.[22] This contrasts with *Shigella*, where only a few organisms are sufficient to induce disease.[23] The experimental infective dose of rotavirus is unknown. The target organ of cholera, *E. coli*, and rotavirus is the small intestine. *Shigella* primarily affects the large intestine, although there is indirect evidence that it may

Table III. Mechanism of Disease Pathogenesis

Etiologic agent	Experimental infective dose	Target organ (Intestine)	Toxin	Tissue invasion	Fluid electrolyte loss	Hospitalization rate
V. cholerae	10^8	Small	Enterotoxin	0	++++	+++
E. coli	10^8	Small	Enterotoxin (LT,ST)	0	++	++
Rotavirus	?	Small	?	+	+++	+++
Shigella	10^1	Large Small?	Cytotoxin Enterotoxin?	+	+	+

also affect the small intestine. Cholera and *E. coli* cause disease primarily via enterotoxins, although there are enteropathogenic *E. coli* organisms that cause invasive disease.[20] *E. coli* organisms may elaborate one or both toxins (heat labile, LT; heat stable, ST). LT toxin is similar to cholera toxin in its genetic code, antigenicity, and mode of action. Like cholera toxin, LT toxin stimulates adenyl cyclase, while ST toxin stimulates the guanyl cyclase system, which, in turn, causes the same pattern of aberrant sodium and chloride movement across the intestinal cells seen in cholera.[24] Rotavirus infects primarily villus tip cells and induces mucosal inflammation, villus shortening, and crypt hypertrophy, but the full mechanism of its pathogenesis is uncertain.[25,26] *Shigella* apparently elaborate a cytotoxin that inhibits protein synthesis in the epithelial cells of the large intestine. Cell death, inflammation, bloody diarrhea, and invasion into the systemic circulation are all possible outcomes.[27] *Shigella* may also elaborate an enterotoxin, but this has yet to be substantiated.

In contrast to the acute diarrheas, knowledge of the epidemiology and pathophysiology of the "chronic diarrheas" is extremely scanty. Chronic diarrhea is a syndrome of a constellation of symptoms characterized by anorexia, apathy, weight loss, and prolonged, intractable diarrhea. The factors or agents responsible for this syndrome are unclear and have been underinvestigated. The depth of this ignorance is matched by the significance of the syndrome in precipitating or worsening malnutrition and in causing death.

MECHANISM OF DIARRHEA AND MALNUTRITION

The pathogenesis of clinical diarrhea is better understood than other pathophysiologic consequences of the diarrheal diseases, particularly those that cause, precipitate, or worsen protein-calorie malnutrition. As shown in Figure 1, the nutritional impact of diarrhea is postulated to operate through at least four basic mechanisms.

Food Intake. Reduction of food intake during diarrhea may be due to child anorexia or maternal food-withholding behavior, or both.[28-32] Child anorexia could be a consequence of clinical disturbances, including dehydration, electrolyte imbalance, fever, vomiting, or abdominal discomfort. Food-withholding behavior by mothers could be a response to child anorexia or culturally ingrained changes of dietary practices either in response to illness or as an active component of disease management. In many situations, the net outcomes are the cessation of breast-feeding, compromises in the quality and quantity of weaning foods, and in some cases, reduction of food intake by lactating mothers themselves.

Mata reported a strong inverse correlation between infectious disease and calorie intake in the second year of life when Guatemalan children were being weaned.[4,32] Martorell found that diarrhea in Guatemalan children was associated with an average reduction in daily food intake of nearly 20%, equivalent to 175 kcal and 4.8 grams of protein.[31] Comparison among three groups of matched children in a rural treatment unit in Bangladesh (a control group, a group with acute diarrhea, and a group with acute diarrhea encouraged to eat) showed a reduction in calorie and protein intake of sick children. The control children consumed 129.9 kcal/kg and 0.96 g protein/kg. Intensive efforts to promote food intake by having mothers encourage children with diarrhea to eat more failed, suggesting that child anorexia operated as a major barrier to improved feeding practices.[30,33] Moreover, the study showed that breast-

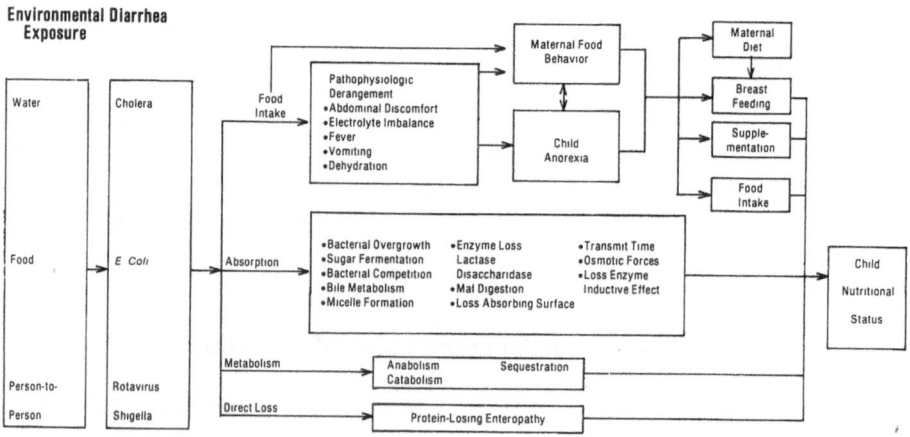

Figure 1. Mechanisms of diarrheal disease.

fed children were better protected against reduced intake during diarrhea than completely weaned children.

Absorption. Many studies have documented the malabsorption of macro- and micronutrients during acute diarrhea.[34-37] Malabsorption of sugars (glucose, xylose, lactose) and fats is well substantiated, and solid evidence exists for malabsorption of nitrogen, amino acids, and protein. Certain water- and fat-soluble vitamins (A, B_{12}, folate) and trace minerals (magnesium, zinc) are also malabsorbed.

The mechanism by which diarrhea produces malabsorption has not been clearly elucidated. Pancreatic malfunction resulting in compromised digestion is possible but has not been investigated. Bacterial overgrowth, another hypothesized mechanism, could set in motion a variety of events, including bacterial fermentation of sugars, bacterial competition for certain nutrients (e.g. vitamin B_{12}), and disturbed bile metabolism with abnormal deconjugation of bile salts, resulting in impaired micelle formation and fat malabsorption.[36,37] Disaccharidase enzymes in the brush border, the most prominent and sensitive of which is lactase, have been shown to be reduced during acute disease.[38,39] Certain diarrheal diseases may also be associated with morphological changes. Cell death or the reduction of the absorbing surface of the intestinal tract could contribute to lower absorptive capacity. Furthermore, diarrhea hastens transit time, compromising the time available for absorption, and may generate osmotic forces against the movement of substances from the lumen into the circulation. Finally, if carbohydrates are withheld during acute disease, certain intestinal enzymes may be reduced because of the absence of the inductive effects of dietary sugars and amino acids.[40]

Quantitative studies on the magnitude of nutrient malabsorption are few in number. Chung investigated, in 1948, the absorption of nitrogen and fat in six infants with diarrhea who ate normal or reduced diets.[41,42] It was found that absolute absorption was improved on the higher intake even though fecal loss increased. Whereas normal absorption of nitrogen and fat exceeded 90%, Chung noted that nitrogen absorption averaged 67% and fat absorption 52% among children on high intakes during diarrhea. Metabolic studies in Bangladesh by the Mollas showed that the absorption of nitrogen, fat, and carbohydrates was reduced during acute disease in comparison to the convalescent period in children with diarrheas caused by cholera, *E. coli*, and other agents.[10]

Metabolism. Systemic infections disturb virtually all normal metabolic and endocrine functions.[43-50] The response is stereotypic (not dependent on the infectious agent) and involves both anabolism and catabolism.[13] In the prefebrile phase, anabolic processes predominate, reflected by the secretion of ACTH, growth hormone, and the adrenal glucocorticoids. Hepatic protein synthesis is stimulated, and there is increased neutrophil production and neutrophil enzymatic activity. Catabolism overshadows anabolism during clinical disease. In general, the magnitude of nutrient loss associated with catabolism is related to the severity and duration of fever.[51] Catabolic processes are expressed as increased gluconeogenesis, glycogenolysis, and the secretion of insulin and glucagon. These processes appear to reflect an effort to increase energy availability to the host. The availability of triglycerides, cholesterol, and lipoproteins is increased. There is also increased secretion of aldosterone, ADH, and thyroid hormone. Obligatory losses of nitrogen and intracellular electrolytes in urine, sweat, and feces are increased.

Quantitative estimates of metabolic losses during diarrhea are scanty. Pollack concluded that the usual 20-day course of typhoid would give total losses of approximately 130 grams of body nitrogen roughly equivalent to 4 kg of body mass.[48] Reviewing work by du Bois and Beisel, Briscoe estimated that each degree of fever implied a basal metabolic increase of 5.0 to 8.2%.[44-46] In a review of metabolic studies on patients with acute infections, Powanda noted that diarrhea of infectious origin induced an average daily negative nitrogen balance of 0.9 g/kg/day.[49] Furthermore, the recovery phase may last two to four times longer than the acute stage.[4,12,32,50]

Direct Loss. While rarely investigated, there is some evidence of direct loss of protein and other nutrients in the gastrointestinal tract during certain diarrheal diseases. Dossetor reported frank protein-losing enteropathy during acute measles enteritis.[52] Diarrhea capable of causing morphological damage would be expected to be associated with greater than normal loss of protein and other nutrients. More subtle losses have been investigated by Rahaman and colleagues in Bangladesh.[10] Using alpha-antitrypsin as a nondigestible serum protein marker in stool, Rahaman has observed increased stool clearance of this protein marker in a variety of diarrheas, including those caused by cholera and *E. coli*, which had heretofore been considered noninvasive, enterotoxic diseases. The magnitude of protein losses directly into the gastrointestinal tract has not been quantified.

INTERVENTIONS

The framework of diarrhea and malnutrition in Figure 1 identifies critical linkages of disease pathogenesis potentially amenable to interventions. These may be categorized in three groups according to the aim of the intervention (Table IV). Environmental measures aim to interrupt

Table IV.   Classification of Interventions against Diarrhea
According to the Aims of the Intervention Measure

Interrupting transmission	Improved host defenses	Disease therapy
Water	Immunization	Rehydration
Sanitation	Measles	Intravenous
Household hygiene	Cholera	Oral
Personal hygiene	Nutrition	Antibiotics
Weaning food	Breast-feeding	Acute
Quarantine	Diet/feeding	Prophylactic
Isolation		Antisecretory agents
Disinfection		Feeding practices
		Acute feeding
		Convalescent feeding

the transmission of the infectious agent. The goal of immunoprophylaxis is to improve the defense capacity of the host. The objective of disease therapy is to reduce the severity and duration of disease, to ameliorate the negative nutritional consequences of diarrhea, and to prevent diarrhea-related mortality.

Environmental measures against disease transmission and the reduction of exposure customarily involve the provision of clean drinking water, institution of the safe disposal of human excreta, and improved personal, household, and community hygiene. Other interventions include quarantine, isolation, and disinfection.[16,17] Given the probable multiple routes of transmission of diarrhea disease, particularly person-to-person transmission, it becomes evident that simplistic, unidimensional environmental measures cannot prevent disease transmission. High rates of asymptomatic infections neutralize the effectiveness of quarantine, isolation, and disinfection. In Bangladesh the provision of clean drinking water alone failed to reduce the incidence of cholera, an entirely waterborne disease, because of multiple sources of contamination.[53] Safe management of human excreta and improved hygiene are shaped by human behavior deeply ingrained by cultural, economic, social, and environmental realities.[17,54]

It has been customary to assume that the eventual control of the diarrheal diseases in most poor communities will come about only with the introduction of clean water and safe disposal of human excreta. This assumption has been important in generating large-scale investments in water sanitation facilities in many settings. While probably correct, as confirmed by the experience of industrial countries, the introduction of new water and sanitation technologies may not be the only, or most appropriate, approach for many poor contemporary societies. Clean water at its source may be nullified by intrahousehold contamination and multiple sources of household bacteria exposure. In-depth research suggests that improvements of household and personal hygiene, breast-feeding, proper management of weaning food, and more effective use of household technologies and resources hold enormous promise for low-cost, culturally acceptable, effective prevention.

No satisfactory immunoprophylaxis technology against the diarrheal diseases is currently available. Whole-cell cholera vaccine provides only limited protection of brief duration.[16] Effective antigens have not been developed for *E. coli*, rotavirus, or *Shigella*. The recent *in vitro* isolation and culture of rotavirus holds promise for an effective vaccine in the future, and several new products are potential candidates for cholera immunoprophylaxis. One vaccine, not directed specifically against diarrhea, is worthy of mention because of its significance. Measles is often associated with diarrhea and is a major cause of childhood malnutrition and mortality. Effective immunization with measles vaccine therefore can exert a significant impact on diarrhea-associated morbidity and mortality.

The nutritional status of the host before infection is a most important determinant of host defense capacity. Immunocompetence is compromised by severe malnutrition, and various forms of mild to moderate deficiencies may also affect host defense capacity. Although recent evidence suggests that disease incidence may not be influenced by nutritional status, improved nutrition would be expected to result in reduced disease duration, severity, prevalence (secondary to shorter duration), and most important, lowered case-fatality rates.[55] Differences in the nutritional and mortality impact of rotavirus and measles between well-nourished and chronically malnourished populations provide indirect evidence of the importance of nutrition in host defense.[33,56]

The past two decades have witnessed remarkable advances in the treatment of the diarrheal diseases. Intravenous fluids are highly effective against dehydration, electrolyte imbalance, and acidosis.[6,19,20,57,58] The revolutionary development of oral glucose-electrolyte fluids makes possible the wide-scale dissemination of this simple, inexpensive, and effective medical technology.[57,60-63] Antibiotics are rarely indicated in watery diarrhea. Tetracycline can shorten the duration of choleric diarrhea and reduce excretion of vibrios into the environment, but it is essentially worthless for *E. coli* and rotavirus diarrheas.[64] Antibiotics are indicated for *Shigella* diarrhea, but wide-scale resistance against the common antibiotics is prevalent. There have also been proposals to employ antibiotics prophylactically (low-dose, nonabsorbable forms), but little firm evidence exists with regard to their efficacy, potential side effects, and applicability on a large scale.

Previous clinical research may have overemphasized the symptom of diarrhea, rather than the nutritional consequences of diarrheal infections. Improved caloric and protein intake during acute disease in one therapeutic goal deserving more attention. Efforts that improve appetite and the quality of feeding during acute disease have the documented benefit of increased net absorption of macronutrients[41,42] and also have the potential benefits of inducing intestinal enzyme activity, sparing protein loss in the catabolic process, and, overall, minimizing the loss of body mass.[40,65] Because lactose and carbohydrate intolerance is common,[26,66,67] some controversy exists with regard to the wisdom of feeding during acute disease. It is possible that the feeding issue is etiology-specific. Evidence suggests little deleterious consequence of feeding during enterotoxic and large-bowel invasive diarrheal diseases, whereas feeding during rotavirus diarrhea, where carbohydrate malabsorption may be a serious problem, deserves further investigation before firm conclusions are possible. Irrespective of feeding practices during acute disease, there is consensus that compensatory feeding during convalescence is indicated for all infections.[6,34,56,68,69] Higher intake of calories and protein during convalescence facilitates catch-up growth, hastens the restoration of immunocompetence, and fortifies the child against the onslaught of the next infection.

DISCUSSION

The most salient aspect of recent advances is the conclusion that diarrhea is not a single disease entity but rather a common clinical manifestation of a variety of pathological processes. In this respect it resembles the respiratory diseases, wherein viral or bacterial infections may all be manifested by cough and sputum. There may exist important geocultural differences in the pattern and significance of various diarrheal agents. Since the transmision pattern and pathogenesis of the diarrheal diseases depends upon an interaction of the agent and host, future research clearly needs to be etiology-specific.[70,71] Although firm evidence is lacking, it is possible that the nutritional impact of the diarrheal diseases varies among infectious agents. Fortunately, in terms of therapeutic action, water and electrolyte treatment appears to be equally effective for all forms of dehydrating diarrheas.[72]

Epidemiological field studies of the diarrheal diseases have been handicapped by several problems. First, the definition of diarrhea varies among individuals and geocultural settings. It would be difficult indeed, if not impossible, to establish a definition of diarrhea applicable to all settings. Second, field studies that depend upon client reporting of diarrhea suffer the common problem of recall omissions and biases. Validity and reliability standardizations are scarce. Third, because of lack of technical resources, new diagnostic methods of identifying enteropathogens have rarely been integrated into field studies. Thus, most of the available data are not etiology-specific.

Finally, clear definitions and concepts have not been adequately applied in field studies. Diarrhea incidence, prevalence, severity, duration, and case-fatality are clearly different epidemiologic characteristics. When epidemiological studies of diarrhea are linked to nutritional field studies, the matter becomes even more complex. Most studies demonstrate associative or correlative relationships—causality, hardly ever. Moreover, the problem of extraneous variables or multicollearity has rarely been included in field studies. Finally, since diarrhea and malnutrition are mutually interactive, time-specific or simultaneous equation methodologies are required to isolate the relative significance of each of the bidirectional relationships.

One of the most puzzling aspects of pathogenesis is the cluster of factors responsible for the spectrum of illness, from severe disease to asymptomatic infections. Disease severity presumably reflects an outcome of a still poorly understood interaction of the invading organism and host defense system. Experimental evidence suggests that even mild disease, such as Norwalk viral diarrhea, is associated with malabsorptive and perhaps catabolic consequences.[73]

Another puzzling issue has been the significance of repeated exposure to enteropathogens. It has been hypothesized that repeated asymptomatic infections is one cause of the "subclinical malabsorption" syndrome commonly observed in the tropics.[35,74,75] The nutritional signifance of this disorder is controversial and uncertain.

Still another dimension of pathogenesis about which we have insufficient information is the time relationship between acute diarrhea and other pathophysiological processes. Studies have demonstrated that the loss of disaccharidase enzymes and the malabsorption of xylose and folate correlate well beyond the diarrheal phase of the disease. Moreover, certain diarrheas and malabsorptive problems become chronic. The sequence of events leading to chronic diarrhea and malabsorption remains unclear.[74,76]

Although four specific mechanisms have been identified in the diarrhea–malnutrition relationship, it is important to recognize that these mechanisms are interactive and interdependent. It has been demonstrated, for example, that a major contributor to the malnutrition of tropical sprue is not only malabsorption but also secondary anorexia and reduced food intake.[75] Similarly, the withdrawal of food during acute diarrhea could influence absorptive and catabolic processes through the absence of an inductive effect of dietary sugars on brush border disaccharidase enzymes and perhaps through increased protein losses during catabolism.[40,65] During convalescence, it is possible that the efficiency of the absorptive and nutrient utilization processes are increased above baseline levels, facilitating catch-up growth.[50,68,77,78]

In terms of interventions, there appears to be solid justification for integrating the dual objectives of diarrhea prevention and treatment with improved nutritional status. Efforts that interrupt disease transmission and prevent exposure to infectious agents are likely to generate important nutritional benefits in addition to diarrhea prevention. Host defense capacity depends in some measure on nutritional status, and the success of immunoprophylaxis, if appropriate antigens are eventually developed, may depend upon the nutritional status of the host for their effectiveness.

These dual objectives have several components. First, it should be recognized that breast-feeding not only is important for nutriture but also confers immunological defenses.[79] At the same time, it is during the weaning period that enteropathogens are introduced to previously unexposed children. The role of contaminated weaning foods in transmitting E. coli has been well documented. Second, although the replacement of fluids and electrolytes and adequate feeding during acute disease have been conceptualized as separate actions, it may be advantageous to integrate them. Large volumes of oral fluid replacement may generate a problem of excess bulk in the stomach, compromising the space available for oral nutrient intake. It is possible that a protein-calorie-enriched electrolyte solution may be the most appropriate form of oral therapy for the diarrheal diseases.[29,80]

Third, more clinical studies are indicated to ensure that therapy is directed equally to the mechanisms of malnutrition as well as to stool losses of water and electrolytes. Antibiotics, for example, may be indicated to shorten absorptive and other nutritional defects rather than to treat the diarrhea, which may not be influenced by this form of therapy. Finally, the convalescent period should be conceptualized as a time for nutritional restoration and catch-up growth as well as diarrheal disease prevention, for without the latter, there would be insufficient opportunity for the former.

REFERENCES

1. United Nations. *World Population and Its Age-Sex Composition by Country, 1950–2000: Demographic Estimation and Projection as Assessed in 1978.* Population Division, Department of International Economic and Social Affairs, United Nations, New York, January 1980.
2. Chen, L. C., Rahaman, M., and Sarder, A. M. Epidemiology and causes of death among children in a rural area of Bangladesh. *Int. J. Epidemiol.* **9**:25–33, 1980.
3. Puffer, R. R., and Serrano, C. V. *Patterns of Mortality in Childhood*, Sci. Public. No. 262. Pan American Health Organization, Washington, D.C. 1973.
4. Mata, L. J. *The Children of Santa María Cauqué: A Prospective Field Study of Health and Growth.* M.I.T. Press, Cambridge, Massachusetts, and London, England, 1978.
5. Mata, L. J., Urrutia, J. J., and Gordon, J. E. Diarrhoeal disease in a cohort of Guatemalan village children observed from birth to age 2 years. *Trop. Geogr. Med.* **19**:247–257, 1967.
6. Rohde, J. E. Preparing for the next round: Convalescent care after acute infection. *Am. J. Clin. Nutr.* **31**:2258, 1978.
7. Rohde, J. E., and Northrup, R. E. Taking science where the diarrhea is in acute diarrhea in childhood. *CIBA Foundation Symposium 42.* Elsevier/Excerpta Medica, Amsterdam, 1976.
8. Fox, J. P., Hall, C.E., Cooney, M. K., Luce, R. E., and Kronmal, R. A. The Seattle virus watch. II. Objectives, study population and its observation, data processing and summary of illnesses. *Am. J. Epidemiol.* **96**:270–285, 1972.
9. Scrimshaw, N. S., Taylor, C. E., and Gordon, J. E. *Interactions of Nutrition and Infection*, World Health Organization Monograph Series No. 57. WHO, Geneva, 1968.
10. *Annual Report, 1979.* International Centre for Diarrhoeal Disease Research, Bangladesh, Dacca, 1980.
11. Martorell, R., Habicht, J. P., Yarbrough, C., Lechtig, A., Klein, R. E., and Western, K. A. Acute morbidity and physical growth in rural Guatemalan children. *Am. J. Dis. Child.* **129**:1296, 1975.
12. Mata, L. J., Urrutia, J. J., Albertazzi, C., Pellecer, O., and Arellano, E. Influence of recurrent infections on nutrition and growth of children in Guatemala. *Am. J. Clin. Nutr.* **25**:1267–1275, 1972.
13. Rowland, M. G. M., Cole, T. J., and Whitehead, R. G. A quantitative study into the role of infection in determining nutritional status in Gambian village children. *Br. J. Nutr.* **37**:441–450, 1977.
14. Black, R. E., Huq, I., Merson, M. H., Alim, A. R. M. A., and Yunus, M. Incidence and severity of rotavirus and *Escherichia coli* diarrhea in rural Bangladesh: Implications for vaccine development. *Lancet* **I**:141–142, 1981.
15. Black, R. E., Merson, M. H., Rahman, A. S. M. M., Yunus, M., Alim, A. R. M. A., Huq, I., Yolken, R. H., and Curlin, G. T. A two year study of bacterial, viral, and parasitic agents associated with diarrhea in rural Bangladesh. *J. Infect. Dis.* **142**:660–664, 1980.
16. Barua, D., and Burrows, W. (Eds.). *Cholera.* W.B. Saunders, Philadelphia, 1974.
17. Mosley, W. H. *Biological contamination of the environment by man.* Paper presented at the IUSSP Seminar on Biological and Social Aspects of Mortality and Length of Life, Fuiggi, Terme, Italy, May 13–16, 1980.
18. Tallett, S., MacKenzie, C., Middleton, P., Keraner, B., and Hamilton, R. Clinical, laboratory, and epidemilogic features of a viral gastroenteritis in infants and children. *Pediatrics* **60**:217–222, 1977.

19. Field, M. Mechanisms of action of cholera and *Escherichia coli* enterotoxins. *Am. J. Clin. Nutr.* **32**:189–196, 1979.
20. Guerrant, R. L., Moore, R. A., Kirschenfeld, P. M., and Sande, M. A. Role of toxigenic and invasive bacteria in acute diarrhea of childhood. *N Engl. J. Med* **293**:567–573, 1975.
21. Field, M., Fromm, D., Al-Awqati, A., and Greenough, W. B. Effect of cholera enterotoxin on ion transport across isolated ileal mucosa. *J. Clin. Invest.* **51**:796, 1972.
22. Dupont, H. L. Pathogenesis of enteric diarrhea and gut immune mechanisms in defense against enteric infection. In: *Proceedings of the XIV International Congress of Pediatrics*, Buenos Aires, Argentina, October 1974, p. 96.
23. Levine, M. M., DuPont, H. L., Formal, S., Hornick, R. B., Takeuchi, A., Gangarosa, E. J., Snyder, M. J., and Libonati, J. P. Pathogenesis of *Shigella dysenteriae I* (Shiga) dysentery. *J. Infect. Dis.* **127**:261, 1973.
24. Hughes, J. M., Murad, F., Chang, B., and Guerrant, R. L. Role of cyclic GMP in the action of heat-stable enterotoxin of *Escherichia coli. Nature* **271**:755, 1978.
25. Rodriquez, W. J., Kim, H. W., Arrobio, J. O., Brandt, C. D., Chanock, R. M., Zapikian, A. Z., Wyall, R. G., and Parrott, R. H. Clinical features of acute gastroenteritis associated with human reovirus-like agent in infants and young children. *J. Pediatr.* **91**:188–193, 1977.
26. Sack, D. A., Rhoads, M., Molla, A., Molla, A. M., and Wahed, M. A. The role of carbohydrate malabsorption in determining the severity of rotavirus diarrhea. International Centre for Diarrhoeal Disease Research, Bangladesh, 1981.
27. Keusch, G. T., Grady, G. F., Mata, L. J., and McIver, J. The pathogenesis of *Shigella* diarrhea. I. Enterotoxin production by *Shigella dysenteriae 1. J. Clin. Invest.* **51**:1212, 1972.
28. Creed, H. M., and Graham, G. G. Determinants of growth among poor children. I. Food and nutrient intake. *Am. J. Clin. Nutr.* **33**:715–722, 1980.
29. Hirschhorn, N., and Denny, K. M. Oral glucose-electrolyte therapy for diarrhea: A means to maintain or improve nutrition? *Am. J. Clin. Nutri.* **28**:189, 1975.
30. Hoyle, B., Yunus, M., and Chen, L. C. Breast-feeding and food intake among children with acute diarrheal disease. *Am. J. Clin. Nutr.* **33**:2365–2371, 1980.
31. Martorell, R., Yarbrough, C., Yarbrough, S., and Klein, R. E. The impact of ordinary illnesses on the dietary intakes of malnourished children. *Am. J. Clin. Nutr.* **33**:345–350, 1980.
32. Mata, L. J., Kronmal, R. A., Urrutia, J. J., and Garcia, B. Effect of infection on food intake and nutritional state: Perspectives as viewed from the village. *Am. J. Clin. Nutr.* **30**:1215, 1977.
33. Murray, M. J., and Murray, A. B. Anorexia of infection as a mechanism of host defense. *Am. J. Clin. Nutr.* **32**:593–596, 1979.
34. Einstein, L. P., McKay, D. M., and Rosenberg, I. H. Pediatric xylose malabsorption in East Pakistan: Correlation with age, growth retardation, and weanling diarrhea. *Am. J. Clin. Nutr.* **25**:1230, 1972.
35. Lindenbaum, J. Malabsorption during and after recovery from acute intestinal infection. *Br. Med. J.* **2**:326, 1965.
36. Rosenberg, I. H., and Scrimshaw, N. S. (Eds.). Workshop on malabsorption and nutrition, Parts I and II. *Am. J. Clin. Nutr.* **25**:1046; 1226, 1972.
37. Rosenberg, I. H., Solomons, N. W., and Schneider, R. E. Malabsorption associated with diarrhea and intestinal infections. *Am. J. Clin. Nutr.* **30**:1248–1253, 1977.
38. Brown, K. H., Parry, L., Khatum, M., and Ahmed, M. G. Lactose malabsorption in Bangladeshi children: Relation with age, history of recent diarrhea, nutritional status, and breast-feeding. *Am. J. Clin. Nutr.* **32**:1962–1969, 1979.

39. Hirschhorn, N., Molla, A., and Molla, A. M. Reversible jejunal disaccharidase deficiency in cholera and other acute diarrheal diseases. *Johns Hopkins Med. J.* **125**:291–300, 1969.
40. Rosensweig, N. S. Diet and intestinal enzyme adaptation: Implications for gastrointestinal disorders. *Am. J. Clin. Nutr.* **28**:648–655, 1975.
41. Chung, A. The effect of oral feeding at different levels on the absorption of foodstuffs in infantile diarrhea. *J. Pediatr.* **33**:1–13, 1948.
42. Chung, A., and Viščorová, B. The effect of early oral feeding versus early oral starvation on the course of infantile diarrhea. *J. Pediatr.* **33**: 14–22, 1948.
43. Beisel, W. R. Metabolic response to infection. *Ann. Rev. Med.* **26**:9, 1975.
44. Beisel, W. R. Nutrient wastage during infection. In: *Proceedings of the Ninth International Congress of Nutrition* **2**:160, 1970.
45. Beisel, W. R., Sawyer, W. D., Ryll, E. D., and Crozier, D. Metabolic effects of intracellular infections in man. *Ann. Intern. Med.* **67**:744, 1967.
46. Briscoe, J. The quantitative effect of infection on the use of food by young children in poor countries. *Am. J. Clin. Nutr.* **32**:648, 1979.
47. Feigin, R. D. Interaction of nutrition and infection: Plans for future research. *Am. J. Clin. Nutr.* **30**:1553, 1977.
48. Pollack, H., and Sheldon, D. R. The factor of disease in the world food problem. *J. Am. Med. Assoc.* **212**:598, 1970.
49. Powanda, M. C. Changes in body balances of nitrogen and other key nutrients: Description and underlying mechanisms. *Am. J. Clin. Nutr.* **30**:1254–1268, 1977.
50. Scrimshaw, N. S. Effect of infection on nutrient requirements. *Am. J. Clin. Nutr.* **30**:1536–1544, 1977.
51. Keusch, G. T. The consequences of fever. *Am. J. Clin. Nutr.* **30**:1211–1214, 1977.
52. Dossetor, J. F. B., and Whittle, H. C. Protein-losing enteropathy and malabsorption in acute measles enteritis. *Br. Med. J.* **2**:592, 1975.
53. Spira, W. M., Saeed, Y. A., Khan, M. V., and Satar, M. A. Microbiological surveillance of intra-neighborhood E1 Tor cholera transmission in rural Bangladesh. *Bull WHO* **58**:731–740, 1980.
54. White, G. F., Bradley, D. J., and White, A. V. *Drawers of Water: Domestic Water Use in East Africa.* University of Chicago Press, Chicago, 1972.
55. Palmer, D. L., Koster, F. T., Alam, A. K. M. J., and Islam, M. R. Nutritional status: A determinant of severity of diarrhea in patients with cholera. *J. Infect. Dis.* **134**:8, 1976.
56. Koster, F. T., Aziz, K. M. A., Haque, A., and Curlin, G. T. Measles in Bangladesh: Synergy between measles, diarrhea, and malnutrition. In press, 1981.
57. Cash, R. A., Nalin, D. R., Rochat, R., Reller, L.B., Haque, Z. A., and Rahaman, A. S. M. M. A clinical trial of oral therapy in a rural cholera treatment center. *Am. J. Trop Med. Hyg.* **19**:653, 1970.
58. Mahalanabis, D., Wallace, C. K., Kallen, R. J., Mondal, A., and Pierce, N. F. Water and electrolyte losses due to cholera in infants and children: A recovery balance study. *Pediatrics* **45**:374–385, 1970.
59. Kielmann, A. A., and McCord, C. Home treatment of childhood diarrhea in Punjab villages. *J. Trop. Pediatr. Environ. Child Health* **23**:195, 1977.
60. Mahalanabis, D., Choudhuri, A. B., Bagchi, N. G., Battacharya, A. K., and Simpson, T. W. Oral fluid therapy of cholera among Bangladesh refugees. *Johns Hopkins Med. J.* **132**:197, 1973.
61. Morley, D. *Paediatric Priorities in the Developing World.* Butterworths, London, 1973.
62. Nalin, D. R., Cash, R. A., and Rahaman, A. S. M. M. Oral (or nasogastric) maintenance therapy for cholera patients in all age groups. *Bull. WHO* **43**:361, 1970.

63. Walsh, J. A., and Warren, K. S. Selective primary health care: An interim strategy for disease control in developing countries. *N. Engl. J. Med.* **301**:967–974, 1979.
64. Lindenbaum, J., Greenough, W. B., and Islam, M. R. Antibiotic therapy of cholera in children. *Bull. WHO* **37**: 529, 1967.
65. Blackburn, G. F., Flatt, J. P., Clowes, G. H. A., O'Donnell, T. F., and Hensle, T. E. Protein-sparing therapy during periods of starvation with sepsis or trauma. *Ann. Surg.* **177**:588–594, 1973.
66. Lifshitz, F., Coelle-Ramirez, R., and Contreras-Gutierrez, M. L. The response of infants to carbohydrate oral loads after recovery from diarrhea. *J. Pediatr.* **79**:612, 1971.
67. Lugo-de-Rivera, C., Rodriguez, H., and Torres-Pinedo, R. Studies on the mechanism of sugar malabsorption in infantile infectious diarrhea. *Am. J. Clin. Nutr.* **25**:1248–1253, 1972.
68. Whitehead, R. G. Protein and energy requirements of young children living in the developing countries to allow for catch-up growth after infections. *Am. J. Clin. Nutr.* **30**:1545–1547, 1977.
69. World Health Organization. *Energy and Protein Requirements,* Report of an FAO/WHO Ad Hoc Expert Committee, WHO Tech. Rep. Ser. No. 522. WHO Geneva, 1973.
70. Merson, M. H., Sack, R. B., Kibria, A. K. M. G., Mahmood, A., Adamed, O. S., and Huq, I. The use of colony pools for diagnosis of enterotoxigenic *Escherichia coli* diarrhea. *J. Clin. Microbiol.* **9**:493–497, 1979.
71. Yolken, R. H., Wyatt, R. G., and Kapikian, A. Z. ELISA for rotavirus. *Lancet* **ii**:819, 1977.
72. Sack, D. A., Chowdhury, A. M. A. K., Eusof, A., Ali, M. A., Merson, M. H., Islam, S., Black, R. E., and Brown, K. H. Rehydration in rotavirus diarrhea: A double blind comparison of sucrose with glucose electrolyte solution. *Lancet* **ii**:280–284, 1978.
73. Blacklow, N. R., Dolin R., Fedson, D. S., DuPont, H., Northrup, R. S., Hornick, R. B., and Chansck, R. M. Acute infectious non-bacterial gastroenteritis: Etiology and pathogenesis. *Ann. Intern. Med.* **76**:993, 1972.
74. Keusch, G. T. Subclinical malabsorption in Thailand. I. Intestinal absorption in Thai children. *Am. J. Clin. Nutr.* **25**:1062–1066, 1972.
75. Klipstein, F. A., and Corcino, J. J. Factors responsible for weight loss in tropical sprue. *Am. J. Clin. Nutr.* **30**:1703–1708, 1977.
76. Baker, S. J., and Mathan, V. I. Tropical enteropathy and tropical sprue. *Am. J. Clin. Nutr.* **25**:1047–1055, 1972.
77. Ashworth, A. Growth rates in children recovering from protein-calorie malnutrition. *Br. J. Nutr.* **23**:835, 1969.
78. Ashworth, A., Bell, R., James, W. P. T., and Waterlow, J. C. Calorie requirements of children recovering from protein-calorie malnutrition. *Lancet* **ii**:600, 1968.
79. Chandra, R. K. Immunological aspects of human milk. *Nutr. Rev.* **36**:265–272, 1978.
80. World Health Organization. Report of a field trial by an international study group. A positive effect on the nutrition of Philippine children of an oral glucose-electrolyte solution given at home for the treatment of diarrhea. *Bull. WHO* **55**:87, 1977.

Diarrhea Pathophysiology and Epidemiology

Pathophysiology of the Enterotoxic and Viral Diarrheas

Richard L. Guerrant

Introduction

As amply documented in other papers in this volume, there is no doubt that diarrheal diseases are the world's biggest health problem. They constitute the commonest cause of death among young children in the most populous developing countries (Tables I–III).[1,2] Although more difficult to quantify, even greater is the impact of 3 to 12 severe, dehydrating illnesses per year on the physical and mental development of those children who survive. Also alarming is the recent "modernization" trend toward reduced breast-feeding in areas where very poor socioeconomic conditions result in a significant lag in the development of adequate water supply and sanitation facilities. The findings in northeastern Brazil of Nations-Shields suggest that the striking mortality of 15 to 25% in the first 5 years of life will likely increase even further as this trend proceeds (M. Nations-Shields, personal communication, 1981).

The nutritional impact of what should be an acute, self-limited derangement of water and electrolyte balance is further accentuated by the transient malabsorption state and by reduced oral intake, while catabolic demand may be increased during the acute phase of diarrheal illness. The leading etiologies are enterotoxigenic *Escherichia coli*, rotaviruses, *Shigella*, and *Campylobacter jejuni*. The frequency and severity of *Giardia* and amoebic infections vary with the setting.

RICHARD L. GUERRANT • Division of Geographic Medicine, University of Virginia School of Medicine, Charlottesville, Virginia. The University of Virginia's Division of Geographic Medicine is supported in part by the Rockefeller Foundation. Much of this work derives from projects supported by the Kellogg Foundation, the Pan American Health Organization, and the World Health Organization.

Table I. Mortality in First 5 Years of Life
in Northeastern Brazil[a]

Total	14.7%
Diarrhea	
as 1° cause, or 35% of all deaths	5.1%
as associated cause	2.6%
Respiratory disease	
as 1° cause	1.8%
as associated cause	5.8%
Measles	1.6%

[a]Source: reference 1.

Table II. Causes of Death in Fortaleza, Brazil (1976–1977)[a]

Diarrheal disease	2129	(22.4%)
Malignancy	1394	(14.6%)
Perinatal mortality	1185	(12.4%)
Cerebrovascular disease	1119	(11.8%)
Cardiac disease	825	(8.7%)
Pneumonia	677	(7.1%)
Motor vehicle accidents	655	(6.9%)
Ischemic heart disease	549	(5.8%)
Other	989	(10.4%)

[a]Source: Dr. Ana Rosa dos Santos, Division of Epidemiology and Biostatistics, Secretary of Health, Ceará, Brazil.

Table III. Age-Specific Mortality, Fortaleza, Brazil (1976–1977)[a]

	<1	1–4	5–14	15–24	25–44	45–64	>65
Diarrhea	1828	196	30	3	9	16	47
Malignancy	22	16	39	47	236	545	489
Perinatal	1185	—	—	—	—	—	—
Cerebrovascular	5	1	9	28	98	290	688
Cardiac	10	17	14	19	94	240	431
Pneumonia	331	155	31	12	24	33	91
Motor vehicle	—	29	104	117	216	122	67
Ischemic heart disease	—	—	—	4	47	165	333

[a]Source: Dr. Ana Rosa dos Santos, Division of Epidemiology and Biostatistics, Secretary of Health, Ceará, Brazil.

It is useful, both conceptually and in practical field diagnosis, to separate acute diarrheal illnesses into two groups according to pathogenesis
and site of disease in the intestinal tract. The first, arising from the action
of enterotoxins or viral agents that impair absorption and elicit net isotonic fluid secretion in the upper small bowel, results in a noninflammatory, often watery, diarrhea. The second type arises from destruction
or invasion of the distal small bowel or colonic mucosa by organisms
such as *Shigella* or *Campylobacter*, or by cytotoxins, that produce an inflammatory dysentery in which the stool may contain blood or pus. Keusch
(chapter 3, this volume) focuses on the latter inflammatory colitides.
After brief mention of enteric host defenses and microbial virulence factors, I will confine my comments to the former, more common, noninflammatory diarrheas caused primarily by bacterial enterotoxins, or by
viral infections of the upper small bowel.

Types of Acute Diarrhea

	1. Noninflammatory	2. Inflammatory
Mechanism: ⟵⟶	Enterotoxin or reduced absorptive surface	Mucosal invasion
Site:	Small bowel	Colon
Type:	Watery	Dysenteric
Diagnosis:	No fecal leukocytes	Polymorphonuclear leukocytes in feces

ENTERIC HOST DEFENSES

Several host factors influence the outcome of enteric infections,
among which poor personal hygiene and unavailability of sanitary facilities are contributing factors. Space permits only a cursory mention of
the normal host gastrointestinal defense mechanisms, including gastric
acidity, normal microflora, motility, mucus, and humoral and cellular
immunity.

Appropriate hygienic measures and sanitary facilities should limit
the ingestion of the large inocula of 10^5 to 10^8 bacteria usually required
for an infectious dose of bacteria (with the exception of *Shigella*). Second,
normal gastric acidity provides an important barrier to bacterial and parasitic infection. Its neutralization by antacids or, perhaps, food results in
increased attack rates or increased severity of infections ranging from
cholera and salmonellosis to giardiasis.[3] The importance of normal

microflora in preventing infections is often overlooked. That antibiotics predispose to increased risk of infection in experimental animals has been known for some time, and this relationship is increasingly being recognized as significant for humans.[4-6]

Likewise, inhibition of normal gastrointestinal motility enhances susceptibility to infection and impedes rather than helps normal absorptive processes.[7,8] Mucus throughout the gastrointestinal tract probably plays a far greater role than currently appreciated, whether by binding organisms or toxins or by protecting the mucosa from toxins or microbial invasion. The major roles of humoral, secretory, and cell-mediated immunity in protection from enteric infection are beyond the scope of this paper.

Microbial "Virulence" Factors

As our understanding of the etiology and pathogenesis of enteric infections develops, it becomes increasingly apparent that the capacity of many microbes to cause disease may be determined by variable gene codes, frequently transmissible among organisms, as well as by the species itself. For example, E. coli may be enterotoxigenic like Vibrio cholerae, invasive like Shigella, or harmless normal flora, depending on the gene code they happen to carry.

Among the virulence traits felt to be important in pathogenesis of diarrhea are colonization factors, enterotoxin production, cytotoxin production, and invasiveness. While several traits may be present in the same organism, the focus of this paper is on the extent of colonization required for enterotoxigenic organisms to act in the upper small bowel, the mechanism of action of the enterotoxins, and specific attack on certain intestinal epithelial cells by viral agents.

Bacterial Adherence to Upper Small Bowel

Numerous surface fimbriate and fibrillar adhesins have been described for E. coli, Salmonella, Shigella, Klebsiella, and Proteus, as well as for Bordetella, Corynebacteria, and Mycoplasma.[9,10] Among the best understood fibrillar adhesins are those required for colonization of enterotoxigenic E. coli in porcine, bovine, and human small bowel. These plasmid-encoded adhesins appear to be species-specific, such as K88, K99, and

Table IV. Effect of K88 and ENT Plasmids
on *E. coli* Capacity to Cause Porcine
Diarrhea[a]

Plasmids	Diarrheal attack rate (No. Ill/Total No. Fed)
K88⁻ENT⁻	0/8
K88⁻ENT⁺	0/11
K88⁺ENT⁻	6/20
K88⁺ENT⁺	20/25

[a]Source: reference 11.

CFA/I for piglets, calves, and humans, respectively, and are probably necessary for colonization and thus·production of disease.

Even colonization alone (without enterotoxin) may occasionally cause mild or chronic diarrhea, as described in piglets studied by Smith and co-workers (Table IV).[11] It has been suggested that these adhesins may adhere by lectinlike interactions with specific carbohydrates. They are detected by immunoassay, specific hemagglutination patterns, or bioassay *in vitro*.[10,12,13] The concepts of developing specific immunity to these adhesins, or of exploiting carbohydrate or lectin competition for their adherence in the upper small bowel, hold great promise. However, it is becoming increasingly apparent that human enterotoxigenic *E. coli* exhibit multiple antigenic and biologic types of adhesins, such as colonization factor antigen/I, colonization factor antigen/II, type I fimbriae, and probably several others.[13,14]

There have been recent descriptions of a close, disruptive adherence of classical enteropathogenic *E. coli* to villous brush border with associated reduction in disaccharidase activities.[15] Whether the less tightly associated colonizing, fimbriate coliform organisms, enterotoxigenic or not, or their metabolites or products are responsible for the well-recognized morphological, enzyme deficiency, and clinical manifestations of malabsorption associated with acute diarrheal illnesses of bacterial, or even viral or parasitic, etiology is unclear.[16-21]

NORMAL SMALL BOWEL PHYSIOLOGY

In order to understand the small bowel secretory derangement caused by enterotoxins or by rotaviruses, or possibly by both simultaneously, one must first examine the normal physiology of upper small bowel electrolyte absorption and secretion.

The small bowel is a remarkable and complex organ, the function of which determines our nutritional and hydration status, and, to a significant degree, our quality of life. It is in the upper small bowel that most macro- and micronutrients are absorbed. These include calcium, magnesium, iron, glucose, and other carbohydrates, often after the action of small bowel disaccharidase enzymes. Water-soluble vitamins and, depending on normal hepatic and pancreatic function, fat-soluble vitamins and essential long chain fatty acids are also absorbed. Furthermore, excessive bacterial overgrowth in the small bowel can alter the intact absorption of substances such as bile salts or vitamin B_{12} farther distally in the colon.

Integrally linked to the micronutrient absorptive function of the small bowel are constant, large, bidirectional fluxes of electrolytes and water. It is a relatively slight shift in this delicate balance toward secretion that results in diarrhea. Shown in Figure 1 are the striking bidirectional fluxes measured in ligated canine jejunum with separate sodium isotopes simultaneously placed intraluminally (^{22}Na) and intravenously (^{24}Na) (R. L. Guerrant and J. E. Rohde, unpublished observations, Cholera Research Laboratory, Dacca, Bangladesh, 1970). In the normal (control) state, the absorptive flux slightly exceeds the secretory flux, resulting in net absorption. From these types of data one might expect the equivalent of 40 to 50 liters per day of isotonic fluid to be exchanged in each direction across the normal human small bowel.

Although specific studies are difficult because of the dynamic status of rapid cell turnover, the small bowel is a complex organ that clearly has regional and subcellular specialization for secretion and absorption. These specialized regions have particular relevance for current hypotheses about the effects of cyclic AMP and cyclic GMP nucleotides

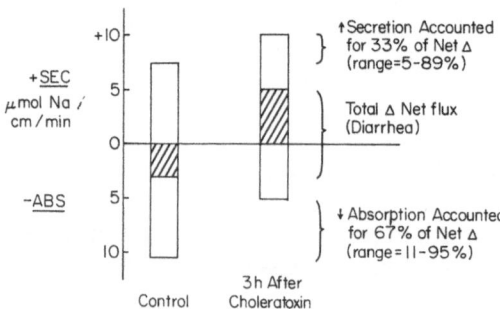

Figure 1. Effect of cholera toxin on unidirectional sodium fluxes in ligated canine jejunal segments (N = 22). (Source: R. L. Guerrant and J. E. Rohde, unpublished observations from the Cholera Research Laboratory, Dacca, Bangladesh, 1970.)

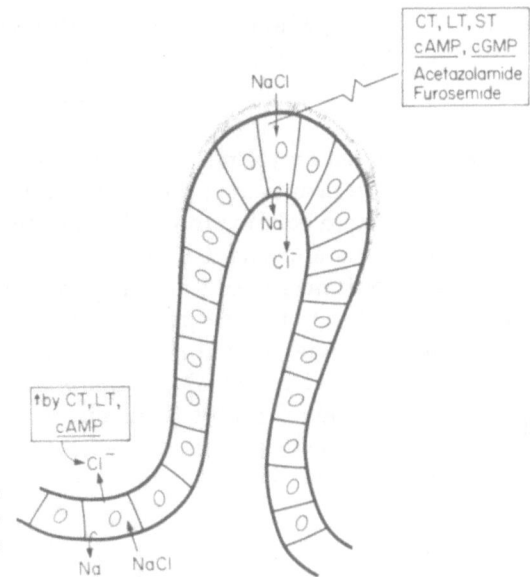

Figure 2. Specialization of villus tip and crypt cells in the small intestinal mucosa and postulated sites of enterotoxin action.

and possible interactions with viral infections of specific cells such as those in villus tips (Figure 2).

The cuboidal crypt cells multiply and provide a continuous supply of differentiating cells that migrate toward the villus tip, where they specialize for absorption by developing microvillous brush borders and producing enzymes such as disaccharidases and alkaline phosphatase. Based largely on studies with enterotoxin probes of ion transport in short-circuit current chambers, current data suggest regional differences in absorptive and secretory function, with villus tip cells being primarily absorptive and intervillus crypts being primarily secretory.

The driving force both for the electrically neutral sodium chloride absorption in villus tip cells and for the electrogenic chloride secretion in crypts may well be the same contralumenal sodium-potassium-activated ATPase-linked sodium pump that extrudes sodium from the cell.[22] The different effects of the same sodium pump that cause neutral sodium chloride absorption or electrogenic chloride secretion can be explained by relative differences in the location of the neutral sodium chloride coupled transport. For electrically neutral absorption of sodium in villus tips, the pump may extrude sodium to the lumenal membrane, while for electrogenic chloride secretion in the villus crypts, the pump may extrude sodium through the contralumenal membrane.

Mechanism of Action of Cholera
Enterotoxin and Heat-Labile Enterotoxin of
E. COLI

As predicted by John Snow over a century ago, the entire syndrome of clinical cholera appears to result from the action of an enterotoxin that shifts the delicate balance toward secretion of isotonic fluid in the upper small bowel. As shown in Figure 3, the effect of cholera toxin on net water (and sodium) fluxes following even a brief experimental exposure results in a net secretory response that occurs after a 30- to 60-minute lag period and becomes maximal at 2 to 3 hours. On the basis of similar effects of dibutyryl cyclic AMP, theophylline, and cholera toxin on ion fluxes across isolated rabbit ileal mucosa in short-circuited chambers,[23] several other investigators and we have explored the effects of cholera toxin on intestinal mucosal adenylate cyclase activity. This secretory

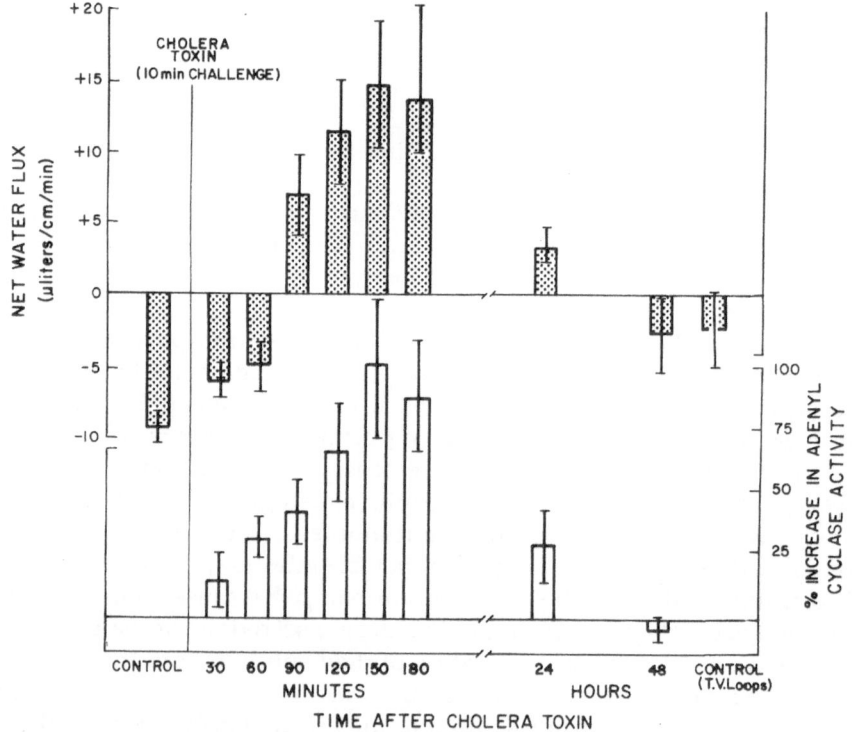

Figure 3. Time course of cholera toxin effects on net fluid transport and on mucosal adenylate cyclase in canine jejunum. (Source: reference 24.)

response parallels precisely the activation of intestinal mucosal adenylate cyclase (Figure 3).[24] Cholera toxin is thus a unique pharmacologic agent that activates intestinal mucosal adenylate cyclase and, after a lag period, causes fluid secretion for longer than 24 hours after exposure, despite removal of the toxin. Only after 48 hours, a time sufficient for renewal of most mucosal epithelial cells, do absorptive function and adenylate cyclase activity return to normal levels.

Unidirectional sodium flux measurements in ligated canine jejunal segments with ^{22}Na given intraluminally and, in some instances, simultaneously with intravenous ^{24}Na, have shown that, in each of 22 consecutive studies, the net secretory response to cholera toxin was due, in part, to an increase in unidirectional sodium secretion (accounting for a mean of 33% of the net change) *and* reduced unidirectional sodium absorption (accounting for an average of 67% of the net change) (Figure 1) (R. L. Guerrant and J. E. Rohde, unpublished observations from the Cholera Research Laboratory, Dacca, Bangladesh, 1970). The increased short-circuit current and secretory response to cholera toxin and cyclic AMP appear to result from two effects: There is reduced neutral NaCl absorption, primarily in villus tips,[25] *and* an increase in the electrogenic secretory flux of chloride and possibly bicarbonate, presumably from crypt cells.[26-28] As noted above, the driving force for both active chloride absorption with electrically neutral sodium-coupled transport in "leaky" epithelia in many species and even for the electrogenic chloride secretion, may be the same Na-K-dependent, ATPase-linked sodium pump in the lateral and basal membranes.

Three lines of indirect evidence suggest that the secretory effect of cholera toxin and cyclic AMP probably arises from crypt cells. First, selective damage of villus tip tissue with hypertonic saline does not impede the cholera toxin-induced secretory response.[29] Second, studies of marine teleost intestine that, like the gall bladder, has no crypt tissue, show that cyclic AMP and theophylline cause only reduced absorption and no net secretion.[26] Third, DeJonge and co-workers showed that a 5-minute exposure of rat intestine to cholera toxin resulted in activation of only villus tip adenylate cyclase and reduced absorption. In contrast, a 30-minute exposure to cholera toxin resulted in crypt as well as villus tip adenylate cyclase activation and a secretory response.[30]

Cholera toxin is a polypeptide with binding (B) and active (A) subunits. The binding portion contains five identical units and appears to be responsible for the avid association of cholera toxin with the monosialoganglioside (G_{M1}) receptor on epithelial cell surfaces (Ka = 10^{-9}M).[31] As shown by Gill, the A_1 subunit (after being split from A_2 by reduction of a disulfide bond), in the presence of NAD, cell cytosol, and ATP, is

capable of activating adenylate cyclase directly in broken cell preparations.[32,33] Prior work had shown that cholera toxin, in addition to activating adenylate cyclase, actually enhances the responsiveness to other hormones such as epinephrine (Table V).[34] From the outstanding work of
Cassel and Selinger,[35,36] it now appears that the active subunit of cholera
toxin, by ADP-ribosylating the GTP-binding component of adenylate
cyclase (? a GTPase), blocks the normal turnoff reaction for activated adenylate cyclase (Figure 4). This explains the enhanced responsiveness to
other hormones and the prolonged activation of adenylate cyclase by
cholera toxin, possibly for the life of the intestinal epithelial cell.

This secretory effect of cholera toxin leaves the glucose and amino
acid-coupled sodium transport mechanism intact, thus providing the
basis for oral glucose-electrolyte therapy.

Table V. Effect of Cholera Toxin on the Response of Rat Fat Cell Membranes
to Epinephrine[a]

| | Adenylate cyclase activity (mol/min per mg protein) | | |
	Basal	+ epinephrine	∇ in response to epinephrine
Control	32.2	124.5	+ 92.3
Cholera toxin	100.8	361.0	+260.2

[a]Source: reference 34.

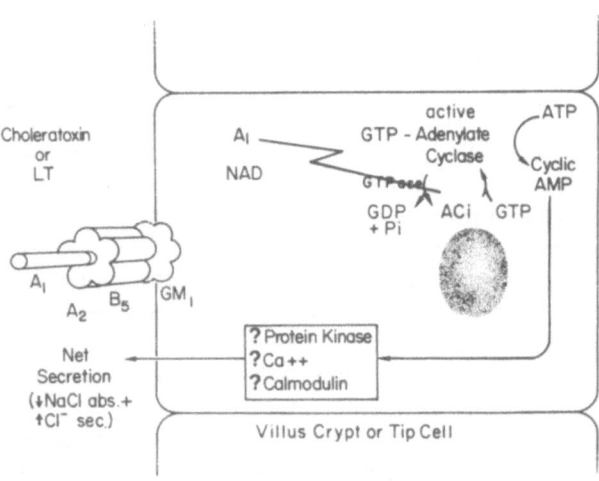

Figure 4. Proposed mechanism of cholera toxin and LT action.

The heat-labile enterotoxin (LT) of *Escherichia coli,* and probably of other Enterobacteriaceae (including *Klebsiella, Citrobacter,* and *Salmonella*), is remarkably similar to cholera toxin in its genetic code, antigenicity, and mechanism of action. Although there appear to be subtle differences in the nature of the binding subunits, both cholera toxin and heat-labile toxin activate adenylate cyclase in a similar fashion in many mammalian cell types. It is this promiscuous activation of adenylate cyclase in multiple cell types that has been exploited in the development of tissue culture bioassay methods, such as the Chinese hamster ovary (CHO) cell[37,38] and Y-1 adrenal cell assays[39,40] for LT and cholera toxin. The precise intracellular mechanism by which both cholera toxin and LT cause fluid secretion after intracellular cyclic AMP is formed remains unclear at present. Whether this is related to the phosphorylation of protein in crypt cell basolateral plasma membranes, as shown by DeJonge,[41] resulting in increased lumenal chloride conductance, remains conjectural. A calcium/calmodulin-dependent step appears to be involved, inferred from indirect studies with lanthanum chloride and chlorpromazine inhibition of cholera toxin-induced secretion (Figure 4).[42,43] Furthermore, calcium ionophore[44] and hormones such as serotonin[45] cause a calcium-dependent secretory response independently of changes in cyclic nucleotides.

MECHANISM OF ACTION OF *E. COLI* HEAT-STABLE ENTEROTOXIN (ST)

Initally known to cause diarrhea in piglets and calves, ST-producing *E. coli* are now recognized as common causes of human diarrhea in adults and children.[46-49] Although its genetic code may coexist on the same plasmid with LT, ST is quite different from LT both antigenically and biologically. ST is a much smaller molecule (molecular weight 1,500 to 4,400).[50,51] In contrast to cholera toxin and LT,[38,52] ST effects are not inhibited by ganglioside G_{M1},[53] ST is inactive in nonintestinal tissue culture assay systems,[37,39] and it requires the suckling mouse assay or calf or piglet ligated segments for its detection. It now appears that there is a family of heat-stable enterotoxins, some of which, such as STb, may be inactive in mice but active in piglets.[54] The role of STb in human disease and its mechanism of action are unknown.

Initial data suggested that early effects of ST- plus LT-containing culture filtrates were associated with an immediate, measurable effect on fluid secretion and on apparent increased intestinal adenylate cyclase activity, in addition to the more prolonged activation of adenylate cyclase by whole enterotoxigenic *E. coli* cultures.[52,55] However, in retrospect, this early effect was most likely caused by ST and the now-recognized ability of activated guanylate cyclase to form some cyclic AMP *in vitro*.[56] Indeed, after ST exposure, intestinal tissue concentrations of cyclic GMP are increased without significant changes in cyclic AMP concentrations, and the 8-bromo analogue of cyclic GMP induces a magnitude and time course of secretory responses in the suckling mouse identical to those of ST.[56]

Thus, the effect of cholera toxin (CT) and LT on cyclic AMP, and the effects of ST on cyclic GMP cause the same (net secretory) rather than the opposite direction of response (Figure 5). ST has been shown to activate guanylate cyclase rapidly, to increase short-circuit current, and to reduce sodium and chloride absorption in rabbit ileal mucosa.[57]

Other studies have shown that ST specifically activates only the particulate, *intestinal* guanylate cyclase,[53,58] an effect that appears primarily to occur in jejunum and ileum.[59] This is in striking contrast to the widespread effect of cholera toxin and LT in many different tissues, and it has sharply limited the development of new bioassay methods for ST.

Particulate guanylate cyclase activity and cyclic GMP in intestinal mucosa are located primarily in the mucosal brush border at the apical regions of villous tips where they are associated with disaccharidase and alkaline phosphatase enzymes.[60-62] This localization is consistent with the principal effect on ion fluxes of decreased absorption with ST and cyclic GMP, rather than the increased chloride secretion seen with cholera toxin, LT, or cyclic AMP. Thus, the effect of ST appears to be reduced villus tip electrolyte absorption, an effect that could be additive with crypt adenylate cyclase-activating toxins.

The activation of guanylate cyclase by ST is quite different from the activation of adenylate cyclase by LT or CT. Free radicals can activate guanylate cyclase,[60] and the free radical scavenger, butylated hydroxyanisole (BHA), significantly reduces the activation of guanylate cyclase as well as the fluid secretory response to ST.[53] Furthermore, both indo-

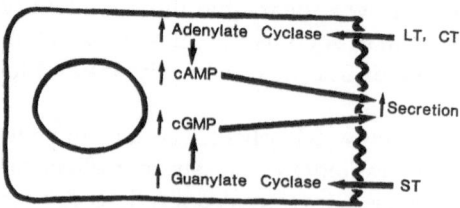

Figure 5. Effect of both adenylate and guanylate cyclase activating enterotoxins (cholera toxin or LT and ST, respectively) on net small intestinal secretion.

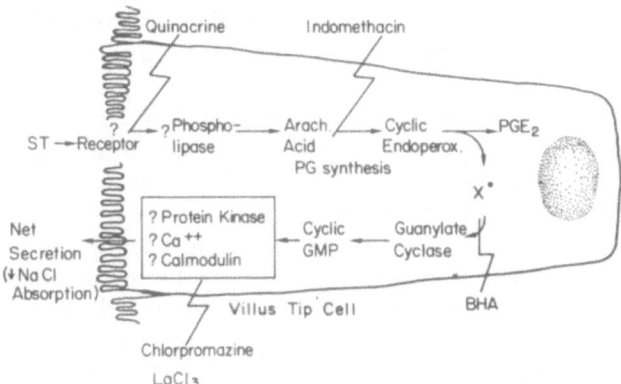

Figure 6. Possible pathways of ST effects on particulate small intestinal villous tip guanylate cyclase and reduced absorption (to cause net secretion).

methacin and antimalarial compounds such as quinacrine and amodiaquine significantly inhibit ST responses before activation of a guanylate cyclase.[63]

As shown in Figure 6, one possible interpretation of these data would be that ST involves initial membrane phospholipase activation (that is altered by quinacrine), followed by the prostaglandin synthesis pathway (that is inhibitable by indomethacin),[58,64] both before formation of a free radical that would activate guanylate cyclase. Recent work by R. N. Greenberg in our laboratory has shown that chlorpromazine and lanthanum synergistically inhibit ST- or 8 Br-cyclic GMP-induced secretion.[64,65] These findings suggest that calmodulin- and lanthanum-sensitive calcium pools may be involved in cyclic GMP-induced net secretion. Thus, cholera toxin and LT may share with ST some of the final, calcium-dependent secretory mechanisms in the small bowel (see Figure 4 and 6).

PATHOGENESIS OF VIRAL ENTERITIS

Although several enteroviral and other viral illnesses may be associated with diarrhea, the principal viral agents now recognized as common causes of diarrhea are the small, 27-nm Norwalk-like parvoviral agents and the 70-nm rotaviruses. Norwalk-like agents typically cause winter vomiting disease[66] and are associated with delayed gastric emptying,[67] reduced small bowel brush border disaccharidases,[21] and transient fat and xylose malabsorption,[68] without changes in jejunal adenylate cyclase activity.[69]

Rotavirus are much more easily detected than Norwalk-like viruses by electron microscopy or by enzyme-linked immunosorbent assay (ELISA), and are associated with diarrheal illnesses in 11 to 50% of cases in children less than 2 years of age throughout the world, with peaks in cooler, drier months.[70,71] With fecal shedding often exceeding 10^{11} per gram, rotaviruses are commonly acquired and occasionally produce symptoms in adult contacts as well.[72] Rotavirus diarrhea may be severe, often with vomiting and low-grade fever at the onset. The diarrhea is usually noninflammatory and watery, with slightly increased fecal sodium excretion and reduced brush border disaccharidase and Na-K ATPase activities.[73] Increased fecal reducing substances have also been described during rotavirus diarrhea (Table VI)[74] that might, theoretically, when challenged with a carbohydrate load during severe rotavirus infection, result in an acidic stool or clinically significant malabsorption, or worsened acidosis.[75]

A potential explanation for the watery diarrhea and carbohydrate malabsorption is suggested by the original studies of rotavirus diarrhea in which duodenal biopsies were taken from infected children.[20] Patchy, irregular mucosal changes were noted, with short and blunted villi and intracytoplasmic rotaviral particles in the villous epithelial cells. Normal columnar epithelium at villus tips was replaced by irregular, cuboidal cryptlike epithelial cells. As would be expected from this histopathology, brush border disaccharidase enzymes were abnormally low in seven of eight children studied. These transient abnormalities have been confirmed by several other investigators, who have shown the rotaviral infection to be localized to the duodenal and upper jejunal villous epithelial cells.[76,77] The degree of microvillous and mucosal damage appears to parallel the severity of clinical diarrhea and dehydration.[78]

Table VI. Stool-Reducing Substances on Hospital Admission for Diarrhea[a]

	Rotavirus (N = 52 patients)	Tox+ E. coli or Shigella (N = 10)
Prehydrolysis	189 mg/dl	64 mg/dl
Posthydrolysis	3063 mg/dl	1139 mg/dl

[a]Source: reference 74.

Similar findings have been noted in infections with the closely related agent of epizootic diarrhea in infant mice (EDIM), and in experimental infection of gnotobiotic, colostrum-deprived calves with human rotaviruses.[79] In the calf model, denuded villus tips are replaced with cuboidal epithelial cells. It has been postulated that the brush border enzyme, lactase, plays a role as a receptor and as an uncoating enzyme, because beta-galactosidase removes the outer capsid layer of rotaviruses *in vitro*.[80] However, lactase-deficient populations remain clearly susceptible to rotavirus infections.[81]

Hamilton and his colleagues have suggested that the pathogenesis of human rotaviral diarrhea may be similar to that of transmissible gastroenteritis (TGE), a coronavirus infection of piglets. In a number of studies of this process, these investigators have shown that TGE viral infection occurs first in the villus tip epithelial cells, and that this is followed by shedding of infected cells and blunting of villi that are replaced by cuboidal, cryptlike epithelial cells with increased thymidine kinase and decreased sucrase activities.[82-85] These morphological abnormalities progress over the first 40 hours of experimental infection and are associated with reduced Na-K ATPase activity, reduced sodium efflux from epithelial cells, and impaired glucose-coupled sodium transport, without changes in adenylate cyclase activity. In these studies, abnormalities disappeared within 6 days.

Similar findings have been described in 8- to 10-day-old weaned piglets infected with human rotaviruses.[86] Eleven animals developed diarrhea or intestinal fluid accumulation within 72 hours after infection, at which point the small intestinal mucosa showed shortened villi, reduced sucrase activity, increased thymidine kinase activity, and no change in cyclic AMP concentration. Although net sodium and chloride fluxes measured in short-circuited chambers were not significantly altered from those in controls, the absorptive response to glucose was blunted in jejunum from infected animals.

When understood in light of the proposed normal small bowel physiology mentioned earlier, the hypothesis that villus tip cell destruction results in a predominantly secretory epithelium could explain the diarrhea caused by rotavirus infection. Such a hypothesis might also pertain to other infections with bacterial or parasitic agents that primarily damage villus tip cell morphology or function. One might also expect accentuated secretory responses to cholera toxin or *E. coli* LT, or impaired glucose or sucrose-coupled absorption in patients with rotavirus infections. The impact of rotaviral and combined infections on nutritional status and on the efficacy of oral glucose, sucrose, or amino acid and electrolyte therapy remains to be determined. The roles of protection against rotaviruses by type-specific local intestinal or breast-milk antibodies are being actively explored now with the recent successful propagation of a human rotavirus in cell culture.[87]

In summary, whether through specific alteration of normal ion fluxes by enterotoxins or through nonspecific but selective damage to villous tip epithelium by viral, parasitic, or bacterial agents (or their toxic products), acute and chronic diarrheal illnesses present major problems for the maintenance of proper nutrition and childhood development throughout tropical developing areas. In some infections, such as rotaviruses, specific nutrient absorptive defects may accompany the electrolyte absorptive defect. In others, the dehydration and tendency to withdraw food from children with diarrhea may be the major factors contributing to malnutrition. Further studies of the nutritional impact of controlling dehydration with early glucose–electrolyte oral therapy, or of controlling certain infections with specific pharmacologic therapy or vaccine prophylaxis, will further elucidate the complex interaction of infectious diarrheas with malabsorption and undernutrition.

References

1. Puffer, R. R., and Serrano, C. V. *Patterns of Mortality in Childhood*. Pan American Sanitary Bureau, Regional Office, World Health Organization, Washington, D.C., 1973.
2. Gordon, J. E., Chitkara, I. D., and Wyon, J. B. Weanling diarrhea. *Am. J. Med. Sci* 245:345, 1963.
3. Giannella, R. A., Broitman, S. A., and Zamcheck, N. Influence of gastric acidity on bacterial and parasitic enteric infections: A perspective. *Ann. Intern. Med.* 78:271, 1973.
4. Bohnhoff, M., Miller, C. P., and Martin, W. R. Resistance of the mouse's intestinal tract to experimental Salmonella infections. *J. Exp. Med.* 120:805, 1964.
5. Mentzing, L. O., and Ringertz, O. Salmonella infection in tourists. 2. Prophylaxis against salmonellosis. *Acta Pathol. Microbiol. Scand.* 74:405, 1968.
6. Bartlett, J. G. Antibiotic-associated pseudomembranous colitis. *Rev. Infect. Dis.* 1:530, 1979.
7. Formal, S. B., Abrams, G. D., Schneider, H., and Sprinz, H. Experimental Shigella infections VI. Role of the small intestine in an experimental infection in guinea pigs. *J. Bacteriol.* 85:119, 1963.
8. Higgens, J. A., Code, C. F., and Orvis, A. L. The influence of motility on the rate of absorption of sodium and water from the small intestine of healthy persons. *Gastroenterology* 31:708, 1956.
9. Jones, G. W. The attachment of bacteria to the surfaces of animal cells. In: *Microbial Interactions: Receptors and Recognition*, Series B, Vol. 3, J. L. Reissig (Ed.), pp. 139–176 Chapman & Hall, London, 1977.
10. Guerrant, R. L., and Bergman, M. J. Attachment factors among enterotoxigenic *Escherichia coli*. In: *Frontiers of Knowledge in the Diarrheal Diseases*, H. D. Janowitz and D. B. Sachar (Eds.). Projects in Health, Montclair, New Jersey, 1979.

11. Smith, H. W., and Linggood, M. A. Observations on the pathogenic properties of the K88, HLY and ENT plasmids of *Escherichia coli* with special reference to porcine diarrhea. *J. Med. Microbiol.* **4**:467–485, 1971.

12. Evans, D. G., and Evans, D. J., Jr. New surface-associated heat-labile colonization factor of enterotoxigenic *Escherichia coli* isolated from adults with diarrhea. *Infect. Immun.* **19**:727–736, 1978.

13. Bergman, M. J., Updike, W. S., Wood, S. J., Brown, S. E., III, and Guerrant, R. L. Attachment factors among enterotoxigenic *Escherichia coli* from patients with acute diarrhea from diverse geographic areas. *Infect. Immun.* **32**:881–888, 1981.

14. Levine, M. M. and Rennels, M. B. *E. coli* colonization factor antigen in diarrhea. *Lancet* ii:534, 1978.

15. Ulshen, M. H., and Rollo, J. L. Pathogenesis of *Escherichia coli* gastroenteritis in man— Another mechanism. *N. Engl. J. Med.* **302**:99–101, 1980.

16. Guerrant, R. L. Yet another pathogenic mechanism for *E. coli* diarrhea? *N. Engl. J. Med* **302**:113–114, 1980.

17. Kent, T. H., and Lindenbaum, J. Correlation of jejunal function and morphology in patients with acute and chronic diarrhea in East Pakistan. *Gastroenterology* **52**:972, 1967.

18. Hirschhorn, N., and Molla, A. Reversible jejunal disaccharidase deficiency in cholera and other acute diarrheal diseases. *Johns Hopkins Med. J.* **125**:291, 1969.

19. Lifshitz, F., Coello-Ramierz, P., and Gutierrez-Topete, G. Carbohydrate intolerance in infants with diarrhea. *J. Pediatr.* **79**:760, 1971.

20. Bishop, R. F., Davidson, G. P., Holmes, I. H., and Ruck, B. J. Virus particles in epithelial cells of duodenal mucosa from children with acute nonbacterial gastroenteritis. *Lancet* ii:1281, 1973.

21. Agus, S. G., Dolin, R., Wyatt, R. G., Tousimis, A. J., and Northrup, R. S. Acute infectious nonbacterial gastroenteritis: Intestinal histopathology, histologic and enzymatic alterations during illness produced by Norwalk agent in man. *Ann. Intern. Med.* **79**:18, 1973.

22. Frizzell, R. A., Field, M., and Schultz, S. G. Sodium-coupled chloride transport by epithelial tissues. *Am. J. Physiol.* **236**:F1–F3, 1979.

23. Field, M., Plotkin, G. R., and Silen, W. Effects of vasopressin, theophylline, and cyclic adenosine monophosphate on short-circuit current across isolated rabbit ileal mucosa. *Nature (London)* **217**:469–471, 1968.

24. Guerrant, R. L., Chen, L. C., and Sharp, G. W. G. Intestinal adenylcyclase activity in canine cholera: Correlation with fluid accumulation. *J. Infect. Dis.* **125**:377–381, 1972.

25. Nellans, H. N., Frizzell, R. A., and Schultz, S. G. Coupled sodium-chloride influxes across the brush border of rabbit ileum. *Am. J. Physiol.* **225**:467–475, 1973.

26. Field, M., Cholera toxin, adenylate cyclase, and the process of active secretion in the small intestine: The pathogenesis of diarrhea in cholera. In: *Physiology of Membrane Disorders*, T. E. Andreoli, J. F. Hoffman, and D. D. Fanestil (Eds.), pp. 877–899. Plenum, New York, 1978.

27. Nellans, H. N., Frizzell, R. A., and Schultz, S. G. Effect of acetazolamide on sodium and chloride transport by *in vitro* rabbit ileum. *Am. J. Physiol.* **228**:1808–1814, 1975.

28. Klyce, S. D., and Wong, R. K. S. Site and mode of adrenaline action on chloride transport across the rabbit corneal epithelium. *J. Physiol.* **266**:77–799, 1977.

29. Roggin, G. M., Banwell, J. G., Yardley, J. H., and Hendrix, T. H. Unimpaired response of rabbit jejunum to cholera toxin after selective damage to villus epithelium. *Gastroenterology* **63**:981–989, 1972.

30. DeJonge, H. R. The response of small intestinal villus and crypt epithelium to cholera

toxin in rat and guinea pig. Evidence against a specific role of the crypt cells in choleragen-induced secretion. *Biochim. Biophys. Acta* **381**:128–143, 1975.

31. Holmgren, J., and Lonnroth, I. Structure and function of enterotoxins and their receptors. In: *Cholera and Related Diarrheas*, O. Ouchterlony and J. Holmgren (Eds.), 43rd Nobel Symposium. S. Karger, Basel, 1980.

32. Gill, D. M., and King, C. A. The mechanism of action of cholera toxin in pigeon erythrocyte lysates. *J. Biol. Chem.* **250**:424–432, 1975.

33. Gill, D. M. Multiple roles of erythrocyte supernatant in the activation of adenylate cyclase by *Vibrio cholerae* toxin *in vitro*. *J Infect. Dis.* **133**:S55–S63, 1976.

34. Hewlett, E. L., Guerrant, R. L., Evans, D. J., Jr., and Greenough, W. G. III. Toxins of *Virbro cholerae* and *Escherichia coli* stimulate adenyl cyclase in rat fat cells. *Nature* **249**:371–373, 1974.

35. Cassel, D., and Selinger, Z. Mechanisms of adenylate cyclase activation by cholera toxin: Inhibition of GTP hydrolysis at the regulatory site. *Proc. Natl. Acad. Sci. (U.S.)* **74**:3307–3311, 1977.

36. Cassel, D., and Pfeuffer, T. Mechanism of cholera toxin action: Covalent modification of the guanyl nucleotide-binding protein of the adenylate cyclase system. *Proc. Nat. Acad. Sci. (U.S.)* **75**:2669–2673, 1978.

37. Guerrant, R. L., Brunton, L. L., Schnaitman, T. C., Rebhun, L. I., and Gilman, A. G. Cyclic adenosine monophosphate and alteration of Chinese hamster ovary cell morphology: A rapid, sensitive *in vitro* assay for the enterotoxins of *Vibrio cholerae* and *Escherichia coli*. *Infect. Immun.* **10**:320–327, 1974.

38. Guerrant, R. L., and Brunton, L. L. Characterization of the Chinese hamster ovary cell assay for the enterotoxins of *Vibrio cholerae* and *Escherichia coli* and for antitoxin: Differential inhibition by gangliosides, specific antisera, and toxoid. *J. Infect. Dis.* **135**:720–728, 1977.

39. Donta, S. T., and King, M. Induction of steroidogenesis in tissue culture by cholera enterotoxin. *Nature (New Biol.)* **243**:246–247, 1973.

40. Donta, S. T., Moon, H. W., and Whipp, S. C. Detection of heat-labile *Escherichia coli* enterotoxin with the use of adrenal cells in tissue culture. *Science* **183**:334–335, 1974.

41. DeJonge, H. R. Cyclic nucleotide-dependent phosphorylation of intestinal epithelium proteins. *Nature* **262**:590–593, 1976.

42. Leitch, G. H., and Amer, M. S. Lanthanum inhibition of *V. cholerae* and E. coli enterotoxin-induced enterosorption and its effects on intestinal mucosa cyclic adenosine 3′, 5′-monophosphate levels. *Infect. Immun.* **11**:1038–1044, 1975.

43. Holmgren, J., Sange, S., and Lonnroth, I. Reversal of cyclic AMP-mediated intestinal secretion in mice by chlorpromazine. *Gastroenterology* **75**:1103–1108, 1978.

44. Bolton, J. E., and Field, M. Ca Ionophore-stimulated ion secretion in rabbit ileal mucosa; Relation to actions of cyclic 3′, 5′-AMP and carbamylcholine. *J. Membr. Biol.* **35**:159–173, 1977.

45. Donowitz, M., Asarkof, N., and Pike, G. Calcium dependence of serotonin-induced changes in rabbit ileal electrolyte transport. *J. Clin. Invest.* **66**:341–353, 1980.

46. Sack, D. A., Merson, M. M., Wells, J. C., Sack, R. B., and Morris, G. K. Diarrhea associated with heat-stable enterotoxin-producing strains of *Escherichia coli*. *Lancet* **ii**:239–244, 1975.

47. Ryder, R. W., Wachsmuth, I. K., Buxton, A. E., Evans, D. G., DuPont, H. L., Mason, E., and Barrett, F. F. Infantile diarrhea produced by heat-stable enterotoxigenic *Escherichia coli*. *N. Engl. J. Med* **295**:849–853, 1976.

48. Hughes, J. M., Rouse, J. D., Barada, F. A., and Guerrant, R. L. Etiology of summer diarrhea among the Navajo. *Am. J. Trop. Med. Hyg.* **29**:613–619, 1980.

49. Guerrant, R. L., Rouse, J. D., and Hughes, J. M. Turista among the Yale Glee Club in Latin America: Studies of enterotoxigenic bacteria, *E. coli* serotypes and rotaviruses. *Am. J. Trop. Med. Hyg.* **29**:895–900, 1980.

50. Staples, D. J., Asher, S. E., and Giannella, R. A. Purification and characterization of heat-stable enterotoxin produced by a strain of *E. coli* pathogenic for man. *J. Biol. Chem.* **255**:4716–4721, 1980.

51. Alderete, J. G., and Robertson, D. C. Purification and chemical characterization of the heat-stable enterotoxin produced by porcine strains of enterotoxigenic *Escherichia coli. Infect. Immun.* **19**:1021–1030, 1978.

52. Pierce, N. F. Differential inhibitory effects of cholera toxoids and gangliosides on the enterotoxins of *Vibrio cholerae* and *Escherichia coli. J. Exp. Med* **137**:1009–1023, 1973.

53. Guerrant, R. L., Hughes, J. M., Chang, B., Robertson, D. C., and Murad, F. Activation of rat and rabbit intestinal guanylate cyclase by the heat-stable enterotoxin of *Escherichia coli*: Studies of tissue specificity, potential receptors and intermediates. *J. Infect. Dis.* **142**:220–228, 1980.

54. Burgess, M. N., Bywater, R. J., Cowley, C. M., Mullan, N. A., and Newsome, P. M. Biological evaluation of a methanol-soluble, heat-stable *Escherichia coli* enterotoxin in infant mice, pigs, rabbits, and calves. *Infect. Immun.* **21**:526–530, 1978.

55. Guerrant, R. L., Ganguly, U. Casper, A. G. T., Moore, E. J., Pierce, N. J., and Carpenter, C. C. J. Effect of *Escherichia coli* on fluid transport across canine small bowel: Mechanism and time course with enterotoxin and whole bacterial cells. *J. Clin. Invest.* **52**:1707–1714, 1973.

56. Hughes, J. M., Murad, F., Chang, B., and Guerrant, R. L. Role of cyclic GMP in the action of heat-stable enterotoxin of *Escherichia coli. Nature* **271**:755–756, 1978.

57. Field, M., Graf, L. G., Jr., Laird, W. F., and Smith, P. L. Heat-stable enterotoxin of *Escherichia coli: In vitro* effects on guanylate cyclase activity, cyclic GMP concentration, and ion transport in small intestine. *Proc. Nat. Acad. Sci. (U.S.)* **75**:2800–2804, 1978.

58. Hughes, J. M., Murad, F., and Guerrant, R. L. Studies to elucidate the mechanism of action of heat-stable enterotoxin of *Escherichia coli. Clin. Res.* **26**:524A, 1978.

59. Rao, M. C., Guandalini, S., Laird, W. J., Smith, P. L., and Field, M. Heat-stable enterotoxins: Mechanism of action (Proceedings of the Fifteenth Joint Conference of the U.S.–Japan Cooperative Medical Science Program of Cholera), NIAID, NIH, Bethesda, Maryland, 1979, *NIH Publ. No.* 80:2003, 1980.

60. Kimura, H., and Murad, F. Subcellular localization of guanylate cyclase—Minireview. *Life Sci.* **17**:837–743, 1975.

61. Ong, S-H., Whitley, T. H., Stowe, N. W., and Steiner, A. L. Immunohistochemical localization of 3′:5′-cyclic AMP and 3′:5′-cyclic GMP. *Proc. Nat. Acad. Sci. (U.S.)* **72**:2022–2026, 1975.

62. DeJonge, H. R. The localization of guanylate cyclase in rat small intestinal epithelium. *FEBS Lett.* **53**:237–242, 1975.

63. Greenberg, R. N., Guerrant, R. L., Chang, B., Robertson, D. C., and Murad, F. *Inhibition of E. coli heat-stable enterotoxin (ST) by quinacrine. Biochem. Pharmacol.* **31**:2005–2009, 1982.

64. Greenberg, R. N., Murad, F., Chang, B., Robertson, D. C., and Guerrant, R. L. Inhibition of *Escherichia coli* heat-stable enterotoxin by indomethacin and chlorpromazine. *Infect. Immun.* **29**:908–913, 1980.

65. Greenberg, R. N., Murad, F., and Guerrant, R. L. Lanthanum chloride inhibition of secretory response to *Escherichia coli* heat-stable enterotoxin *Infect. Immun.* **35**:483–488, 1982.

66. Blacklow, N. R., Dolin, R., Fedson, D. S., DuPont, H., Northrup, R. S., Hornick, R. B., and Chanock, R. M. Acute infectious nonbacterial gastroenteritis: Etiology and pathogenesis. *Ann. Intern. Med.* **76**:993–1008, 1972.

67. Meeroff, J. C., Schreiber, D. S., Trier, J. S., and Blacklow, N. R. Abnormal gastric motor function in viral gastroenteritis. *Ann. Intern Med.* **92**:370–373, 1980.
68. Schreiber, D. S., Blacklow, N. R., and Trier, J. S. The mucosal lesion of the proximal small intestine in acute infectious nonbacterial gastroenteritis. *N. Engl. J. Med.* **288**:1318–1323, 1973.
69. Levy, A. G., Widerlite, L. Schwartz, C. J., Dolin, R., Blacklow, N. R., Gardner, J. D., Kimberg, D. V., and Trier, J. S. Jejunal adenylate cyclase activity in human subjects during viral gastroenteritis. *Gastroenterology* **70**:321–325, 1976.
70. Kapikian, A. Z., Kim, H. W., Wyatt, R. G., Cline, W. L., Arrobio, J. O., Brandt, C. D., Rodriguez, W. J., Sack, D. A., Chanock, R. M., and Parrott, R. H. Human reovirus-like agent as the major pathogen associated with "winter" gastroenteritis in hospitalized infants and young children. *N. Engl. J. Med.* **294**:965, 1976.
71. Black, R. W., Merson, M. H., Huq, I., Alim, A. R. M. A., and Yunus, M. D. Incidence and severity of rotavirus and *Escherichia coli* diarrhea in rural Bangladesh: Implications for vaccine development, *Lancet* i:141–143, 1981.
72. Wenman, W. M., Hinde, D., Feltham, S., and Gurwith, M. Rotavirus infection in adults: Results of a prospective family study. *N. Engl. J. Med.* **301**:303–306, 1979.
73. Tallett, S., MacKenzie, C., Middleton, P., Kerzner, B., and Hamilton, R. Clinical, laboratory, and epidemiological features of a viral gastroenteritis in infants and children. *Pediatrics* **60**:217–222, 1977.
74. Sack, D. A., Chowdhury, A. M. A. K., Eusof, A., Ali, M. A., Merson, M. H., Islam, S., Black, R. E., and Brown, K. H. Oral hydration in rotavirus diarrhea: A double-blind comparison of sucrose with glucose electrolyte solution. *Lancet* ii:280–283, 1978.
75. Torres-Pinedo, R., Lavastida, M., Rivera, C. L., Rodriguez, H., and Ortiz, A., Studies on infant diarrhea. I. A comparison of the effects of milk feeding and intravenous therapy upon the composition and volume of the stool and urine. *J. Clin. Invest.* **45**:469–479, 1966.
76. Middleton, P. J., Szymanski, M. T., Abbott, G. D., Bortolussi, R., and Hamilton, J. R. Orbivirus acute gastroenteritis of infancy. *Lancet* i:1241–1244, 1974.
77. Davidson, G. P., Goller, I., Bishop, R. F., Townely, R. R. W., Holmes, P. H., and Ruck, B. J. Immunofluorescence in duodenal mucosa of children with acute enteritis due to a new virus. *J. Clin. Pathol.* **28**:263–266, 1975.
78. Davidson, G. P., and Barnes, G. L. Structural and functional abnormalities of the small intestine in infants and young children with rotavirus enteritis. *Acta Paediatr. Scand.* **68**:181–186, 1979.
79. Mebus, C. A., Wyatt, R. G., Sharpee, R. L., Sereno, M. M., Kalica, A. P., Zapikian, A. Z., and Twiehaus, M. J. Diarrhea in gnotobiotic calves caused by the reovirus-like agent of human infantile gastroenteritis. *Infect. Immun.* **14**:471–474, 1976.
80. Holmes, I. H., Rodger, S. M., Schnagl, R. D., Ruck, B. J., Gust, I. D., Bishop, R. F., and Barnes, G. L. Is lactase the receptor and uncoating enzyme for infantile enteritis (ROTA) viruses? *Lancet* i:1387, 1976.
81. Schoub, B. D., Jenkins, T., and Robins-Browne, R. M. Rotavirus infection in high-incidence lactase-deficiency population. *Lancet* i:328, 1978.
82. Hamilton, J. R., Gall, D. G., Butler, D. G., and Middleton, P. J. Viral gastroenteritis: Recent progress, remaining problems. *Ciba Founda. Symp.* **42**:209, 1976.
83. Kerzner, B., Kelly, M. H., Gall, D. G., Butler, D. G., and Hamilton, J. R. Transmissible gastroenteritis: Sodium transport and the intestinal epithelium during the course of viral enteritis. *Gastroenterology* **72**:457–461, 1977.
84. Gall, D. G., Chapman, D., Kelly, M., and Hamilton, J. R. Na+ transport in jejunal crypt cells. *Gastroenterology* **72**:452–456, 1977.

85. Shepherd, R. W., Butler, D. G., Cutz, E., Gall, D. G., and Hamilton, J. R. The mucosal lesion in viral enteritis: Extent and dynamics of the epithelial response to virus invasion in transmissible gastroenteritis of piglets. *Gastroenterology* **76**:770–777, 1979.
86. Davidson, G. P., Gall, D. G., Petric, M., Butler, D. G., and Hamilton, J. R. Human rotavirus enteritis induced in conventional piglets: Intestinal structure and transport. *J. Clin. Invest.* **60**:1402–1409, 1977.
87. Kapikian, A. Z., Wyatt, R. G., Greenberg, H. B., Kalica, A. R., Wha, K. H., Brandt, C. D., Rodriguez, W. J., Parrott, R. H., and Chanock, R. M. Approaches to immunization of infants and young children against gastroenteritis due to rotaviruses. *Rev. Infect. Dis.* **2**:459, 1980.

The Epidemiology and Pathophysiology of Invasive Bacterial Diarrheas

With a Note on Biological Considerations in Control Strategies

GERALD T. KEUSCH

INTRODUCTION

A fundamental distinction among enteric bacterial pathogens involves the capacity of some, but not all, to invade intestinal epithelial cells and multiply within the gut mucosa.[1] This property not only affects the epidemiology of these infections and their clinical presentation but also imposes biological constraints on attempts to control their spread among susceptible populations. This paper will consider the epidemiology, pathogenesis, clinical manifestations, and potential nutritional consequences of four distinctive invasive bacterial agents of gastroenteritis, the shigellas, the salmonellas (including the causative agents of the enteric fever syndrome), *Yersinia enterocolitica*, and *Campylobacter jejuni*, and will attempt to evaluate control strategies based on the biological attributes of the organisms.

GERALD T. KEUSCH • Division of Geographic Medicine, Tufts University School of Medicine, Boston, Massachusetts.

Epidemiology

In some respects the epidemiology of these various infections is bor-
ing, an inexorable circle from oral ingestion to anal excretion to oral
ingestion. However, the organisms differ in so many ways, as, for example, host range, that the epidemiological circle is far from stereotyped,
there being an almost infinite variety of routes of transmission deviating
through foods, fluids, fingers, feces, flies, fomites, and even fornication.
These are not random pathways, but actually represent an expression of
the biological properties of the organisms (Table I).

For example, the shigellas are highly host-adapted bacteria; they are
natural pathogens only for the human and certain species of higher primates.[2] Domestic animals, poultry, dogs, cats, turtles, etc., do not harbor
the organism. As a consequence, one human infection is always traceable
to another human (or on occasion to a monkey), although the actual
transmission may involve a food vehicle, or water- or milk-borne transmission.[3-5] The features that determine this host specificity, however, are
not known.

Another feature of clear importance but unknown mechanism is the
capacity of small inocula to cause symptomatic infection. Experimental
infections in human volunteers with as few as 10 to 100 viable *Shigella
dysenteriae* 1 is actually easily accomplished.[6] For this reason, the principal route of infection for these organisms turns out to be person-to-person contact spread.[2] Since convalescent or asymptomatic carriers usually
pass 10^2 to 10^3 bacteria per gram of stool,[7] it is easy to see how anal–oral
spread can occur. This is well documented among household contacts of
cases, with attack rates of 30 to 40% percent reported among children,
and 15 to 20 percent among adults[8,9]. Recent studies also document direct
transmission among homosexuals as the result of oral–anal sex practices[2].

In contrast, gastroenteritis strains of *Salmonella* are not at all particular about host; for most, it seems that whatever host is convenient and

Table I.   Epidemiological Characteristics of the Invasive Enteric Pathogens

Genus	Host range	Infectious dose	Environmental survival
Shigella	Narrow	Low	Poor
Salmonella			
Gastroenteritis strains	Broad	Moderate	Excellent
Enteric fever strains	Narrow	Moderate	Poor
Yersinia enterocolitica	Narrow	Unknown	?
Campylobacter jejuni	Broad	? Moderate	Good

available is acceptable. There are three species of *Salmonella: S. typhi, S. cholerasuis,* and *S. enteritidis.* The latter contains almost 2,000 distinct serotypes, the majority being non-host-adapted. The majority are also potential causes of gastroenteritis, but actually the major portion of these infections are caused by a short list of 10 to 20 serotypes of *S. enteritidis,* the most prevalent of all being *S. enteritidis* serotype *typhimurium* (*S. typhimurium*). While these infections may be traced directly to another human host, most often food, especially poultry and eggs, milk, or water are implicated.[10] Salmonellosis is usually a food-borne gastroenteritis (commonly classified as "food poisoning") with fever. One reason for this in the well-sanitized highly industrialized nations is that large-scale, intensive farming practices force animals to live intimately with their own feces, facilitating spread of *Salmonella* by direct contact or through animal feed and water sources. Introduction of a strain from any source into a *Salmonella*-free herd or flock can therefore rapidly infect large numbers of animals and become entrenched in the environment. This is especially true of poultry and swine rearing, two of the most common sources of human salmonellosis. In addition, the lack of strict host preference of the organisms involved, and the mass production of processed foods and worldwide distribution networks will rapidly disseminate contaminated items through the food chain on an international scale. Outbreaks of common source salmonellosis have been documented for a number of foodstuffs, including dried and whole milk, milk chocolate, poultry, pork, shellfish, eggs, cake mixes, and even oral pancreatic enzyme preparations used for replacement therapy, or carmine red dye used in hospitals to mark stool collection periods for various diagnostic studies.[10-15]

In contrast, *S. typhi* and the other causes of enteric fever (*S. enteritidis* serotypes *paratyphi* A, B, and C) are highly host-adpated to humans. The epidemiological route is thus always traceable to another human, whether case or carrier, but again many interesting, intricate, and ingenious routings may be involved in carrying the organism to a susceptible new human host. Indeed, a food or water vehicle usually is the direct carrier of the infecting dose.

The minimum oral infectious dose of *S. typhi* and gastroenteritis strains of *Salmonellae* in normal adult volunteers is around 10^5 organisms,[16,17] but 10^8 to 10^9 are needed to infect the majority of subjects. Host factors, including gastric acidity, composition of the normal bacterial flora, and age of the host, influence this, while certain vehicles involved in natural infections (such as capsules of carmine red dye, chocolate, and pancreatic enzyme preparations) may permit infection with far fewer bacteria (44 to 15,000).[18-20] Hypochlorhydric subjects or postgastrectomy patients are clearly at risk of *Salmonella* infection.[21,22] While grossly contaminated food or water accounts for most outbreaks, person-to-person spread certainly occurs, especially in individuals at the extremes of life, or those debilitated with underlying illness, and may also be important in sporadic cases.[23]

The genus *Campylobacter fetus* is composed of three subspecies (ss *fetus*, ss *jejuni*, ss *intestinalis*) of primarily animal-adapted organisms.[24] *C. fetus* ss *fetus*, which causes abortion and sterility in cattle, is not a human pathogen.[24] The other two organisms, ss *intestinalis* and ss *jejuni*, are found in a variety of domestic animals (cattle, sheep, goats, swine, dogs, cats, chickens, turkeys, and other birds). The former is associated with rare episodes of septic abortion or septicemic disease in humans.[25] The latter is a recently defined cause of human gastroenteritis, involved in 5 to 10% or more of etiologically defined acute enteritis in infants, children, and young adults in many areas around the world.[26-30] These cases have generally been attributed to contact with infected dogs with acute diarrhea,[27] drinking unpasteurized milk,[28] or contact with infected poultry,[29] but in the majority the route is unknown. Infection with *C. jejuni* is thus probably a zoonosis, although outbreaks, possibly caused by person-to-person transmission, have been reported in day care nurseries.[31] The infectious dose is not known, but one volunteer ingesting 10^6 organisms became ill in three days.[32]

Yersinia enterocolitica has only recently been classified in the family Enterobacteriaceae, along with *Y. pseudotuberculosis*, having formerly been designated as *Pasteurella* species.[33] *Y. enterocolitica* can be further subdivided by serologic criteria into 34 O-antigen types, with further distinctions made on the basis of 19 H-antigens, phage typing (five types), and biotypes (five distinct patterns). Most human infections, however, are caused by only three O-antigen types, 0:3, 0:9, and 0:8.

The prevalence of the individual serotypes varies from country to country and within a given area, sometimes from region to region.[33-35] Serotype 0:8 is common in the United States and unusual in neighboring Canada, where 0:3, phage type 9B, biotype 4 predominates. Over 90% of infections in Sweden are caused by 0:3, phage type 8, biotype 4, while in adjacent Finland, serotype 0:9 accounts for 40% of human isolates. In Japan, 0:3, phage type 8 prevails, while in South Africa it is 0:3, phage type 9A. It may well be this circumscribed distribution of distinctive *Y. enterocolitica* strains that accounts for differences in clinical manifestations of yersiniosis from country to country—for example, the prevalence of erythema nodosum in Scandinavia. Of the common serogroups in human infections, only 0:3 is frequently found in animals, being recovered from feces, cecal contents, and mesenteric lymph nodes of swine.[36] In some situations transmission fron animal to human has been suggested.[37]

Y. enterocolitica has also been isolated from unchlorinated mountain stream or well water, unpasteurized milk, pasteurized chocolate milk and ice cream, and raw or vacuum-packed meat.[34,38-41] Most of these isolates have been non-human-assocated serotypes; however, some of these sources (well or mountain stream water and chocolate milk) have been implicated as the cause of documented infections.[38,40] Human-to-human transmission is thought to account for spread of infection during outbreaks in families, between families, or in institutions (hospitals) as well.[42] The role of asymptomatic fecal carriers in transmission is unknown, but such individuals have been identified.[43] The infectious dose is not known.

PATHOGENESIS

The ability of each of the organisms considered here to invade intestinal epithelial cells and to cause tissue pathology appears to underlie some aspects of pathogenesis of disease.[1] The evidence for tissue penetration and its importance is incontrovertible for shigellas and salmonellas, and highly suggestive for both *Campylobacter jejuni* and *Yersinia enterocolitica* (Table II).

THE ROLE OF EPITHELIAL CELL INVASION

Invasive properties of *Shigellae* have been well studied by Formal and co-workers in animal models of diarrhea and dysentery in the Rhesus monkey and guinea pig, experimental infections in humans, infections of guinea pig, rabbit, or rat cornea, or in cell culture.[44-48] In all models, there is a strong correlation between invasion and gastrointestinal virulence of the isolate. Spontaneous transformation of *Shigella* during *in vitro* culture from a translucent colonial form to an opaque colony

Table II. Evidence for Tissue Invasion by Enteric Pathogens *in Vivo*

			Fecal cells	
Genus	Tissue biopsy	Bacteremia	RBC	WBC
Shigella sp.	I,N,B[a]	Rare	Common	Common
Salmonella sp.	I,B	Common	Occasionally	Common
Yersinia enterocolitica	I,B	? Unusual	Occasionally	? Occasionally
Campylobacter jejuni	I	? Common	? Common	? Common

[a]I = inflammation, N = necrosis, B = bacteria demonstrable by histologic examination and/or microbiological culture techniques.

has been shown to be associated with conversion from invasive to non-invasive, and from virulent to avirulent.[6,45,46,49,50] In *S. sonnei*, this conversion has recently also been ascribed to the loss of a large, ~ 120 Mdal plasmid coding for smoth lipopolysaccharide (LPS) (Form I).[51] The plasmid-deleted avirulent Form II rough colony can be restored to the virulent colonial type by mobilizing the 120 Mdal DNA with another plasmid, R386, tagged with the transposon Tn5. But inasmuch as noninvasive Form I colonies have been isolated, this antigen marker cannot be the only determinant of invasiveness of *S. sonnei*. A rough mutant *S. flexneri* 2a has also been isolated that is able to invade tissue culture cells, but not to evoke keratoconjunctivitis in guinea pigs.[52] These data suggest that multiple virulence factors may be involved in invasiveness of *Shigellae.*

Other experiments indeed point to involvement of other attributes of the bacterial cell surface in cellular invasion. For example, in *S. flexneri* 2a, the translucent-to-opaque transformation is associated with alterations in bacterial electrophoretic mobility and detergent sensitivity, and also with quantitative changes in glycerol kinase activity.[53-55] In addition, if *E. coli* 0-8 chromosomal material is inserted into virulent *Shigella* recipients by hybridization techniques that convert the somatic O-antigen specificity from *S. flexneri* 2a to *E. coli* 0-8 (which share the common immunodominant sugar, rhamnose), invasiveness is maintained in the hybrid.[56] If, however, *E. coli* 0-25, which has a different immunodominant sugar, is employed instead, then invasive properties are lost and the resulting hybrid is avirulent. It is of interest that the few *Shigella*-like, naturally invasive *E. coli* strains that cause *Shigella*-like disease are of a limited number of 0-serotypes, and frequently share distinct *Shigella* surface antigens,[57] further indicating the importance of these surface properties in the invasive process. It is fair to state, however, that the actual mechanism of penetration is unknown at this time.

Some *E. coli–Shigella flexneri* 2a hybrids have been found to penetrate the gut epithelium, but instead of multiplying they are cleared within a few hours and no clinical manifestations of infection ensue.[47] Some, but not all, hybrid strains are also inhibited in their growth on minimal media *in vitro.*[58,59] These observations suggest that multiplication of penetrating shigellas is required for virulence as well, a concept supported by the finding that streptomycin-dependent variants, unable to multiply in the absence of the antibiotic, are also avirulent.[60] For this reason, streptomycin-dependent organisms have been employed experimentally as an attenuated live oral vaccine strain with considerable success.[61]

Following invasion of colonic epithelium, shigellas multiply intracellularly, resulting in lateral cell-to-cell spread of organisms, epithelial cell death, the formation of microulcers on the mucosal surface, and a marked inflammatory reaction. This has been found during infection in both humans and monkeys.[6,46,48,49,62] In the latter species, the small intestine is spared, and the infection specifically results in an invasive bacterial colitis.[63] Consistent with this, colonic pathology is found by endoscopy in human patients, and by histologic examination of biopsy and postmortem specimens[62] (Figures 1 and 2). But in spite of these extensive mucosal lesions, *Shigellae* are not usually recovered from blood culture,[63,64] in part because these are not generally obtained, and also in part because most strains appear to be readily killed by the serum comple-

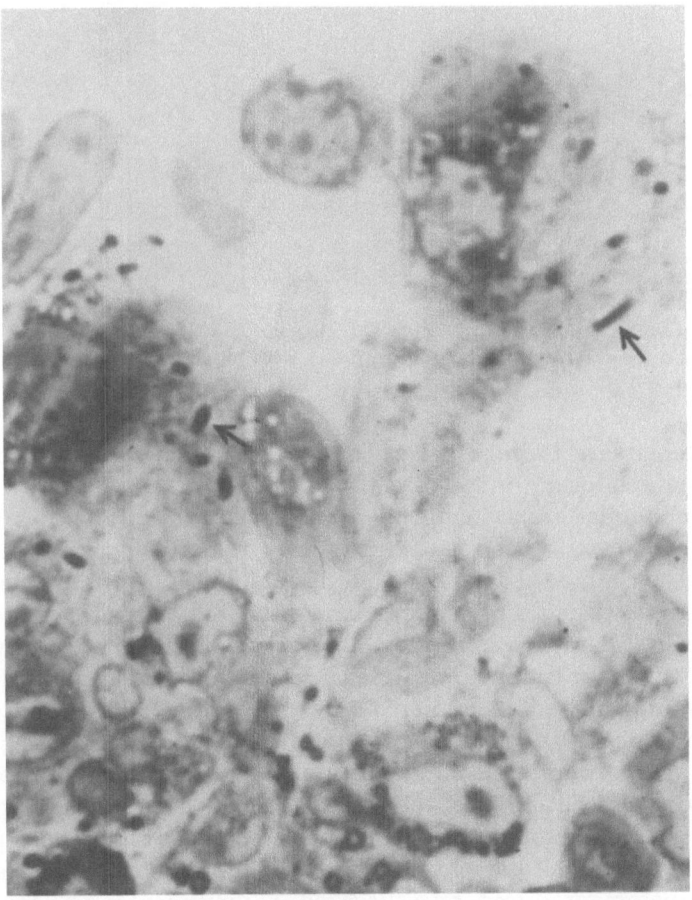

Figure 1. Colonic biopsy during acute shigellosis demonstrating the presence of intracellular bacteria (arrows); Giemsa stain, 400 ×.

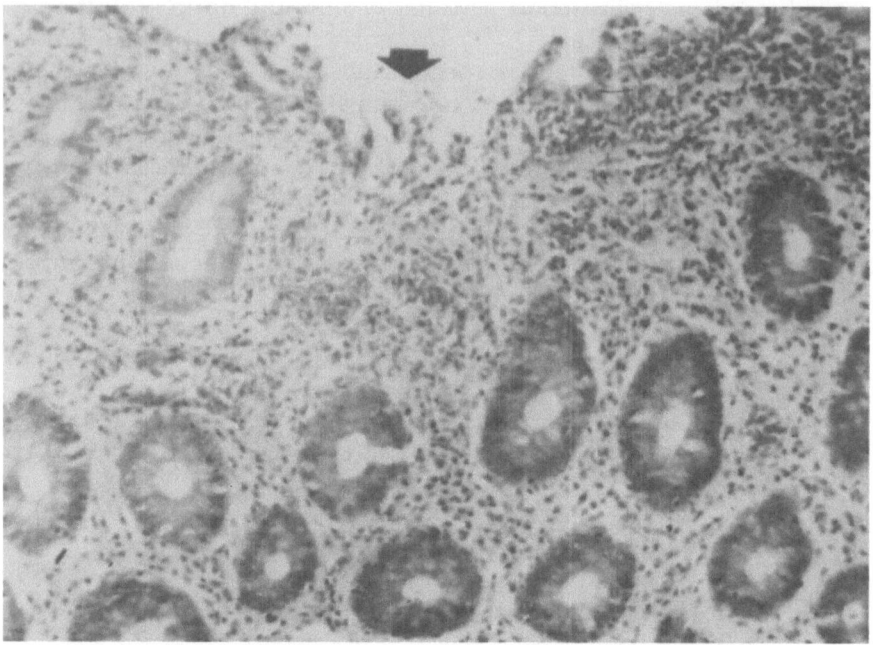

Figure 2. Colonic biopsy during acute shigellosis demonstrating microulcer formation (arrow) and the intense inflammatory response with hemorrhage in the lamina propria; H&E stain, 400 ×.

ment-dependent bactericidal system.[65] The genus should therefore be classified as a locally invasive pathogen.

Salmonellas are systemically invasive; culture of blood early in the course of *Salmonella* gastroenteritis will regularly yield positive results,[1,10] whereas sustained bacteremia is the hallmark of both the enteric (typhoid) fever and septicemic (*S. cholerasuis*) syndromes.[66] While *S. typhi* invades in the upper gastrointestinal tract and initially enters the bloodstream, the organism is rapidly cleared by mononuclear phagocytic cells in liver and spleen.[67] In human studies with the Quailes strain, an inoculum of at least 10^5 organisms is required to produce disease.[16] Further events are determined by the ability of the organism to multiply intracellularly, and the ability of the host to activate bactericidal mechanisms against the intracellular pathogen. This latter process depends upon activation of the macrophage by cell-mediated immune mechanisms involving mediators produced by sensitized T-lymphocytes.[68,69] Dose-dependence of disease production is thus an expression of the race between multiplication and killing of the intracellular bacterial population, for it seems that whenever a critical number of bacteria are present, they will break out into the bloodstream, initiating the clinical phase of the disease.[70] The greater the inoculum, the sooner this happens; at the other extreme, with a small enough dose bacteremia never occurs and no clinical disease results. This secondary bacteremia also leads directly to two critical events in typhoid fever—invasion of the gall bladder and Peyer's patches of the gut, both of which cause positive stool cultures by the second week of the clinical disease.[67] When the ensuing local inflammatory response is severe, necrotizing cholecystitis or intestinal hemorrhage or perforation may follow.

Studies of *Salmonella* gastroenteritis in experimental animals, summarized recently by Turnbull,[10] indicate that the ileum is the major site of infection, but that cecal and colonic lesions occur as well. The invasion process has been studied by Takeuchi and co-workers using *S. typhimurium* in a guinea pig model.[71,72] When the organisms closely approach the epithelial cell brush border (<35 nm), the microvilli appear to melt away and organisms enter the cells in a membrane-bound vesicle. Turnbull and Richmond have also demonstrated invasion of *S. enteritidis* into cecal epithelial cells in the day-old chick, also within vesicles.[73] In both models, organisms penetrate into the lamina propria, from which they can presumably enter the bloodstream to produce early bacteremia.

The evidence that *C. jejuni* or *Y. enterocolitica* are virulent because they are invasive is less well established than is the case for *Shigella* or *Salmonella*. For both organisms clinical evidence of intestinal mucosal damage, the frequency of positive cultures from tissues or bloodstream, experimental animal studies, and assays of *in vitro* invasive properties in cell culture all indicate that virulent strains are invasive.[29,33,42,74–76] However, only limited data are available to indicate that noninvasive strains are avirulent, and it is not yet possible to convert avirulent strains to virulence by selecting for (or genetically creating) invasive variants.

Carter has demonstrated that intragastric inoculation of a human clinical isolate of *Y. enterocolitica* is SPF mice (CD-1) will produce an illness having many features in common with the human disease.[77] Within 24 hours there is evidence of penetration of the organism into Peyer's patches in the ileum, and a neutrophilic infiltration is found at the site. Within the next few days infection spreads to the mesenteric lymph nodes, resulting in intramedullary abscesses. Following this, more generalized spread occurs, manifesting as suppurative lesions of liver, spleen, and lung. Intravenous inoculation gives rise to liver, spleen, and lung involvement, but not intestinal lesions; hence, oral inoculation is necessary to cause ulcerative enteritis of the ileum. This indicates the need for local contact and invasion in pathogenesis. Progression beyond the gut mucosa is related at least in part to inoculum size, and if this is sufficiently large, infection spreads systemically to mesenteric nodes, and from there to the various parenchymal organs.

Endoscopy and histological examination of human biopsy materials suggest a similar sequence of events.[78,79] Patients with diarrhea often manifest nonspecific intestinal inflammatory changes, with cellular infiltration and ulceration of bowel mucosa. Terminal ileitis is often found at laparotomy in *Y. enterocolitica*-infected patients with mesenteric adenitis who present with the "pseudo-appendicitis (right lower quadrant) syndrome."[80] Furtheremore, dissemination to the liver and spleen can occur in some human patients with yersinial sepsis.[81]

Clinical manifestations are also consistent with an invasive process, at least in some patients. Diarrheal disease, most commonly in young children (and the most common presentation of *Y. enterocolitica* in them), can vary in severity from extremely mild to fulminant ulcerative enteritis involving the entire intestinal tract.[33,35,40,42,43,78,82] Fever is frequently noted and may be prominent and spiking, but it can also be entirely absent.[35,79] Occasionally, blood is present in stool (gross or occult), but bleeding may become massive in a few patients.[42,78,79] Finally, the presence of fecal leukocytes is described, although its frequency is uncertain because it is not always looked for.[35,42,79,82,83]

In vitro studies of clinical *Y. enterocolitica* isolates in cell culture employing HeLa or Hep-2 cells demonstrate a high frequency of invasiveness,[76,83,84] particularly serogroups 0:3, 0:8, and 0:9. Invasive properties can also be demonstrated with serotype 0:8 isolates in a Sereny test in guinea pig cornea.[75] Pai *et al.*[85] have shown that clinical isolates of the 0:3 serogroup will cause a symptomatic, acute enteritis in baby (500 to 800 g) rabbits, involving both small and large bowel, but predominantly in the ileum. The early lesion consists of bacterial invasion of the mucosa with subsequent extension to form deep crypt abscesses composed of a nidus of bacteria surrounded and admixed with inflammatory cells, including neutrophils, macrophages, and eosinophils. Adjacent crypts often show focal necrosis and degeneration with minute areas of overlying mucosal ulceration. An isolate from raw fish, serotype 0:6, unable to invade HeLa cells and negative for heat-stable enterotoxin, was clinically avirulent in this model and caused no lesions by histological examination.

C. jejuni produces a fairly characteristic diarrheal illness with a predilection for young adults in industrialized nations and young children in developing countries.[29,30,74] There is often a prodromal period with fever, nausea, malaise, headache, myalgia, backache, and abdominal pain.[29,74,86] After a day or so, the abdominal pain becomes colicky and watery diarrhea begins. In some patients, fresh blood or mucus may be grossly visible in the stools; however, on microscopic examination the majority of samples contain both erythrocytes and leukocytes.[29,74,86] Blood cultures are frequently positive for the organism.[29,74] The fever usually promptly subsides, the diarrhea may continue for 3 to 4 days, while abdominal pain and tenderness persist.[74] Recurrence of fever, diarrhea, and/or abdominal symptoms occurs in up to 10% of patients.[29,74] The prominence of the abdominal condition may result in exploratory laparotomy.[87] Diffuse bowel inflammation and mesenteric adenitis are usually found in such patients. Occasionally, involvement of the colon can be so severe as to lead to toxic dilatation, but more often in patients subjected to sigmoidoscopy one observes erythema, edema, granularity, focal contact bleeding, and exudation of the mucosa.[88-90] Biopsy is consistent with a nonspecific colitis.[89,90]

Experimental C. jejuni infection in 10-day-old chick embryo cell cultures results in extensive invasion by 24 hours.[74] The organisms at first are found within membrane vesicles, but over the next 8 hours, as bacterial multiplication occurs, degenerative changes develop in the cytoplasm and the cells die. Oral infection of 3- to 8-day-old chicks leads to colonization of small bowel and cecum, and invasion of intestinal epithelial cells, associated with positive blood cultures in about one-third of the birds.[74,91] The younger chicks also manifest bloody diarrhea.[91]

THE ROLE OF ENTEROTOXINS

Recent studies indicate that invasive pathogens can also produce enterotoxins (Table III). Their role in pathogenesis, however, is uncertain. Let us first consider Shigella, a locally invasive organism. The clinical consequence of the acute invasive bacterial colitis this produces is the classical dysentery syndrome, a triad of abdominal pain and cramps,

Table III. Reported Toxin Effects in Model Systems for Bacterial Enterotoxins

Genus	Rabbit loop (LT-like)	Suckling mouse (ST-like)	CHO cell	HeLa cytotoxicity
Shigella sp.	+[a]	−[b]	+	+
Salmonella sp.	Variable +	+	+	−
Yersinia enterocolitica	+	+	−	?[c]
Campylobacter jejuni	?	Some strains +	?	?

[a] + = reported positive.
[b] − = reported negative.
[c] ? = unreported or equivocal evidence to date.

tenesmus, and frequent passage of scant-volume, bloody-mucoid stools containing many leukocytes.[62] However, the most frequent clinical presentation of shigellosis is not dysentery, but rather simple watery diarrhea.[62,92] What, then, is the cause of the watery diarrhea? An important seminal observation has been provided by Rout et al.,[63] who demonstrated in the infected Rhesus monkey that diarrhea in shigellosis is associated with the secretion of isotonic fluid by the jejunum in the absence of local invasion or histologic abnormalities, but associated with the presence of many bacteria in the jejunal lumen. Kinsey and co-workers[93] further demonstrated that infection produced by intracecal, rather than per oral, inoculation, causes invasive colitis and dysentery, but neither jejunal secretion nor watery diarrhea develops. The latter manifestations thus apparently require local bacterial colonization for pathogenesis, and certainly suggest the possiblity of an enterotoxin effect, as seen in cholera and most E. coli diarrhea.[1]

Recent studies by Keusch et al.[94-96] have demonstrated that all species of Shigella are toxigenic, producing a heat-labile protein toxin that induces fluid secretion in rabbit small bowel. In rabbit ileum this is accompanied by histologic abnormalities similar to those produced by infection in the Rhesus or human colon,[97] but in the rabbit ileum there is no pathologic alteration.[98] Although some evidence suggests that activation of adenylate cyclase and increases in mucosal cyclic AMP may accompany the secretion,[99] other conflicting data have been published,[100] and at the present time the biochemical mechanism is not known.

The toxin appears to be inactive when placed on the surface of Rhesus or rat colon.[101,102] However, a second toxic activity of Shigellae may be relevant to the production of colonic lesions.[103] All species also produce a lethal cytotoxin that has been studied in a variety of in vitro cell culture systems.[95,96,104-107] These data indicate that the cytotoxin acts at an intracellular locus, probably as an inhibitor of cellular protein synthesis.[108] Hale and Formal[50] have demonstrated that Shigella strains invading HeLa cells rapidly turn off protein synthesis by the HeLa cell, while the bacteria continue to metabolize normally, and this is probably related to intracellular toxin production. Pathology in the colon could therefore be secondary to in situ toxin production by the invading organism within the epithelial cell, leading to inhibition of protein synthesis and cell death.[103]

Studies in natural and induced experimental infections in humans with S. dysenteriae 1, S. flexneri strains, and S. sonnei document the production of specific toxin-neutralizing antibody during the course of infection.[95,109] The antibody has been shown to be of the IgM class, to rise rapidly, and to disappear gradually after a year or so.[95,96,109] Altbough antitoxin has been assayed in a cytotoxicity neutralizing assay, all current evidence indicates that this biological activity is associated witb the enterotoxin (rabbit intestinal loop activity) as well.[110,111] These data certainly support the hypothesis that toxin antigen is produced during actual infection of the human host.

Cell-free toxin(s) thus can explain the pathogenesis of the specific, distinctive cellular lesions in acute shigellosis.[62] Toxin may also explain the motor abnormalities of the gut during shigellosis, clinically manifested as waves of cramps and tenesmus.[62] Application of toxin to in situ loops of rabbit bowel is reported to result in significant alterations in myoelectric activity of the gut, including increase in both migrating action potential complexes (activity of single, isolated ring contractions) and repetitive bursts of action potential (multiple, simultaneous ring contractions that may or may not propagate).[112] The effect is similar to that observed in actual infection with either invasive-toxigenic S. dysenteriae 1 or invasive E. coli.[112,113] If toxin, and not invasion, is the key to the proximal small bowel abnormalities in shigellosis, while invasion of colonic epithelia is simply a mechanism to deliver toxin to the cytoplasm of the colonic cell (because colon may lack appropriate cell surface toxin receptors),[114,115] then it remains to be explained why toxigenic, noninvasive opaque colonial mutants of virulent shigellas are totally avirulent. Why is there no diarrheal phase as well as no dysentery? The answer is unknown, but two possibilities come to mind: (1) The transformation of colonial form alters both invasive and colonizing activity of the organism, and/or (2) the altered colony type is more susceptible to elimination in the gut mucosa by normal host defense mechanisms. These are readily testable hypotheses.

With respect to Salmonella gastroenteritis strains, Giannella et al. have shown that, whereas invasion is necessary for virulence, it is not sufficient; the organism must also induce a local polymorphonuclear leukocyte inflammatory response to evoke a secretory process.[116,117] Treatment of rabbits with nitrogen mustard to deplete leukocytes before exposure to Salmonella typhimurium infection blunts the subsequent secretory response.[118] In spite of the inflammation, however, the permeability barrier function of the gut is maintained; intravenous administration of ^{51}Cr-albumin or ^{14}C mannitol does not result in their appearance in the gut lumen in infected Rhesus monekys or in the rabbit ileal loop model.[119,120] However, not all of the invasive inflammation-provoking strains cause secretion.[116] This suggests the possibility that an enterotoxin activity may be present as well. This remains an unproven hypothesis, in spite of reports by Sandefur and Peterson[121] of a heat-labile skin-permeability factor from S. typhimurium, which is also active on Chinese hamster ovary cells in vitro and neutralized by cholera toxin, and by Koupal and Deibel[122] of a factor from S. enteritidis causing fluid secretion in the infant mouse intestine, and by Sedlock and Deibel[123] of positive ligated rabbit ileal loop responses to broth culture supernatants from various gastroenteritis strains of S. enteritidis if the gut is first washed with a mucolytic agent.

Giannella and Kinsey and colleagues[119,120] have shown, in perfused, infected ligated ileal loops in Rhesus monkeys, that gut permeability to monosaccharides is unaltered, even in the presence of histologic damage. Rather, adenylate cyclase is activated and mucosal cyclic-AMP is elevated and this may explain the secretory state of the tissue. Based on the inhibitory effects of indomethacin upon the secretory response, however, these authors have speculated tbat instead of an enterotoxin, prostaglandins may be involved in this process.[124-126] However, difficulties in consistently demonstrating in vitro either a choleralike or an E. coli-like enterotoxin in Salmonella strains does not exclude their production in vivo, or the possibility of a different kind of enterotoxin.

The relationship of the CHO factor of Sandefur and Peterson to a bona fide enterotoxin activity in vivo is, in fact, suggested by the observation that partially purified CHO (delayed permeability) factor causes a positive rabbit loop that is blocked by monospecific cholera antitoxin, as well as by the report that protection against live Salmonella challenge is provided by prior immunization with heated cholera toxin.[127]

Molina and Peterson[128] have recently reported that the CHO factor is inducible in vitro by mitomycin-C treatment of the organism (0.5 μg/ml of culture); under these conditions, five of seven clinical gastroenteritis isolates of S. enteritidis produced detectable CHO factor. Consistent with previous data, this was heat-labile, inhibited by G_{M1} ganglioside, and neutralized by cholera antitoxin. Assuming the specific activity of the salmonella CHO to be equal to that of cholera toxin, one can calculate that the level of toxin production by Salmonellae, even in the presence of mitomycin-C, is many magnitudes of order less than for V. cholerae.[128] The quantitative differences could readily account for the difficulty in demonstrating rabbit loop activity in the salmonella product.

In contrast, it has been relatively easy to demonstrate production of an enterotoxin by strains of Y. enterocolitica, of both buman and non-human-associated serotypes, provided the organism is grown at 22 to 25°C and not at 35 to 37°C.[75,129-132] Mors and Pai[133] reported that 70/88 (79.5%) of Y. enterocolitica of diverse serogroups and 37/40 (92.5%) of human serogroup isolates (0:3, 0:8, 0:9) were positive in the suckling mouse assay. Yersinia enterotoxin shares many properties with E. coli ST. Both are active in the mouse model, both are heat-stable (especially the Y. enterocolitica toxin, which is resistant to even 121°C for 30 minutes), both are acid-stable (the yersinia toxin is in fact reported to be stable to pH 1–11), both are soluble in methanol, and neither is active in Y-l adrenal or CHO cell assays. The *Y. enterocolitica* toxin, like *E. coli* ST, apparently is also able to activate intestinal guanylate cyclase activity, to increase intracellular levels of cyclic guanosine 3′,5′-monophosphate, and to inhibit active chloride absorption.[134,135]

Rao *et al.*[134] have reported that a partially purified yersinia toxin causes a rapid and persistent increase in rabbit ileal electrical potential difference when applied to the luminal side of stripped mucosa mounted *in vitro* in a Ussing chamber, with a rise in short-circuit current and no significant alteration in tissue resistance. Unidirectional and net flux measurements of chloride show that the toxin decreases the mucosa-to-serosa movement and increases the serosa-to-mucosa flux, resulting in a net decrease in chloride absorption. A threefold increase in tissue cyclic-GMP was found, and when higher doses of toxin were employed, a consistent increase in mucosal particulate guanylate cyclase was observed as well. Robin-Browne *et al.*[135] have also reported that 20-fold concentrated *Y. enterocolitica* toxin activates guanylate cyclase in the infant mouse small bowel but does not affect adenylate cyclase.

Unlike *E. coli* ST, however, the role of the yersinia toxin in pathogenesis remains speculative. A major argument against such a role is the consistent finding that toxin is not produced *in vitro* when organisms are grown at temperatures above 30°C. If this is true *in vivo* as well, then a thermally suitable human host would have problems more severe than *Yersinia enterocolitica* infection to deal with. A less convincing argument is the failure to find evidence of toxin production in gut lumen contents in animal models, for this might occur only intracellularly following invasion and therefore be difficult to detect. The ST activity of *Y. enterocolitica* is therefore a toxin in search of a disease.

In a preliminary report, Butzler and Skirrow[74] screened 100 strains of *Campylobacter jejuni* for production of *E. coli* ST-like toxins in the infant mouse model. While 16 were positive, the authors suggested that it was unlikely to be of significance because 84 were negative. However, it is possible that the necessary genetic information is carried on an unstable plasmid easily lost during *in vitro* growth, or that the culture conditions employed were inappropriate. It is therefore premature to draw any conclusions concerning enterotoxigenicity in the genus *Camplyobacter*. Certainly, given the data recently accumulated for other enteroinvasive organisms, it would be unwise to dismiss the possibility of an inducible or intracellular toxin being produced *in vivo*. There is clear evidence for *Shigella* that Fe^{+++} concentration affects toxin production *in vitro*, and many other regulatory factors could be involved to explain the current problems with *in vitro* culture systems.

NUTRITIONAL CONSEQUENCES

The above considerations of pathogenesis indicate that all four groups of pathogens penetrate the intestinal epithelium and result in damage and inflammation of the mucosa, with a predilection for specific sites in the gastrointestinal tract. In addition, there is evidence for *Shigella*, *Salmonella*, and perhaps *Yersinia enterocolitica* infection, that, independent of histologic changes, a secretory mechanism may be activated by cell-free toxic bacterial metabolites, either by up-regulating an active blood-to-lumen transport or down-regulating a lumen-to-blood absorptive process. These are important considerations, for the nutritional consequences of generalized mucosal injury are likely to be much different from those of a selective aberration of an ion transport regulatory system, as in cholera.

Whatever the actual pathogenesis of the four infections, there are several mechanisms through which significant nutritional effects may occur.

First, these agents have a propensity to cause fever, often as the first manifestation of the infection. In the case of *Shigella* infection of young children, the rise in temperature may be so steep and so high that febrile convulsions are induced.[62,64] In the example of *Campylobacter*, fever may be present during the prodrome only, and may disappear when diarrhea begins.[74] Fever has definable metabolic costs,[136] and in addition is clearly associated with a variety of metabolic alterations in the host,[137] including shifts in trace minerals from plasma to an intracellular compartment, increased amino acid flux from muscle to liver, altered priorities for protein synthesis in liver, and dramatic changes in carbohydrate tolerance. The associated anorexia, of uncertain pathophysiology, serves to sharply reduce oral intake of nutrients at precisely the same time, forcing the individual to rely upon tissue (muscle) protein catabolism and gluconeogenesis for energy.[138] Prolonged or repetitive fever has a significant cumulative adverse effect upon host nutriture. This is readily seen in typhoid fever, which is in essence a systemic infection of the mononuclear phagocyte system, producing sustained bacteremia, lasting from 4 to 10 weeks in the untreated patient, and resulting in profound weight loss and debility.[137,138]

Second, all four agents do cause structural abnormalities of some portion of the gut mucosa and an inflammatory response, as the result of either bacterial invasion or toxin production, or both. Tissue destruction in the gut and sloughing of epithlial cells must lead to abnormal fecal losses of nitrogen in the form of denuded epithelium, inflammatory cells, erythrocytes, and some leakage of plasma proteins along with the blood, which, if great or sustained, could directly result in a clinical protein-losing enteropathy.

Third, it has been shown at least for *Shigella* and *Salmonella*, that malabsorption of carbohydrate and possibly of fat or vitamins is often present during and for a time after acute enteritis.[139-141] Disaccharidase deficiency is quite common, in fact. There is no reason to suspect that *Yersinia* or *Campylobacter* are different in this regard, although data are not available at the present time.

Fourth, the enterotoxin of *Shigella dysenteriae* 1 has been experimentally demonstrated to reduce active sugar and amino acid absorption by small bowel mucosa.[142] This may be secondary to the mucosal structural damage the toxin causes. On the other hand, *Salmonella* infection of the ileum in rabbits does not result in leakage of monosaccharide markers from blood to lumen in spite of the acute inflammation present.[119,120] However, these studies were designed to investigate the permeability barrier function of the gut mucosa, which was thus shown to be intact, and they were not intended to reveal nutritionally significant absorptive defects that may be present. *Salmonella* infection has been associated with malabsorption.[140,141]

Fifth, the frequency of intestinal cramps during infection indicates the occurrence of abnormal gut motility. Any alteration of motility that affects the efficient aboral propulsion of intestinal contents can lead to local stasis and bacterial proliferation. Persistent bacterial overgrowth in the small bowel can certainly have a significant impact on nutritional status.[143]

Sixth, all four agents can cause a profound watery diarrhea, directly resulting in electrolyte losses and dehydration. While prodigious choleralike diarrhea and rapid cardiovascular collapse, shock, and death are unusual, significant dehydration requiring appropriate oral or intravenous fluid therapy is not at all uncommon.

Finally, the propensity of *Shigella* and possibly *Campylobacter* infections (and occasionally *Yersinia enterocolitica* as well) to become chronic stretches out over time the potential nutritional impact of infection, and increases the cumulative effects caused by any of the above mechanisms.[2,35,74] At the same time, the multiplicity of distinctive shigellas and salmonellas, and at least for the former, the restricted (homologous) nature of acquired immunity,[61] means that repeated infections with different strains can occur. Indeed, prospective studies in Guatemala and Egypt have both demonstrated an incidence of two *Shigella* infections per person per year in preschool children.[144,145]

Biological Considerations in Control
Strategies

For those noninvasive intestinal pathogens that require a large inoculum (in excess of 10^6 organisms) for clinical virulence, a vehicle in which bacterial multiplication can occur is generally required to amplify the infectious dose. Since smaller numbers of bacteria, whether directly transmitted or carried in food or by water, will not result in disease, a logical strategy is to prevent postcontamination multiplication by appropriate food-handling and storage techniques, particularly proper cold storage. The latter will not suffice for *Yersinia enterocolitica*, however, as this organism can multiply reasonably well at low temperature,[33] and indeed, microbiological isolation of the organism is facilitated by cold enrichment techniques, in which the differential multiplication of the *Yersinia* compared to other *Enterobacteriaceae* significantly increases the isolation rate.[146]

However, proper food-handling will not alter transmission of pathogens that spread by direct person-to-person contact and/or need only a tiny dose to cause infection. The shigellas are a good example of this class of pathogen. Theoretically at least, highly host-adapted organisms such as shigellas can be eradicated from the world by an effective vaccine to prevent person-to-person spread. If the organism cannot indefinitely survive in the carrier state, then it should eventually become an extinct species. Two problems arise with this approach to shigellosis: First, such a vaccine does not exist, and second, primates other than man are acceptable hosts,[2] and therefore there may be a natural sylvatic cycle in the wild in monkeys.

Actually, some of the shigellosis occurring in monkeys in captivity could be acquired from humans and then transmitted from monkey-to-monkey, or monkey-to-man, and the extent of shigellosis in the wild is uncertain. The reality of transmission of *Shigella* infection by a few hundred bacteria also increases the likelihood that fomites are involved wherever adequate handling of human excreta is not possible. On a scale of priorities, however, it is infinitely more important to deal with fecal indiscretion than it is to control flies, since the problem of transmission can certainly be said to begin and end in stool.

Unlike shigellosis, the problem of salmonellosis is complicated by the lack of host adaptation of the major gastroenteritis strains, and the enormous number of animal reservoirs. Eradication strategies therefore will not work, and if the inoculum in food or various dessicated vehicles (in which the organism does not multiply but simply survives) is as low as reported, then similar to the situation with shigellosis, good food-handling will not stop the spread of disease.[10] As a zoonosis of domesticated food animals, the problem could be approachable by exemplary veterinary public health measures. This is not easy, however. If the threat to human health were largely due to clinically ill animals, the veterinarian could conceivably weed these out of the food chain. However, much clinical animal salmonellosis is caused by animal-adapted strains that do not cause human illness, whereas nonadapted human pathogens in animals cause asymptomatic infections.[10] Unless vaccines for these various human strains were available (which is not the case), and economically feasible as well, there is no practical way to approach eradication of the reservoir in animals.

What can be done is to practice simple, high-quality husbandry techniques to prevent introduction of strains into herds or flocks by monitoring the health of new additions to flocks and herds and ensuring that feeds are not contaminated, by containment practices to limit spread of an introduced infection, by avoidance of stress that promotes fecal excretion of *Salmonella*, by minimizing spread of intestinal contents during animal slaughter, and by refrigeration or heat to prevent growth or to kill organisms in unprocessed or processed foods, respectively.[10] These measures will reduce the inoculum reaching the susceptible population and, combined with proper cooking, handling, and storage of food, will reduce the incidence and prevalence of infection. In the most sophisticated industrialized nations this goal may be in part attainable by intensive efforts and surveillance by regulatory agencies, as well as voluntary compliance by farmers, abattoir workers, and the entire food industry, but it is an imposing task. What is the likelihood of success in a developing country, with other, more immediate problems to deal with and a limited budget for either technical support for surveillance or enforcement agents?

However successfully this is accomplished, it will not completely stop transmission of salmonellosis. Other sources of introduction to susceptibles must be considered and stopped as well, including spread in nature by nondomesticated animals, via pets such as turtles, and person-to-person spread within institutions such as hospitals. If these are ignored, and particularly if organisms from such sources can contaminate inadequate sewage or water systems, another cycle of transmission may be established with eventual reintroduction into the food supply system and dissemination once again. Nosocomial infections can be reduced by enforcement of enteric precautions for known cases and good hand-washing practices by staff, and by monitoring food-handlers and other hospital employees with direct patient-contact responsibiltiy during convalescence from acute diarrheal disease.

In some ways, the problem of *Campylobacter* infection appears similar to that of the salmonellas, since a major source of human infection is from farm or household animals.[29,74] For the latter situation, proper education—such as hand-washing after handling pet animals or their excreta and before kitchen work; separate utensils for pets; proper use, preparation, and storage of food (e.g., drinking only pasteurized milk)—should reduce risk. Again, this is more difficult in rural communities in developing countries in which humans and animals live together as one extended family, eating, sleeping, and defecating on the same turf, or indeed in the same room of the house.

At the present time, there is insufficient knowledge of the epidemiology of *Yersinia enterocolitica*, or the biological peculiarities that determine its geographic serotype distribution, to predict the critical factors to consider for emphasis in control measures. Undoubtedly, common sense in environmental sanitation and health practices within households is important, but this is not unique. The one area that seems of special interest is the apparent temperature regulation of certain potential virulence factors,[33] such as motility or toxin production, both of which occur at relatively low temperatures of less than 30°C. This, coupled with the winter peak in incidence and the concentration of documented infection in temperate (or cold) rather than in tropical countries, has suggested that cold enhancement of virulence may be a prerequisite for pathogenicity. In other words, the organism is basically friendly in the 37°C human (asymptomatic carriers) but is converted to a virulent form by growth at low ambient temperature, presumably occurring in the environment. Whether this means that *Yersinia* gastroenteritis is due to ingestion of preformed toxin or other virulence factor is uncertain. It is unknown what the organism is really like *in vivo* at 37°C and whether or not it makes toxin or other virulence factors, and if so what regulates their production. ˙

For all invasive pathogens, whether motile like *Salmonella*, nonmotile like *Shigella*, or like *Yersinia enterocolitica*, motile or not, depending on growth conditions, there must be a critical interaction at the cell surface for invasion to occur. Since there is clear site specificity for this process and localization to certain areas of the gut, some sort of recognition mechanism must be operative in addition to whatever is involved in the phagocytosis of these bacteria by the "nonprofessional" phagocytic intestinal epithelial cells. If this involves a receptor–ligand type of complementary binding interaction, then it is possible to consider receptor-oriented strategies, such as blockade, modification, or elution therapy.[103,115] If the specificity involves simple carbohydrate determinants that do not mediate other essential functions, then such ecological control measures can be considered. If this is not the case, and this is more likely so, then development of an insoluble, nonabsorbable receptor analogue for oral administration might be feasible to compete for the attachment to the natural cell receptor. Favorable results have recently been reported for cholera in which the toxin receptor, G_{M1} ganglioside, was coupled to charcoal and administered per os, with significant reduction in diarrhea in treated patients.[147]

If cell penetration is essential to pathogenesis, no matter what happens after that step to initiate disease, the first level of biological control is to interfere with the invasion step itself. Phenotypic variation in either host cell or bacterium could conceivably modulate invasiveness, and such variation could be related to alterations in glycosylation of surface components or metabolite suppression of biosynthetic pathways. While there are no advances in this regard to report at present, it seems reasonable to raise the level of interest now, since there is considerable ongoing research attempting to define the nature of the relevant cell–cell interactions and to understand their regulation and modulation. This is an example of the identity of basic and applied science interests that is most likely to lead to progress without excessively channeling scientific creativity.

REFERENCES

1. Grady, G. F., and Keusch, G. T. Pathogenesis of bacterial diarrhea. *N. Engl. J. Med.* **285**:831–845; 891–900, 1971.
2. Keusch, G. T. Shigellosis. In: *Bacterial Infections of Humans: Epidemiology and Control*, A. S. Evans and H. Feldman (Eds.), Plenum, New York, 1982.
3. Rosenberg, M. L., Weissman, J. B., Gangarosa, E. J., Reller, L. B., and Beasley, R. P. Shigellosis in the United States: Ten year review of nationwide surveillance. *Am. J. Epidemiol.* **104**:543–551, 1976.
4. Donadio, J., and Gangarosa, E. J. Foodborne shigellosis. *J. Infect. Dis.* **119**:666–668, 1969.
5. Black, R. E., Graun, G. F., and Blake, P. A. Epidemiology of common-source outbreaks of shigellosis in the United States, 1961–1975. *Am. J. Epidemiol.* **108**:47–52, 1978.
6. Levine, M. M., DuPont, H. L., Formal, S. B., Hornick, R. B., Takeuchi, A., Gangarosa, E. J., Snyder, M. J., and Libonati, J. P. Pathogenesis of *Shigella dysenteriae* 1 (Shiga) dysentery. *J. Infect. Dis.* **127**:261–270, 1973.
7. Dale, D. C., and Mata, L. J. Studies of diarrheal disease in Central America. XI. Intestinal bacterial flora in malnourished children with shigellosis. *Am. J. Trop. Med. Hyg.* **17**:397–403, 1968.
8. Hardy, A. V., and Watt, J. Studies of acute diarrheal diseases. XVIII. Epidemiology. *Public Health Rep.* **63**:363–378, 1948.
9. Thomas, M. E. M., and Tillett, H. E. Dysentery in general practice: A study of cases

and their contacts in Enfield and an epidemiological comparison with salmonellosis. *J. Hyg. (Cambridge)* **71**:373–389, 1973.

10. Turnbull, P. C. B. Food poisoning with special reference to salmonella—Its epidemiology, pathogenesis, and control. *Clin. Gastroenterol.* **8**:663–714, 1979.

11. Lang, D. J., Kinz, L. J., Martin, A. R., Schroeder, S. A. O., and Thomas, L. A. Carmine as a source of nosocomial salmonellosis. *N. Engl. J. Med.* **276**:829–832, 1967.

12. Craven, P. C., Mackel, D. C., Baine, W. B., Barker, W. H., and Gangarosa, E. J. International outbreak of *Salmonella eastbourne* infection traced to contaminated chocolate. *Lancet* **1**:788–792, 1975.

13. Clark, G. McC., Kaufmann, A. F., Gangarosa, E. J., and Thompson, M. Epidemiology of an international outbreak of *Salmonella agona*. *Lancet* **ii**:490–493, 1973.

14. Lipson, A., and Meikle, H. Porcine pancreatin as a source of salmonella infection in children with cystic fibrosis. *Arch. Dis. Child.* **52**:569–572, 1977.

15. Cohen, M. L., and Gangarosa, E. J. Non-typhoid salmonellosis. *South. Med. J.* **71**:1540–1555, 1978.

16. Hornick, R. B., Greisman, S. E., Woodward, T. E., DuPont, H. L., Dawkins, A. T., and Snyder, M. J. Typhoid fever: Pathogenesis and immunological control. *N. Engl. J. Med.* **283**:686–691; 736–746, 1970.

17. Giannella, R. A., Broitman, S. A., and Zamcheck, N. Salmonella enteritis. I. Role of reduced gastric secretion in pathogenesis. *Am. J. Digest. Dis.* **16**:1000–1016, 1971.

18. Bohnhoff, M., and Miller. C. P. Enhanced susceptibility to salmonella infection in streptomycin-treated mice. *J. Infect. Dis.* **111**:117–127, 1962.

19. Bohnhoff, M., Miller, C. P., and Martin, W. R. Resistance of the mouse intestinal tract to experimental salmonella infection. I. Factors which interfere with the initiation of infection by oral inoculation. *J. Expt. Med.* **120**:805–816, 1964.

20. D'Aoust, J. Y., and Pivnick, H. Small infectious doses of salmonella, *Lancet* **i**:866, 1976.

21. Waddell, S. R., and Kunz, L. J. Association of salmonella enteritis with operations on the stomach, *N. Engl. J. Med.* **255**:555–559, 1956.

22. Giannella, R. A., Broitman, S. A., and Zamcheck, N. Influence of gastric acidity on bacterial and parasitic enteric infections. A perspective. *Ann. Int. Med.* **78**:271–276. 1973.

23. Lowenstein, M. S. An outbreak of salmonellosis propagated by person-to-person transmission on an Indian reservation. *Am. J. Epidemiol.* **102**:257–262, 1975.

24. Simbert, R. M. The genus *Campylobacter*. *Ann. Rev. Microbiol.* **32**:673–709, 1978.

25. Guerrant, R. L., Lahita, R. G., Winn. W. C., and Roberts, R. B. Campylobacteriosis in man: Pathogenic mechanisms and review of 91 bloodstream infections. *Am. J. Med.* **65**:584–592, 1978.

26. Butzler, J. P. Related vibrios in Africa. *Lancet* **ii**:858, 1973.

27. Blaser, M. J. Cravens, J., Powers, B. W., and Wang, W. L. L. *Campylobacter* enteritis associated with canine infection. *Lancet* **ii**:979–981, 1978.

28. Blaser, M. J., Cravens, J., Powers, B. W., LaForce, F. M., and Wang, W. L. L. *Campylobacter* enteritis associated with unpasteurized milk. *Am. J. Med.* **67**:179–185, 1978.

29. Blaser, M. J., Berkowitz, I. D., LaForce, F. M., Cravens, J., Reller, L. B., and Wang, W. L. L. *Campylobacter* enteritis: Clinical and epidemiologic features. *Ann. Int. Med.* **91**:179–185, 1979.

30. Blaser, M. J., Glass, R. I., Huq, I., Stoll, B., Kibriya, G. M., and Alim, A. R. Isolation of *Campylobacter fetus* ssp *jejuni* from Bangladeshi children. *J. Clin. Microbiol.* **12**:744–747, 1980.

31. Itoh, T., Saito, K., Maruyama, T. Sakai, S. Ohashi, M., and Oka, A. An outbreak of acute enteritis due to *Campylobacter fetus* ssp *jejuni* at a nursery school in Tokyo. *Microbiol. Immunol.* **24**:371–379, 1980.

32. Steele, T. W., and McDermott, S. *Campylobacter* enteritis in South Australia. *Med. J. Aust.* **2**:404–406, 1978.

33. Bottone, E. J. *Yersinia enterocolitica*: A panoramic view of a charismatic microorganism. *CRC Crit. Rev. Microbiol.* **5**:211–241, 1977.

34. Morris, G. K., and Feeley, J. C. *Yersinia enterocolitica*: A review of its role in hygiene. *Bull. WHO* **54**:79–85, 1976.

35. Wormser, G. P., and Keusch, G. T. *Yersinia enterocolitica*: Clinical observations. In: *Yersinia enterocolitica*, E. J. Bottone (Ed.). CRC Press, Boca Raton, Florida, 1981.

36. Zen-Yoji, H., Sakai, S., Maruyama, T., and Yanagawa, Y. Isolation of *Yersinia enterocolitica* and *Yersinia pseudotuberculosis* from swine, cattle, and rats at an abattoir. *Jpn. J. Microbiol.* **18**:103-05, 1974.

37. Esseveld, H., and Goudzwaard, G. On the epidemiology of *Yersinia enterocolitica* infections: Pigs as the source of infections in man. *Contrib. Microbiol. Immunol.* **2**:99–101, 1973.

38. Harvey. S., Greenwood, J. R., Pickett, M. J., and Mah, R. A. Recovery of *Yersinia enterocolitica* from streams and lakes of California. *Appl. Environ. Microbiol.* **32**:352–354, 1976.

39. Schiemann, D. A., and Toma, S. Isolation of *Yersinia enterocolitica* from raw milk. *Appl. Environ. Microbiol.* **35**:54–58, 1978.

40. Black, R. E., Jackson. R. J., Tsai, T., Medvesky, M., Shayegani, M., Feeley, J. C., MacLeod, K. I. E., and Wakelee, A. M. Epidemic *Yersinia enterocolitica* infection due to contaminated chocolate milk. *N. Engl. J. Med.* **298**:76-79, 1978.

41. Hanna, M. D., Zink, D. L., Carpenter, Z. L., and Vanderzant, C. *Yersinia enterocolitica*-like organisms from vacuum packaged beef and lamb. *J. Food Sci.* **41**:1254–1256. 1976.

42. Gutman, L. T., Ottesen, E. A., Quan, T. J., and Katz. S. L. An interfamilial outbreak of *Yersinia enterocolitica* enteritis. *N. Engl. J. Med.* **288**:1372–1377, 1973.

43. Kohl, S., Jacobsen, J. A., and Nahmias, A. *Yersinia enterocolitica* infections in children. *J. Pediatr.* **89**:77–79, 1976.

44. Formal, S. B., Abrams, G. D., Schneider, H., and Sprinz, H. Experimental *Shigella* infections VI. Role of the small intestine in an experimental infection in guinea pigs. *J. Bacteriol.* **85**:119–125, 1963.

45. LaBrec, E. H., Schneider. H., Magnani, T. J., and Formal, S. B. Epithelial cell penetration is an essential step in the pathogenesis of bacillary dysentery, *J. Bacteriol.* **88**:1503–1518, 1964.

46. Formal, S. B., LaBrec, E. H., and Schneider, H. Pathogenesis of bacillary dysentery in laboratory animals. *Fed. Proc.* **24**:29–34, 1965.

47. Formal, S. B., LaBrec, E. H., Kent, T. H., and Falkow, S. Abortive intestinal infection with an *Escherichia coli-Shigella flexneri* hybrid strain. *J. Bacteriol.* **89**:1374–1382, 1965.

48. Formal, S. B., Kent, T. H., Austin, S., and LaBrec, E. H. Fluorescent-antibody and histological study of vaccinated and control monkeys challenged with *Shigella flexneri*, *J. Bacteriol.* **91**:2368–2376, 1966.

49. Gemski, P., Jr., Takeuchi, A., Washington, O., and Formal, S. B. Shigellosis due to *Shigella dysenteriae* 1: Relative importance of mucosal invasion versus toxin production in pathogenesis. *J. Infect. Dis.* **126**:523–530, 1972.

50. Hale, T. L., and Formal, S. B. Cytotoxicity of *Shigella dysenteriae* 1 for cultured mammalian cells. *Am. J. Clin. Nutr.* **33 (Suppl.)**:2485–2490, 1980.

51. Kopecko, D. J., Washington. O., and Formal, S. B. Genetic and physical evidence for plasmid control of *Shigella sonnei* Form I cell surface antigen. *Infect. Immun.* **29**:207–214, 1980.

52. Okamura, N., Nakaya, R. Rough mutant of *Shigella flexneri* 2a that penetrates tissue culture cells but does not evoke keratoconjunctivitis in guinea pigs. *Infect. Immun.* **17**:4–8, 1977.

53. Corwin, L. M., Rothman, S. W., Kim. R., and Talevi, L. A. Mechanisms and genetics of resistance to sodium lauryl sulfate in strains of *Shigella* and *Escherichia coli. Infect. Immun.* **4**:287–294, 1971.

54. Corwin. L. M., and Talevi, L. A. Mutation in *Shigella flexneri* 2a resulting in an increased electrophoretic mobility. *Infect. Immun.* **5**:798–802, 1972.

55. Kim, R., and Corwin, L. M. Mutation in *Shigella flexneri* resulting in loss of ability to penetrate HeLa cells and loss of glycerol kinase activity. *Infect. Immun.* **9**:916–923, 1974.

56. Gemski, P., Jr., Sheahan, D. C., Washington, O., and Formal, S. B. Virulence of *Shigella flexneri* hybrids expressing *Escherichia coli* somatic antigens. *Infect. Immun.* **6**:104–111, 1972.

57. DuPont, H. L., Formal, S. B., Hornick, R. B., Snyder, M. J., Libonati, J. P., Sheahan, D. G., LaBrec, E. H., and Kalas, J. P. Pathogenesis of *Escherichia coli* diarrhea. *N. Engl. J. Med.* **285**:1–9, 1971.

58. Radoutcheva, T., Veljanov, D., and Bandarenko, V. M. Studies on the energetic metabolism of *Shigella flexneri* X *Escherichica coli* hybrids devoid of penetration ability. IV. Growth characteristics in the presence of some tricarboxylic acid cyclic intermediates. *Zentralbl. Bakeriol. Org.* **A236**:99–104, 1976.

59. Radoutcheva, T., Veljanov, D., and Bondarenko, V. M. On the metabolic characteristics of hybrid *Shigella flexneri* X *Escherichia coli*, devoid of their ability for intracellular multiplication in the epithelial cells. IV. Growth characteristics in the presence of some tricarboxylic acid cyclic intermediates. *Zentralbl. Bacteriol. Org.* **A241**:319–324, 1978.

60. Formal, S. B., LaBrec, E. H., Hornick, R. B., Dupont, H. L., and Snyder, M. J. Attenuation of strains of dysentery bacilli. In: *International Symposium on Enterobacterial Vaccines*, Vol. 15, pp. 73–79. Karger, Basel, 1971.

61. Mel, D. M., Arsić, B. L., Nikolić, B. D., and Radovanović, M. L. Studies on vaccination against bacillary dysentery. 4. Oral immunization with live monotypic and combined vaccines. *Bull. WHO* **39**:375–380, 1968.

62. Keusch, G. T. Shigella infections. *Clin. Gastroenterol.* **8**:645–662, 1979.

63. Rout, W. R., Formal, S. B., Giannella, R. A., and Dammin, G. J. Pathophysiology of shigella diarrhea in the rhesus monkey: Intestinal transport, morphological, and bacteriological studies. *Gastroenterology* **68**:270–278, 1975.

64. Barrett-Connor, E., and Connor, J. D. Extraintestinal manifestations of shigellosis. *Am. J. Gastroenterol.* **53**:234–245, 1970.

65. Reed, W. P., and Albright, E. L. Serum factors responsible for killing of shigella. *Immunology* **26**:205–215, 1974.

66. Saphra, J., and Winter, J. W. Clinical manifestations of salmonellosis in man. An evaluation of 7779 human infections at the New York Salmonella Centre. *N. Engl. J. Med.* **256**:1128–1134, 1957.

67. Mandal, B. K. Typhoid and paratyphoid fever. *Clin. Gastroenterol.* **8**:715–735, 1979.

68. Blanden, R. B., Mackaness, G. B., and Collins, F. M. Mechanisms of acquired resistance in mouse typhoid. *J. Exp. Med.* **124**:573–600, 1966.

69. Mackaness, G. B. Resistance of intracellular infection. *J. Infect. Dis.* **123**:439–445, 1971.

70. Collins, F. M., and Carter, P. B. Growth of *Salmonellae* in orally infected germ-free mice. *Infect. Immun.* 21:41–47, 1978.
71. Takeuchi, A. Electron microscope studies of experimental salmonella infection. 1. Penetration into the intestinal epithelium by *Salmonella typhimurium. Am. J. Pathol.* 50:109–136, 1967.
72. Takeuchi, A., and Sprinz, H. Electron microscope studies of experimental salmonella infection in preconditioned guinea pigs. II. Response of intestinal mucosa to invasion by *Salmonella typhimurium. Am. J. Pathol.* 51:137–161, 1967.
73. Turnbull, P. C. B., and Richmond, J. E. A model of salmonella enteritis: The behavior of *Salmonella enteritidis* in chick intestine studied by light and electron microscopy. *Br. J. Exp. Pathol.* 59:64–75, 1978.
74. Butzler, J. P., and Skirrow, M. B. *Campylobacter* enteritis. *Clin. Gastroenterol.* 8:737–765, 1979.
75. Feeley, J. C., Wells, J. G., Tsai, T. F., and Puhr, N. D. Detection of enterotoxigenic and invasive strains of *Yersinia enterocolitica. Contrib. Microbiol. Immunol.* 5:329–334, 1979.
76. Une, T. Studies on the pathogenicity of *Yersinia enterocolitica*. II. Interaction with cultured cells *in vitro. Microbiol. Immunol.* 21:365–377, 1977.
77. Carter, P. Pathogenicity of *Yersinia enterocolitica* for mice. Infect. Immun. 11:164–170, 1975.
78. Bradford, W. D., Noce, P. S., and Gutman, L. T. Pathologic features of enteric infection with *Yersinia enterocolitica, Arch. Pathol.* 98:17–22, 1974.
79. Vantrappen, G., Agg, H. O., Ponethe, E., Geboes, K., and Bertran, P. H. *Yersinia* enteritis and enterocolitis: Gastrointestinal aspects. *Gastroenterology* 72:220–227, 1977.
80. Sjöström, B. Surgical aspects of infection with *Yersinia enterocolitica. Contrib. Microbiol. Immunol.* 2:137–141, 1973.
81. Rabson, A. R., Hallett, A. F., and Koornhof, H. Generalized *Yersinia enterocolitica* infection. *J. Infect. Dis.* 131:447–451, 1975.
82. Bergstrand, C. G., and Winblad, S. Clinical manifestations of infection with *Yersinia enterocolitica* in children. *Acta Paediatr. Scand.* 63:875–877, 1974.
83. Mäki, M., Grönroos, P., and Versikari, T. *In vitro* invasiveness of *Yersinia enterocolitica* isolated from children with diarrhea. *J. Infect. Dis.* 138:677–680, 1978.
84. Lee, W. H., McGrath, P. P., Carter, P. E., and Eide, E. L. The ability of some *Yersinia enterocolitica* strains to invade HeLa cells. *Can. J. Microbiol.* 23:1714–1722, 1977.
85. Pai, C. H., Mors, V., and Seemayer, T. A. Experimental *Yersinia enterocolitica* enteritis in rabbits. *Infect. Immun.* 28:238–244, 1980.
86. Karmali, M. A., and Fleming, P. C. *Campylobacter* enteritis in children, *J. Pediatr.* 94:527–533, 1979.
87. Skirrow, M. B. *Campylobacter* enteritis: A "new" disease. *Br. Med. J.* 2:9–11, 1977.
88. McKinley, M. J., Taylor, M., and Sangree, M. H. Toxic megacolon with *Campylobacter* colitis. *Conn. Med.* 44:496–497, 1980.
89. Lambert, M. E., Schofield, P. F., Ironside, A. G., and Mandal, B. K. *Campylobacter* colitis. *Br. J. Med.* 1:857–859, 1979.
90. Blaser, M. J., Parsons, R. B., and Wang, W. L. Acute colitis caused by *Campylobacter fetus* ss *jejuni. Gastroenterology* 78:448–453, 1980.
91. Ruiz-Palacios, G. M., Escamilla, E., and Torres, N. Experimental *Campylobacter* diarrhea in chicken. In: *Abstracts of the 20th Interscience Conference on Antimicrobial Agents and Chemotherapy.* American Society for Microbiology, No. 697, 1980.
92. DuPont, H. L., Hornick, R. B., Dawkins, A. T., Snyder, M. J., and Formal, S. B. The response of man to virulent *Shigella flexneri* 2a. *J. Infect. Dis.* 119:296–299, 1969.

93. Kinsey, M. D., Formal, S. B., Dammin, G. J., and Giannella, R. A. Fluid and electrolyte transport in Rhesus monkeys challenged intracecally with *Shigella flexneri* 2a. *Infect. Immun.* **14**:368–371, 1976.

94. Keusch, G. T., Grady, G. F., Mata, L. J., and McIver, J. The pathogenesis of *Shigella* diarrhea. I. Enterotoxin production by *Shigella dysenteriae* 1. *J. Clin. Invest.* **51**:1212–1218, 1972.

95. Keusch, G. T., and Jacewicz, M. Serum enterotoxin-neutralizing antibody in human shigellosis. *Nature (New Biol)* **241**:31-2, 1973.

96. Keusch, G. T., and Jacewicz, M. Pathogenesis of shigella diarrhea. VI. Toxin and antitoxin in *S. flexneri* and *S. sonnei* infections in humans. *J. Infect. Dis.* **135**:552–556, 1977.

97. Keusch, G. T., Grady, G. F., Takeuchi, A., and Sprinz, H. The pathogenesis of *Shigella* diarrhea. II. Enterotoxin-induced acute enteritis in the rabbit ileum. *J. Infect. Dis.* **126**:92–95, 1972.

98. Steinberg, S. W., Banwell, J. G., Yardley, J. H., Keusch, G. T., and Hendrix, T. R. Comparison of secretory and histological effects of shigella and cholera enterotoxins in rabbit jejunum. *Gastroenterology* **68**:309–317, 1975.

99. Charney, A. N., Gots, R. E., Formal, S. B., and Giannella, R. A. Activation of intestinal adenylate cyclase by *Shigella dysenteriae* 1 enterotoxin. *Gastroenterology* **70**:1085–1090, 1976.

100. Flores, J., Grady, G. F., McIver, J., Witkum, P., Beckman, B., and Sharp, G. W. G. Comparison of the effects of enterotoxins of *Shigella dysenteriae* and *Vibrio cholerae* on the adenylate cyclase system of the rabbit ileum. *J. Infect. Dis.* **130**:374–379, 1974.

101. Branham, S. E., Dack, G. M., and Riggs, D. B. Studies with *Shigella dysenteriae* (Shiga) IV. Immunological reactions in monkeys to the toxins in isolated intestinal pouches. *J. Immunol.* **70**:103–113, 1953.

102. Donowitz, M., and Binder, H. J. Effect of enterotoxins of *Vibrio cholerae, Escherichia coli,* and *Shigella dysenteriae* Type 1 on fluid and electrolyte transport in colon. *J. Infect. Dis.* **134**:135–143, 1976.

103. Keusch, G. T. Ecological control of the bacterial diarrheas: A scientific strategy. *Am. J. Clin. Nutr.* **31**:2208–2218, 1978.

104. Vicari, G., Olitzki, A. L., and Olitzki, Z. The action of thermolabile toxin of *Shigella dysenteriae* on cells cultivated *in vitro Br. J. Exp. Pathol.* **41**:179–189, 1960.

105. Keusch, G. T., Jacewicz., and Hirschman, S. Z. Quantitative microassay in cell culture for enterotoxin of *Shigella dysenteriae* 1. *J. Infect. Dis.* **125**:539–541, 1972.

106. Keusch, G. T., and Donta, S. T. Classification of enterotoxins on the basis of activity in cell culture. *J. Infect. Dis.* **131**:58–63, 1975.

107. O'Brien, A. D., Thompson, M. R., Gemski, P., Doctor, B. P., and Formal, S. B. Biological properties of *Shigella flexneri* 2a toxin and its serological relationship to *Shigella dysenteriae* 1 toxin. *Infect. Immun.* **15**:796–798, 1977.

108. Keusch, G. T. Receptor mediated endocytosis of shigella cytotoxin. In: *Receptor Mediated Binding and Internalization of Toxins and Hormones,* J. Middlebrook and L. Kohn (Eds.), pp. 95–110. Academic Press, New York, 1981.

109. Keusch, G. T. Jacewicz, M., Levine, M. M., Hornick, R. B., and Kochwa, S. Pathogenesis of *Shigella* diarrhea. Serum anticytoxin antibody response produced by toxigenic and nontoxigenic *Shigella dysenteriae* 1. *J. Clin. Invest.* **57**:194–202, 1976.

110. Keusch, G. T., and Jacewicz, M. The pathogenesis of *Shigella* diarrhea. V. Relationship of Shiga enterotoxin neutrotoxin and cytotoxin. *J. Infect. Dis.* **131**:S33–S39, 1975.

111. O'Brien, A. D., LaVeck, G. D., Griffin, D. E., and Thompson, M. R. Characterization of *Shigella dysenteriae* 1 (Shiga) toxin purified by anti-shiga toxin affinity chromatography. *Infect. Immun.* **30**:170–179, 1980.

112. Mathias, J. R., Carlson, G. M., Martin, J. L., Shields, R. P., and Formal, S. B. *Shigella dysenteriae* 1 enterotoxin: Proposed role in pathogenesis of shigellosis. *Am. J. Physiol.* **239**:G382–G386, 1980.

113. Burns, T. W., Mathias, J. R., Martin, J. L., Carlson, G. M., and Shields, R. P. Alteration of myoelectric activity of small intestine by invasive *Escherichia coli. Am. J. Physiol.* **238**:G57–G62, 1980.

114. Keusch. G. T., and Jacewicz, M. Pathogenesis of *Shigella* diarrhea VII. Evidence for a cell membrane toxin receptor involving Beta 1→4-Linked N-Acetyl-D-Glucosamine oligomers. *J. Exp. Med.* **146**:535–546, 1977.

115. Keusch, G. T. Specific membrane receptors: Pathogenetic and therapeutic implications in infectious disease. *Rev. Infect. Dis.* **1**:517–529, 1979.

116. Giannella, R. A., Formal, S. B., Dammin, G. J., and Collins, H. Pathogenesis of salmonellosis: Studies of fluid secretrion, mucosal invasion, and morphologic reaction in the rabbit ileum. *J. Clin. Invest.* **52**:441–453, 1973.

117. Fromm, D., Giannella, R. A., Formal, S. B., Quijano, R., and Collins, H. Ion transport across isolated ileal mucosa invaded by salmonella. *Gastroenterology* **66**:215–225, 1974.

118. Giannella, R. A. Importance of tbe intestinal inflammatory reaction in salmonella-mediated intestinal secretion. *Infect. Immun.* **23**:140–145, 1979.

119. Giannella, R. A. Rout, W. R., Formal, S. B., and Collins, H. Role of plasma filtration in the intestinal fluid secretion mediated by infection with *Salmonella typhimurium. Infect. Immun.* **13**:470–474, 1976.

120. Kinsey, M. D., Dammin, G. J., Formal, S. B., and Giannella, R. A. The role of altered permeability in the pathogenesis of *Salmonella* diarrhea in the Rhesus monkey. *Gastroenterology* **71**:429–434, 1976.

121. Sandefur, P. D., and Peterson, J. W. Isolation of skin permeability factors from culture filtrates of *Salmonella typhimurium, Infect. Immun.* **14**:671–679, 1976.

122. Koupal, L. R., and Deibel, R. H. Assay, characterization, and localization of an enterotoxin produced by *Salmonella, Infect. Immun.* **11**:14–22, 1975.

123. Sedlock, D. M., and Deibel, R.H. Detection of *Salmonella* enterotoxin using rabbit ileal loops. *Can. J. Microbiol.* **24**:268–273, 1978.

124. Gots, R. E., Formal, S. B., and Giannella, R. A. Indomethacin inhibition of *Salmonella typhimurium, Shigella flexneri,* and cholera-mediated rabbit ileal secretion. *J. Infect. Dis.* **130**:280–284, 1974.

125. Giannella, R. A., Gots, R. E., Charney, A. N., Greenough, W. B., and Formal, S. B. Pathogenesis of *Salmonella*-mediated intestinal secretion. Activation of adenylate cyclase and inhibition by indomethacin. *Gastroenterology* **69**:1238–1245, 1975.

126. Giannella, R. A., Rout, W. R., and Formal, S. B. Effect of indomethacin on intestinal water transport in *Salmonella*-infected Rhesus monkeys. *Infect. Immun.* **17**:136–139, 1977.

127. Peterson, J. W., and Sandefur, P. D. Evidence for a role for permeability factors in the pathogenesis of salmonellosis. *Am. J. Clin. Nutr.* **32**:197–209, 1979.

128. Molina, N. C., and Peterson, J. W. Cholera toxin-like toxin released by *Salmonella* species in the presence of Mitomycin C. *Infect. Immun.* **30**:224–230, 1980.

129. Pai, C. H., and Mors, V. Production of enterotoxin by *Yersinia enterocolitica. Infect. Immun.* **19**:908–911, 1978.

130. Boyce, J. M., Evans, D. J., Jr., Evans, D. G. and DuPont, H. L. Production of heat-stable, methanol-soluble enterotoxin by *Yersinia enterocolitica. Infect. Immun.* **25**:532–537, 1979.

131. Francis, D. W., Spaulding, P. L., and Lovett, J. Enterotoxin production and thermal resistance of *Yersinia enterocolitica* in milk. *Appl. Environ. Microbiol.* **40**:174–176, 1980.

132. Kapperud, D., Berdal, B. P., and Omland, T. Enterotoxin production by *Yersinia enterocolitica* and *Yersinia enterocolitica*-like microbes at 22°C and 37°C. *Acta Pathol. Microbiol, Scand.* **88**:65–67, 1980.

133. Mors, V., and Pai, C. H. Pathogenic properties of *Yershinia enterocolitica. Infect. Immun.* **28**:292–294, 1980.

134. Rao, M. C., Guandalini, S., Laird, M. J., and Field, M. Effects of heat-stable enterotoxin of *Yersinia enterocolitica* on ion transport and cyclic guanosine 3', 5'-monophosphate metabolism in rabbit ileum. *Infect. Immun.* **26**:878, 1979.

135. Robins-Browne, R. M., Stills, C. S., Miliotis, M. D., and Koornhof, H. J. Mechanism of action of *Yersinia enterocolitica* enterotoxin. *Infect. Immun.* **25**:680–684, 1979.

136. Keusch, G. T. The consequences of fever. *Am. J. Clin. Nutr.* **30**:1211–1214, 1977.

137. Beisel, W. R. Magnitude of the host nutritional responses to infection. *Am. J. Clin. Nutr.* **30**:1236–1247, 1977.

138. Keusch, G. T. Nutrition as a determinant of host response to infection and the metabolic sequellae of infectious disease. *Semin. Infect. Dis.* **2**:265–303, 1979.

139. Lindenbaum, J. Malabsorption during and after recovery from acute intestinal infection. *Br. Med. J.* **2**:326–329, 1965.

140. Rosenberg, I. H., Solomons, N. W., and Schneider, R. E. Malabsorption associated with diarrhea and intestinal infections. *Am. J. Clin. Nutr.* **30**:1248–1253, 1977.

141. Giannella, R. A., Broitman, S. A., and Zamcheck, N. *Salmonella* enteritis II. Fulminant diarrhea in and effects on the small intestine. *Am. J. Digest. Dis.* **16**:1007–1013, 1971.

142. Binder, H. J., and Whiting, D. S. Inhibition of small-intestinal sugar and amino acid transport by the enterotoxin of *Shigella dysenteriae* 1. *Infect. Immun.* **16**:510–512, 1977.

143. Rosenberg, I. H., Hardison, W. G., and Bull, D. M. Abnormal bile-salt patterns and intestinal bacterial overgrowth associated with malabsorption. *N. Engl. J. Med.* **276**:1391–1397, 1967.

144. Higgins, A. R. Floyd, T. M., and Kader, M. A. Studies in shigellosis. II: Observations on incidence and etiology of diarrheal disease in Egyptian village children. *Am. J. Trop. Med. Hyg.* **4**:271–280, 1955.

145. Mata, L. J. *The Children of Santa María Cauqué: A prospective field study of health and growth.* M. I. T. Press, Cambridge, Massachusetts, 1978.

146. Feeley, J. C. Isolation techniques for *Yersinia enterocolitica.* In: *Yersinia enterocolitica,* E. J. Bottone (Ed.), pp. 9–15. CRC Press, Boca Raton, Florida, 1981.

147. Stoll, B. J., Holmgren, J., Bardhan, P. K., Huq, I., Greenough, W. B., III, Fredman, P., and Svennerholm, L. Binding of intraluminal toxin in cholera: Trial of GM1 ganglioside charcoal. *Lancet* ii:888–891, 1980.

4

Epidemiological Aspects of Diarrhea Associated with Known Enteropathogens in Rural Bangladesh

ROBERT E. BLACK, MICHAEL H. MERSON, AND KENNETH H. BROWN

INTRODUCTION

Diarrheal diseases are among the most important causes of death among children in developing countries.[1-3] Furthermore, these highly prevalent illnesses have been found to be major determinants of growth retardation and malnutrition.[4-6]

Previous studies of the epidemiology of diarrheal diseases in children in developing countries were able to detect well-recognized bacterial pathogens such as *Salmonella* and *Shigella* in less than 20% of stool specimens from children with diarrhea.[7-9] This lack of information about the causes of diarrhea precluded complete exposition of the epidemiology of the diarrheal syndromes. Furthermore, it led some to conclude, inaccurately, that a sizable proportion of the diarrhea in children in developing countries was the result of malnutrition rather than a series of infectious illnesses.

ROBERT E. BLACK • Center for Vaccine Development, University of Maryland School of Medicine, Baltimore, Maryland.   MICHAEL H. MERSON • International Centre for Diarrhoeal Disease Reserach, Dacca, Bangladesh.   KENNETH H. BROWN • Division of Geographical Medicine, School of Medicine, Johns Hopkins University, Baltimore, Maryland.

Although classic enteric bacterial pathogens are not isolated from most patients with diarrhea, recent studies indicate that enterotoxigenic *Escherichia coli* (ETEC) and rotaviruses may frequently cause diarrhea.[10,11] Although these agents have been isolated from patients in developing countries, the studies have been brief, and the results do not permit an accurate assessment of the relative importance of the various causative agents. Thus, we assessed the etiology, incidence, and severity of diarrhea in people living in a rural village in Bangladesh, and in those attending a diarrhea treatment center serving this and neighboring villages.[12,13] This paper will summarize the information from these studies, which were done between February 1977 and January 1979.

MATERIALS and METHODS

The studies were done in the field research area of the International Centre for Diarrhoeal Disease Research, Bangladesh (formerly the Cholera Research Laboratory). A central treatment facility, staffed by physicians and paraprofessionals, provided free therapy for patients with diarrhea who came in directly or were brought by speedboat or jeep ambulances stationed in the field area. For a 2-year period, data for all patients who lived in the research area and who were treated for diarrhea were gathered for a study of enteric pathogens. Between February 1977 and January 1978 (year 1), 8139 patients were included in the study, and from February 1978 to January 1979 (year 2) 6352 patients were enrolled. In years 1 and 2, respectively, 43% and 41% of all patients were children less than 2 years of age, 22% each year were children 2 through 9 years old, and 35% and 37% were persons $\geq$ 10 years of age.

When the patient visited the treatment center, a physician or nurse did a standard clinical evaluation of the degree of dehydration on the basis of such signs as skin elasticity, sunken eyes or fontanelle, pulse, respiration, volume of urine, and level of consciousness. Dehydration was classified as none, mild (corresponding to < 5 percent loss of body weight), moderate (5 to 10%), or severe (> 10%).

Patients judged to have mild or no dehydration were treated with oral electrolyte solution (composition in milliequivalents per liter: Na^+, 90; K^+, 20; Cl, 80; HCO_3, 30) containing 20 g of glucose/liter (year 1), or 40 g of sucrose/liter (year 2).[14] Patients with moderate or severe dehydration were given a solution (composition in milliequivalents per liter: Na^+, 134; K^+, 13; Cl, 86; HCO_3, 48) intravenously to replace their estimated fluid deficit and were also given the oral solution for maintenance therapy. Because laboratory findings were not available at the time of admission, the assessment of dehydration and the choice of treatment were not influenced by the identification of an enteropathogen. Only persons whose histories indicated a dysenteric illness were given ampicillin or trimethoprim–sulfamethoxazole on admission.

In one village (Amaukanda) of the field area, a surveillance worker visited all households daily from December 1977 to November 1978 and obtained clinical information and rectal swabs from all persons with diarrhea (defined as four or more liquid stools in 24 hours).

Laboratory Studies. Rectal swabs were taken from all patients on admission to the treatment center or at the time of household visit, and plated directly on *Salmonella–Shigella*, trypticase–tellurite–gelatin, and MacConkey's agars. Part of each specimen was enriched overnight in bile peptone and then plated on trypticase–tellurite–gelatin agar. The plates were examined for *Salmonellae*, *Shigellae*, and vibrios by standard methods.[15] Vibriolike colonies identified on trypticase–tellurite–gelatin plates were further characterized in terms of biochemical, serotypic, and salt-tolerance properties and classified as *Vibrio cholerae* group 0:1, nongroup 0:1 vibrios, *Vibrio parahaemolyticus*, or group F vibriolike organisms.[16,17]

In the treatment center, a sample of patients, stratified by age group, was further studies for ETEC infection. During year 1, studies were performed with 4498 patients (52% of patients less than 2 years of age, 67% of patients 2 to 19 years old, and 79% of patients ≥ 20 years of age). During year 2 the sample was modified because of the results from year 1, and 2042 patients (19% of patients less than 2 years of age. 66% of patients 2 to 19 years old, and 40% of patients ≥ 20 years of age) were studied. From each culture selected for toxin studies, 10 lactose-positive colonies with typical *E. coli* morphology were removed from Mac-Conkey's agar plates and pooled on nutrient agar slants. These pools were tested with the Chinese hamster ovary cell assay for heat-labile toxin (LT) and with the infant mouse assay for heat-stable toxin (ST).[18]

In year 1, fresh stool specimens from 40% of the patients were treated with saline and iodine preparations and examined for intestinal parasites. In this study, only stools containing vegetative-stage *Giardia lamblia* or *Entamoeba histolytica* were considered positive.

Beginning in December 1977, a second rectal swab was taken from each patient and refrigerated in phosphate-buffered saline for less than 1 month (and generally less than 1 week) before being tested by enzyme-linked immunosorbent assay for rotavirus antigen.[19–21] Positive results were confirmed by testing about 30 positive specimens per month with an enzyme-linked immunosorbent assay involving wells coated with immune and nonimmune sera.[22] Of 404 specimens retested, 380 (94%) were confirmed as positive.

All rectal swabs from persons in Amaukanda were tested for ETEC and rotavirus. All rotavirus-positive specimens were confirmed.

Analysis. The frequency with which patients were infected with the pathogens was calculated directly; however, since only subgroups of patients were tested for ETEC and for parasites, those results had to be extrapolated for the entire group of patients. Because rotavirus was tested for only the last 2 months of year 1, we included these data in the analysis of seasonality, degree of dehydration, and hospital death rates, but did not try to determine the overall frequency of infection with rotavirus in year 1. We calculated age-specific incidences of treatment center visits for rotavirus and enterotoxigenic *Escherichia coli* diarrhea from the number of persons with diarrhea associated with each agent and the 1977 and 1978 midyear populations of the field research area (268,880 and 269,605, respectively).[23] For Amaukanda, we calculated age- and pathogen-specific incidence from the midyear population of the village (1245 persons).

RESULTS

Identification of Enteropathogens in Treatment Center Patients with Diarrhea. For both year 1 and year 2, ETEC was the pathogen most frequently isolated from all patients and from adults; however, it was the second most often isolated (after *V. cholerae*) from children 2 to 9 years of age. Most of the ECTE produced only ST, fewer produced both ST and LT, and still fewer produced only LT (Table I).

Rotavirus was found in the stools of 46% of the children less than 2 years of age and in the stools of 12 and 9%, respectively, of older children and adults. *V. cholerae* group 0:1 was rarely identified for children less than 2 years of age but was an important pathogen in older children and adults, while nongroup 0:1 vibrios were found in the stools of 4 to 11% of the patients of each age group for both years of the study. Group F vibriolike organisms were associated with diarrhea for 3% of all patients in year 1, but rarely in year 2. *V. parahaemolyticus* and *Salmonella* were rarely isolated during the study, but *Shigella* was isolated from 5 to 6% of all patients treated at the center for diarrhea. Vegetative *G. lamblia* was identified from 4% of the older children and adults, and vegetative *E. histolyticus* was identified from 13% of the older children and 8% of the adults. For 2039 patients tested for bacterial pathogens, including ETEC, and for rotavirus (but not for parasites) in year 2, an enteropathogen was identified for 70% of the children less than 2 years of age, 47% of the children 2 to 9 years old, and 56% of the adults. Infection with more than one pathogen was found in about 20% of all patients.

Table I.   Percentage of Matlab Treatment Center Patients, by Age, with Diarrhea Associated with Enteric Pathogens during February 1977–January 1978 (Y1) and February 1978–January 1979 (Y2)

Pathogen identified		Age group							
		<2 years		2–9 years		≥10 years		All ages	
		Y1	Y2	Y1	Y2	Y1	Y2	Y1	Y2
Enterotoxigenic									
Escherichia coli	ST	12	17	12	15	16	22	14	18
	ST/LT	6	7	6	7	14	19	9	11
	LT	5	4	3	1	3	2	4	2
	Total	23	28	21	23	33	43	27	31
Rotavirus		—	46	—	12	—	9	—	24
Vibrio cholerae		2	2	29	34	14	14	12	14
Non-O Group I vibrios[a]		8	5	6	4	8	11	7	7
Shigella		4	5	8	10	4	5	5	6
Entamoeba histolytica		1	—	13	—	8	—	4	—
Giardia lamblia		<1	—	4	—	4	—	2	—
Group F organisms		4	<1	2	<1	2	<1	3	<1
Salmonella		<1	<1	<1	<1	<1	<1	<1	<1
Vibrio parahaemolyticus		0	<1	0	0	<1	<1	<1	<1
Negative[b]		—	31	—	53	—	44	—	44

[a]Includes vibrios of Heiberg Groups I, II, V.
[b]Determined for patients tested for bacterial pathogens, including enterotoxigenic *E. coli* and rotavirus in year 2.

The seasonal patterns of occurrence of the three most common enteric pathogens are illustrated in Figure 1. Infections with *V. cholerae* were decidedly seasonal, with a peak occurrence during the hot monsoon period. In contrast, infections with ETEC had two seasonal peaks, one in the hot, dry months, March and April, and the other in August through September. Although the highest number of patients with diarrhea associated with rotavirus were seen in the cool, dry months, December 1977 to January 1978, there was no comparable peak in the second year of study. The number of infections with nongroup 0:1 vibrios and group F vibriolike organisms peaked in April and May, whereas the incidence of *Shigella* infections peaked between June and August. No seasonal pattern could be determined for infections with *G. lamblia* or *E. histolytica*.

The degree of dehydration at the time that patients visited the treatment center during year 1 was tabulated for those infected with *V. cholerae*, ETEC, or rotavirus after data for patients with known mixed infec-

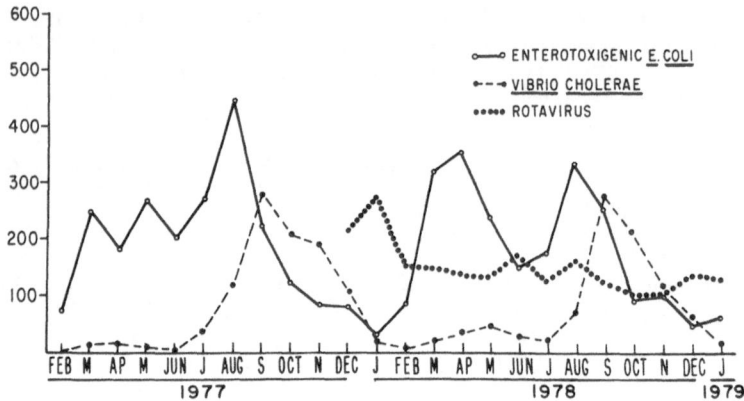

Figure 1. Treatment center visits in rural Bangladesh for diarrhea associated with entero-toxigenic *Escherichia coli, Vibrio cholerae,* or rotavirus.

tions were exluded. Among children less than 2 years of age, moderate or severe dehydration requiring inpatient therapy occurred in 24 (40%) of 60 patients with cholera; this proportion was significantly higher than the 68 (20%) of 340 and 76 (16%) of 473 patients with ETEC and rotavirus diarrhea, respectively (both $p < 0.001$, χ^2). Among adults, moderate or severe dehydration was found in 307 (77%) of 398 patients with cholera, and 269 (43%) of 624 with ETEC diarrhea ($p < 0.001$). There were no significant differences in the levels of dehydration accompanying diarrhea associated with ETEC of different toxin types in children or adults.

For the second year of the study we determined the number of children seen at the treatment center with sufficient (at least 7.5%) dehydration to require intravenous fluid replacement. Assuming that 50% of these children would have died, we calculated the number of deaths that would have been expected if treatment had not been available. We estimate that, during the second year of the treatment center study, 173 deaths would have occurred in children less than 2 years old; 60 of these would have been children with ETEC diarrhea and 73 those with rotavirus diarrhea. Thus, illnesses associated with these two enteropathogens would have accounted for 77% of deaths estimated by treatment center visits and would have resulted in a mortality rate of 6.5 per 1000 children less than 2 years old.

Case-Fatality Rates. In spite of substantial dehydration in patients of all ages, the hospital case-fatality rate for this 2-year period was very low (Table II). Furthermore, there were no significant differences in fatality rates between year 1, when glucose–electrolyte oral therapy was used, and year 2, when a sucrose-base solution was used. The fatality rate for patients with diarrhea associated with *Shigella* was higher than that for patients infected with *V. cholerae*, both group 0:1 (Fisher's exact test, $p <$ 0.01) and nongroup 0:1 ($p < 0.02$), rotavirus ($p < 0.01$), or ETEC ($p <$ 0.001).

Identification of Pathogens in Village Residents with Diarrhea. Daily surveillance in Amaukanda detected 877 episodes of diarrhea in a 1-year period (Table III). Enterotoxigenic *E. coli*, predominantly those producing only ST, were the most common enteropathogens identified in all age groups and in children less than 2 years old; *Shigellae* (predominantly *S. flexneri*) were the second most commonly found enteropathogens, and rotaviruses the third. In the village study, an enteropathogen was identified in 48% of children under 2 years old, in 39% of children 2 to 9 years old, and in 29% of older children and adults with diarrhea.

Incidence of Diarrhea Assessed by Village Surveillance and by Treatment Center Visits. Diarrhea noted by village surveillance was most common at 9 to 11 months of age when a rate of more than four episodes per year was noted (Figure 2). The diarrhea incidence for the first 4 years of life was approximately three episodes per year; however, the incidence decreased with increasing age to less than 200 per 1000 village residents 10 years old or older.

Annual age-specific incidence of ETEC diarrhea noted by village surveillance are given in Figure 3. At ages of peak incidence, ETEC diarrhea was noted nearly once per year per child, and the incidence remained relatively high throughout childhood. Treatment center visits for ETEC diarrhea were most common among children 6 to 11 months of age. Among children less than 2 years old, the incidence of ETEC diarrhea

Table II. Matlab Treatment Center Case Fatality Rate by Pathogen Associated with Diarrhea, February 1977–January 1979

Pathogen identified	Cases	Deaths	Case fatality rate (per 100 cases)
Salmonella	38	1	2.6
Shigella	782	9	1.2
Group F vibrios	245	2	0.8
Vibrio cholerae	1,864	4	0.2
Non-O Group 1 vibrios			
Heiberg Groups I, II, V	1,032	2	0.3
Rotavirus	2,112	5	0.2
Enterotoxigenic *Escherichia coli*	2,279	0	0
All diarrhea	14,499	37	0.3

Table III.   Percentage of Diarrhea Episodes Associated with Enteric Pathogens, by Age, Village of Amaukanda, December 1977–November 1978

	Age group			
Pathogen identified	<2 years 377 episodes	2–9 years 380 episodes	≥10 years 120 episodes	All ages 877 episodes
Enterotoxigenic *Escherichia coli*				
ST	11 (41)[a]	17 (65)	12 (15)	14 (121)
LT	4 (15)	5 (18)	0 (0)	4 (33)
ST/LT	5 (18)	6 (21)	8 (9)	5 (48)
Total	20 (74)	28 (104)	20 (24)	23 (202)
Shigella	15 (57)	8 (32)	4 (5)	11 (94)
Rotavirus	11 (43)	0 (0)	0 (0)	5 (43)
Other[b] and mixed	2 (8)	3 (12)	5 (6)	3 (26)

[a]Percentage (number of episodes).
[b]Includes *Vibrio cholerae*, both O group and I and Non-O group 1, and *Salmonella*.

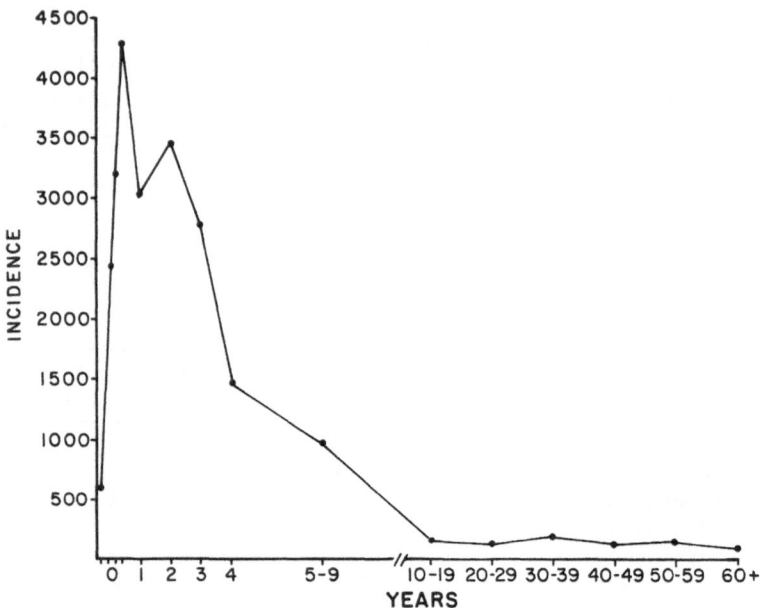

Figure 2. Annual age-specific incidence of diarrhea per 1000 persons assessed by village surveillance, December 1977–November 1978.

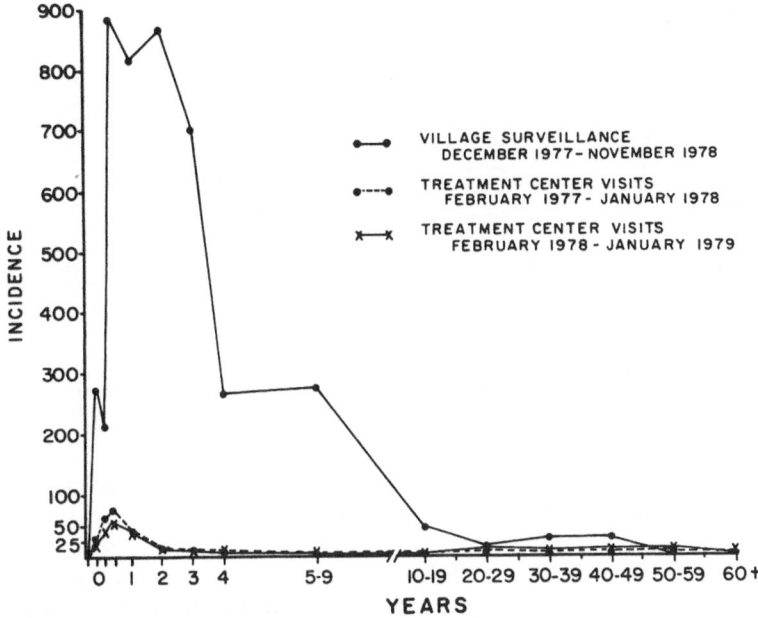

Figure 3. Annual age-specific incidence of enterotoxigenic *Escherichia coli* diarrhea per 1000 persons assessed by village surveillance and by treatment center visits.

assessed by village surveillance was approximately 15 times that determined by treatment center visits, but among children aged 2 to 9, the village incidence was 70 times the incidence of treatment center visits.

In Amaukanda, the incidence of rotavirus diarrhea reached a peak in the second 6 months of life and was high between 3 and 23 months of age; no rotavirus was noted in those older than 24 months (Figure 4). Treatment center visits for rotavirus diarrhea also reached a peak at 6 to 11 months of age, and the number of visits for older children and adults was very low. In contrast to ETEC diarrhea among children under 2 years old, the village incidence of rotavirus diarrhea was only six times the incidence determined by visits to the treatment center.

Occurrence of Dehydration with Diarrhea Associated with Specific Enteropathogens. Children under 2 years old with rotavirus diarrhea were more likely to have experienced dehydration and visited the treatment center than those with ETEC diarrhea (both $p < 0.001$) (Table IV). Dehydration was significantly more common in children with rotavirus diarrhea ($p < 0.001$) and ETEC diarrhea ($p = 0.01$) than in children with diarrhea of other or unknown etiology. Of 41 children under 2 years old with dehy-

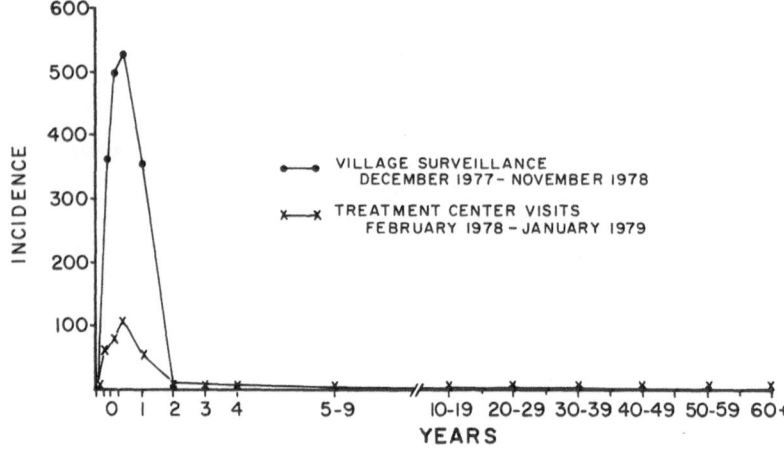

Figure 4. Annual age-specific incidence of rotavirus diarrhea per 1000 persons assessed by village surveillance and by treatment center visits.

Table IV. Percentage of Children Under Two Years with Diarrhea Experiencing Dehydration and Visiting the Treatment Center, Village of Amaukanda, December 1977–November 1978

	Type of diarrhea		
Characteristic	*Rotavirus* 43 episodes	Enterotoxigenic *E. coli* 74 episodes	*Other* 260 episodes
Mild dehydration	35 (15)[a]	12 (9)	4 (11)
Moderate dehydration	9 (4)	1 (1)	0.4 (1)
Total with dehydration	44 (19)	13 (10)	5 (12)
Visiting treatment center	30 (13)	5 (4)	2 (4)

[a]Percentage (number) of children.

dration during a diarrheal episode, 19 (46%) had rotavirus detected, 10 (24%) had ETEC, 3 (7%) had *Shigellae*, and 9 (21%) had no pathogen detected. Of 65 children aged 2 to 4 years with ETEC diarrhea, only 1 had dehydration and none visited the treatment center.

DISCUSSION

In these studies we were able to identify an enteropathogen associated with half of the diarrheal episodes of children less than 2 years old living in a rural community and with 70% of episodes seen in a diarrhea treatment facility. As in previous studies of children in developing countries, only a small fraction of these episodes were associated with the long-accepted bacterial pathogens, *Shigellae*, *V. cholerae*, and *Salmonella*.[7-9] By contrast, a high proportion of the episodes were associated with two recently recognized pathogens: enterotoxin-producing *E. coli* and rotavirus.

Enterotoxigenic *E. coli* have been found in the stools of a substantial proportion of children who have been treated for diarrhea at medical facilities in several developing countries.[13,24,25] Furthermore, in the few studies that also sought ETEC from appropriately selected control children who did not have diarrhea, ETEC were more often isolated from ill children than from controls.[24-26] In the village study, ETEC were the most frequent pathogens identified, and the peak incidence was in children 9 to 11 months of age. Additional studies in rural villages in Bangladesh confirm that the incidence of ETEC diarrhea ranges from one to two episodes per child per year in the first 5 years of life and that additional asymptomatic infections occur.[26] Thus, it is obvious that repeated infections with ETEC occur throughout childhood.

ETEC are thought to be transmitted primarily by food or water. Food-borne outbreaks have been reported in a hospital nursery and on a cruise ship, and ETEC have been isolated from foods in the United States and in Bangladesh.[27-29] Water was the vehicle for an outbreak in a national park in the United States, and ETEC have been found in drinking water.[29,30] In Bangladesh, studies suggest that transmission of ETEC to young children may occur most frequently as a result of consumption of contaminated weaning foods.[31]

Our recovery of *Shigellae* from 15% of specimens from diarrheal episodes is similar to findings of previous studies of children in communities with poor sanitation.[7-9,32] As in these other communities, *S. flexneri* was the predominant serotype. In these settings, transmission is predominantly from person to person, although water- or food-borne transmission is also possible.[33]

In studies of diarrhea in children less than 2 years old in treatment facilities in many developing countries, rotaviruses have been the enteropathogens found most frequently.[13,34,35] This prominence of rotavirus as the cause of diarrhea among hospitalized children is undoubtedly related to the greater degree of dehydration with rotavirus diarrhea than with most other types of diarrhea, a characteristic that has been noted in comparisons of hospitalized children[34,35] and in one previous community-based study.[36] The greater frequency of dehydration with rotavirus diarrhea is evident in our village study, where rotavirus was found in 11% of all diarrheal episodes, but in 46% of episodes associated with dehydration. The incidence of rotavirus diarrhea was high only in the first 2 years of life, with few episodes of rotavirus diarrhea after that age.

Our studies suggest that symptomatic infection with rotavirus occurs one to two times in the first 2 years of life in Bangladeshi children. Additional studies of antirotavirus antibody titers of children in this area further suggest that numerous asymptomatic infections may occur during the first 5 years of life.[37] Although rotavirus infections had a slightly higher incidence in the cool months, transmission was noted year round. Most of this transmission appears to occur from child to child; however, waterborne spread cannot be ruled out.

The demonstration of an enteropathogen associated with the majority of diarrheal episodes permits some observations on the relative importance of illnesses associated with specific bacterial and viral agents. Rotavirus-associated diarrhea may be more likely to result in death from dehydration if treatment is not available. On the other hand, ETEC- and *Shigellae*-associated diarrhea result in more morbidity because of their high incidence and prevalence throughout childhood. Furthermore, ETEC-diarrhea may have the greatest adverse effect on growth because of its high incidence during the first 2 years of life.

Acknowledgments

This study was supported by the International Centre for Diarrhoeal Disease Research, Bangladesh (ICDDR,B), by NIH Grant 5R07110048-17, and by the Center for Vaccine Development, University of Maryland School of Medicine, Baltimore. Drs. Black and Merson performed the work in Bangladesh while assigned to the ICDDR,B from the Bureau of Epidemiology, Center for Disease Control, Atlanta, Georgia. The computer time for this research was supported in part through the facilities of the Computer Science Center of the University of Maryland. We thank the field workers of the MATLAB research area, especially the project supervisors, Miss S. Nahar, Mr. A. Hoque, and Dr. A. Baqui, and the laboratory personnel of the ICDDR,B, including Dr. I. Huq, Mr. A. R. M. A. Alim, Dr. K. A. Al Mahmud, Dr. A. S. M. Hamidur Rahman, Mr. G. Kibriya, Mr. S. Islam, and Mr. S. Huda.

References

1. Chen, L. C., Rahman, M., and Sarder, A. M. Epidemiology and causes of death among children in a rural area of Bangladesh. *Int. J. Epidemiol.* 9:25–33, 1980.
2. Walsh, J. A., and Warren, K. C. Selective primary health care: An interim strategy for disease control in developing countries. *N. Engl. J. Med.* 301:967–974, 1979.

3. Puffer, R. R., and Serrano, C. A. *Patterns of mortality in childhood*. Pan American Health Organization, PAHO Scientific Publication No. 262, Washington, D. C., 1973.
4. Scrimshaw, N. S., Taylor, C. E., and Gordon, J. E. *Interactions of Nutrition and Infection*, WHO Monograph Series No. 57. World Health Organization, Geneva, Switzerland, 1968.
5. Martorell, R., Habicht, J-P., Yarbrough, C., Lechtig, A., Klein, R. E., and Western, K. A. Acute morbidity and physical growth in rural Guatemalan children. *Am. J. Dis. Child.* **129**:1296-1301, 1975.
6. Rowland, M. G. M., Cole, T. J., and Whitehead, R. G. A quantitative study into the role of infection in determining nutritional status in Gambian village children. *Br. J. Nutr.* **37**:441-450, 1977.
7. Gordon, J. E., Guzmán, M. A., Ascoli, W., and Scrimshaw, N. S. Acute diarrhoeal disease in less developed countries: Patterns of epidemiological behaviour in rural Guatemalan villages. *Bull. WHO* **31**:9-20, 1964.
8. Feldman, R. A., Bhat, P., and Kamath, K. R. Infection and disease in a group of South Indian families. IV. Bacteriologic methods and a report of the frequency of enteric bacterial infection in preschool children. *Am. J. Epidemiol.* **92**:367-375, 1970.
9. Mata, L. J. *The Children of Santa Mariá Cauqué: A Prospective Field Study of Health and Growth*, M. I. T. Press, Cambridge, Massachusetts, 1978.
10. Evans, D. G., Olarte, J., DuPont, H. L., Evans, D. J., Jr., Galindo, E., and Portnoy, B. L. Enteropathogens associated with pediatric diarrhea in Mexico City. *Pediatrics* **91**:65-68, 1977.
11. Ryder, R. W., Sack, D. A., Kapikian, A. Z., McLaughlin, A. Z., Chakraborty, J. C., Rahman, A. S. M. M., Merson, M. H., and Wells, J. G. Enterotoxigenic *Escherichia coli* and reovirus-like agents in rural Bangladesh. *Lancet* i:659-663, 1976.
12. Black, R. E., Merson, M. H., Huq, I., Alim, A. R. M. A., and Yunus, M. Incidence and severity of rotavirus and *Escherichia coli* diarrhoea in rural Bangladesh: Implications for vaccine development. *Lancet* **1**:141-142, 1981.
13. Black, R. E., Merson, M. H., Rahman, A. S. M. M., Yunus, M., Alim, A. R. M. A., Huq, I., Yolken, R. H., and Curlin, G. T. A two year study of bacterial, viral and parasitic agents associated with diarrhea in rural Bangladesh. *J. Infect. Dis.* **142**:660-664, 1980.
14. Black, R. E., Merson, M. H., Taylor, P. R., Yolken, R. H., Yunus, M., Alim, A. R. M. A., and Sack, D. A. Comparison of glucose with sucrose in oral rehydration therapy of rotavirus diarrhea in infants and young children. *Pediatrics* **67**:79-83, 1981.
15. Edwards, P. R., and Ewing, W. H. *Identification of enterobacteriaceae*, 3rd ed. Burgess, Minneapolis, 1972.
16. Collwell, R. R. Polyphasic taxonomy of the genus *Vibrio*: Numerical taxonomy of *Vibrio cholerae*, *Vibrio parahaemolyticus*, and related *Vibrio* species. *J. Bacteriol.* **104**:410-433, 1970.
17. Furness, A. L., Lee, J. V., and Donovan, T. J. Group F, a new *Vibrio*, (Letter). *Lancet* ii:565-566, 1977
18. Merson, M. G., Sack, R. B., Kibriya, A. K. M. G., Mahmood, A., Ahmed, Q. S., and Huq, I. The use of colony pools for diagnosis of enterotoxigenic *Escherichia coli* diarrhea. *J. Clin. Microbiol.* **9**:493-497, 1979.
19. Yolken, R. H., Kim, H. W., Chen, T., Wyatt, R. G., Kalica, A. R., Chanock, R. M., and Kapikian, A. Z. Enzyme-linked immunoassay (ELISA) for detection of human reovirus-like agent of infantile gastroenteritis. *Lancet* ii:263-266, 1979.
20. Yolken, R. H., Wyatt, R. G., and Kapikian, A. Z. ELISA for rotavirus. *Lancet* ii:819, 1977.
21. Huq, M. I., Sack, D. A., and Black, R. E. *Working Manual for Assay of E. Coli Enterotoxin*

and ELISA Assay for Rotavirus Antigen. International Centre for Diarrhoeal Disease Research, Bangladesh, ICDDR,B, Special Publication No. 3, Dacca, Bangladesh, 1979.

22. Yolken, R. H., and Stopa, P. J. Analysis of nonspecific reactions in enzyme-linked immunosorbent assay testing for human rotavirus. *J. Clin. Microbiol.* **10**:703–707, 1979.

23. Samad, A., Sheikh, K, Sarker, A. M., Becker, S., and Chen, L. C. *Demographic Surveillance System Matlab*, Vol. 6, *Vital Events and Migration–1977*, Scientific Report No. 18. International Centre for Diarrhoeal Disease Research, Bangladesh, 1979.

24. Guerrant, R. L., Moore, R. A., Kirschenfeld, P. M., and Sande, M. A. Role of toxigenic and invasive bacteria in acute diarrhea of childhood. *N. Engl. J. Med.* **293**:567–573, 1975.

25. Donta, S. T., Wallace, R. B., Whipp, S. C., and Olarte, J. Enterotoxigenic *Escherichia coli* and diarrheal disease in Mexican children. *J. Infect. Dis.* **135**:482–485, 1977.

26. Black, R. E., Brown, K. H., Becker, S., Alim, A. R. M. A., and Huq, I. Longitudinal studies of infectious diseases and physical growth of children in rural Bangladesh. II. Incidence of diarrhea and association with known pathogens. *Am. J. Epidemiol.* **115**:315–324, 1982.

27. Ryder, R. W., Wachsmuth, I. K., Buxton, A. E., Evans, D. G., DuPont, H. L., Mason, E., and Barrett, F. F. Infantile diarrhea produced by heat-stable enterotoxigenic *Escherichia coli. N. Engl. J. Med.* **295**:849–853, 1976.

28. Sack, R. B., Sack, D. A., Mehlman, I. J., Orskov, F., and Orskov, I. Enterotoxigenic *Escherichia coli* isolated from food. *J. Infect. Dis.* **135**:313–317, 1977.

29. Black, R. E., Merson, M. H., Rowe, B., Taylor, P. R., Alim, A. R. M. A., Gross, R. J., and Sack, D. A. Enterotoxigenic *Escherichia coli* diarrhoea: Acquired immunity and transmission in an endemic area. *Bull. WHO* **59**:263–268, 1981.

30. Rosenberg, M. L., Koplan, J. P., Wachsmuth, I. K., Wells, J. G., Gangarosa, E. J., Guerrant, R. L., and Sack, D. A. Epidemic diarrhea at Crater Lake from enterotoxigenic *Escherichia coli:* A large waterborne outbreak. *Ann. Intern. Med.* **86**:714–718, 1977.

31. Black, R. E., Brown, K. H., Becker, S., Alim, A. R. M. A., and Merson, M. H. Contamination of weaning foods and transmission of enterotoxigenic *Escherichia coli* diarrhoea in children in rural Bangladesh. *Trans. Roy. Soc. Trop. Med. Hyg.*, **76**:259–264, 1982.

32. Hughes, J. M., Rouse, J. D., Barada, F. A., and Guerrant, R. L. Etiology of summer diarrhea among the Navajo. *Am. J. Trop. Med. Hyg.* **29**:613–619, 1980.

33. Black, R. E., Craun, G. F., and Blake, P. A. Epidemiology of common-source outbreaks of shigellosis in the United States, 1961–1975. *Am. J. Epidemiol.* **108**:47–52, 1978.

34. Hieber, J. P., Shelton, S., Nelson, J. D., Leon, J., and Mohs, E. Comparison of human rotavirus disease in tropical and temperate settings. *Am. J. Dis. Child.* **132**:853–858, 1978.

35. Kapikian, A. Z., Kim, H. W., Wyatt, R. G., Cline, W. L., Arrobio, J. O., Brandt, C. D., Rodriguez, W. J., Sack, D. A., Chanock, R. M., and Parrott, R. H. Human reovirus-like agent as the major pathogen associated with "winter" gastroenteritis in hospitalized infants and young children. *N. Engl. J. Med.* **294**:965–972, 1976.

36. Wyatt, R. G., Yolken, R. H., Urrutia, J. J., Mata, L., Greenberg, H. B., Chanock, R. M., and Kapikian, A. Z. Diarrhea associated with rotavirus in rural Guatemala: A longitudinal study of 24 infants and young children. *Am. J. Trop. Med. Hyg.* **28**:325–328, 1979.

37. Black, R. E., Greenberg, H. B., Kapikian, A. Z., Brown, K. H., and Becker, S. Acquisition of serum antibody to Norwalk virus and rotavirus and relation to diarrhea in a longitudinal study in rural Bangladesh. *J. Infect. Dis.* **145**:483–489, 1982.

5

Epidemiology of Childhood Diarrhea in The Gambia

M. G. M. ROWLAND

INTRODUCTION

The data discussed in this paper are derived from a study of young children in three neighboring subsistence farming villages in a rural area of The Gambia. Their general relevance will be discussed later. The original aim of the survey was to determine the main dietary and disease causes of growth-faltering known to affect children particularly severely in the first 3 years of life. More specific studies of diarrheal disease were undertaken because it was identified as the major nondietary cause of growth impairment,[1] leading, on average, to a halving of the expected monthly weight gain in infants and young children.[2] With good accessibility between subjects and medical survey facilities, acute diarrheal mortality was insignificant but there was a definite though declining mortality in association with protracted diarrhea and malnutrition (weanling diarrhea syndrome).

MATERIALS AND METHODS

The survey was started in 1974 and data are included up to 1978. Growth and morbidity data were collected at sick children clinics and at routine "call" clinics held every 4 to 6 weeks on children entering the survey between birth and 6 months of age until they left at between 18 and 36 months (the range arising from slightly different target groups at different periods of the survey).

M. G. M. ROWLAND • Medical Research Council Laboratories, Fajara, Banjul, The Gambia, West Africa.

Virtually all children from the three villages of Keneba, Kanton-kunda, and Manduar were included in the survey, yielding some 60 to 70 births annually, of which two-thirds were from Keneba. Thus, the basic cohort study involved longitudinal monitoring of several hundred children. More detailed microbiological studies were undertaken on children in 1975–1977, confined largely to the main annual "diarrhea season," and environmental hygiene was studied in 1977.

More details of the survey population and methods are listed in various publications. In general, it should be noted that the frequency with which children are affected by diarrheal illness is expressed as the number of days with symptoms during a given period expressed as "percentage time ill" or "prevalence." The term *incidence* has deliberately been avoided, as the pattern of disease at its height makes it difficult to identify the true end-point of one attack and the start of another.

THE HOST

AGE

Young children of Keneba and neighboring villages, when they are 3 months to 3 years of age, suffer diarrheal symptoms on average for 1 day in 8. The peak age prevalence occurs at around 9 months of age; in this group the infants have diarrhea for 25% of the time during the rainy season,[3] the prevalence falling off slowly during the next few years.[4]

In an earlier study in the coastal village of Sukuta, Marsden[5] noted a slightly later peak in age distribution at around 1 year, with no cases before 6 months, but numbers in this study were much smaller.

It is clear from the Keneba study that diarrhea may be seen even in early infancy before weaning commences, but it is relatively less common and rarely associated with growth-faltering,[6] which is the hallmark of the disease in slightly older children, a feature also noted by Marsden in his study.[5]

SEX

In neither study were the data analyzed on the basis of the sex of the subjects, but there is no evidence of the markedly discriminative weaning practices between boys and girls that have been described in some other cultures.

NUTRITIONAL STATUS

Diarrheal disease is the major nondietary cause of growth impairment in children under 3 years and at certain times appears to account for most of the growth deficit observed.

Different approaches to analysis of our data suggest that diarrhea leads to impaired nutritional status rather than vice versa,[1] though it is commonly stated that poor nutritional status leads to increased diarrheal morbidity. The two statements are not incompatible, and we are simply identifying which of the two interrelations has priority in our study community. On a general basis, it may be noted that at the season of optimal nutritional status in Gambian children (May, June), diarrheal prevalence starts to rise. When nutritional status has plummeted some 5 months later, diarrheal rates are substantially lower.[7]

There does, however, seem to be one specific instance when nutritional status relates to subsequent diarrheal experience: birth weight appears to be an important prognosticator for the severity of diarrheal morbidity experienced in infancy. Watkinson[6] has shown that children of higher birth weight receive greater quantities of breast milk and experience less diarrhea-induced growth-faltering during infancy than their lower-birth-weight counterparts.

FEEDING PRACTICES

The method of infant feeding observed in Keneba is highly traditional.[8] The feeding bottle is virtually unknown and commercial milk products play no significant role in the diet. All children are breast-fed well into the second year of life, the pattern being one of demand feeding by day and by night, with a suckling frequency of around 10 to 20 times per day being commonplace.[9] Breast milk intake is complemented, usually between 2 to 5 months of age, with local cereal gruels or paps, with a gradual change to more adult foods around 1 year of age.

This uniformity of practice provides little opportunity for comparison other than that already noted in relation to birth weight and quantity of breast milk consumed. It is clear, however, that the amount and severity of diarrhea experienced rises, as in other communities, with the onset of the weaning process. In fact, the whole pattern of the disease observed (which will be expanded in the course of this chapter) indicates that the term *weanling diarrhea*, as described by Gordon and colleagues in 1963,[10] is highly appropriate for these children.

In view of the uniformly extended period of regularly sustained breast-feeding, the absence of "commerciogenic malnutrition," and the use of a traditional complementary feed that is cooked, it is perhaps surprising that these village children suffer so much from diarrhea and its effects. The question arises as to whether the enviromental contamination to which they are exposed is so gross as to swamp the various protective mechanisms, including factors in breast milk, or whether mothers' milk may in some way be deficient in protective factors, perhaps due to maternal undernutrition and other stresses.

We have attempted to correlate the *in vitro* grade of anti-*Escherichia coli* activity[11] of mothers' milk with the amount of diarrhea suffered by the recipient infant.[12] In doing this, we make two broad assumptions: first, that the level of challenge for different infants is very similar, and second, that *E. coli* are important causes of infant diarrhea in The Gambia. A group of mothers (about 10%) were identified who produced breast milk of very high antibacterial activity (similar to that of colostrum) sustained for substantial periods, some into the second half of infancy. Their offspring suffered little or no diarrhea during these periods. There was, however, no significant relationship between the amount of morbidity and other grades of *in vitro* activity of the milk received. It seems now that this group of mothers were good antibody-producers in general (Dolby, personal communication), but this characteristic was related neither to nutritional status during lactation (as measured by subcutaneous fat) nor to the volumes of milk produced.[12] Moreover, the most active milks were unusually potent compared with findings in the United Kingdom. Thus, it seems that we cannot ascribe the generally excessive amount of diarrhea experienced by most Gambian children to some deficiency in breast milk content, though we may ask why all mothers did not produce equally "supersafe" milk.

Two practices can be identified as likely to be dangerous. All children are given a regular "top-up" through the day with crude well water, albeit in small volumes, from birth onward, sometimes as a substitute for colostrum in the early days of life. The dose of pathogens to which a child may be exposed in this way is unlikely to be high, but it seems to be an entirely unnecessary risk. Second, the heavy imposition of farming duties on women during much of the year leads to increasing separation and prolonged intervals between breast-feeds for the mother and her infant.[13] This must tend to impair the effectiveness of at least some of the protective factors in milk, such as the IgA component.

In summary, despite generally good feeding practices, it is the weanling village child (i.e., age 6 to 18 months or more) who suffers the highest diarrheal morbidity to an extent that is quite incompatible with normal health and growth.

The Disease/Agent

Definition

Many attempts have been made to achieve some precision in the use of the term *diarrhea,* usually encompassing at least stool frequency, consistency, and color. It is well recognized that all these factors may vary considerably between one normal individual and another. Ultimately, it is a *change* from the individual's normal pattern toward more frequent or watery stools, with or without other features, on which the diagnosis hinges. For children in their home environment, the person most competent to observe and relate that change (often the only person) is the mother. In the local language, diarrhea has a clear and unequivocal translation,[3] and for these reasons we have based our data largely on the mothers' account of their children's symptoms. It is important to note, however, that in the course of 4 years of intensive observation and investigation, many stool specimens have been seen and collected, and these have vindicated to our satisfaction our largely historical definition of the disease.

Duration

Most of the recognizably acute diarrheal episodes have a mean duration of around 3 days in children less than 6 months and 4 days after that age. In the older age group, also, the range of duration of symptoms was much greater, with considerable numbers of children having attacks lasting longer than 2 weeks (unpublished results).

Prevalence

Even below 6 months of age, between 40 and 75% of infants suffered some diarrhea in any 2-month period, and the figures rose to between 40 to 100% thereafter, according to season. In the children affected, the number of attacks experienced appeared to vary between one and four, but the difficulty of defining an attack when symptoms are frequent has already been alluded to. Prolonged attacks appeared to contribute notably to high prevalence figures (unpublished results).

Seasonality

One of the most conspicuous features of childhood diarrhea in The Gambia is its close association with the 5 months of the annual rainy

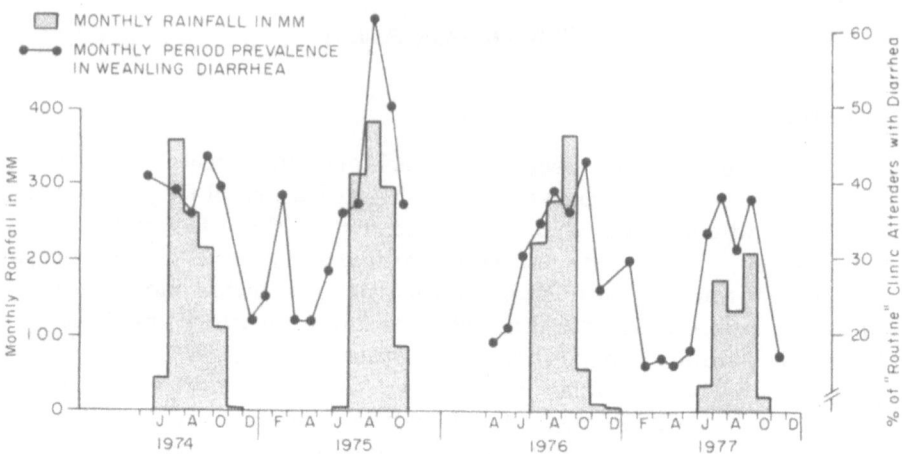

Figure 1. Monthly rainfall and diarrheal prevalence in weanlings in Keneba and neighboring survey villages, 1974–1977. (Source: *Transactions of the Royal Society of Tropical Medicine and Hygiene* **74**:663–665, 1980, with permission of the Royal Society. See reference 15.)

season, the peak prevalence coinciding largely with the time of peak precipitation ([14,15]) (Figure 1). Apparently unrecognized before our study was the regular occurrence of a smaller, cool, dry-season epidemic in which more severe acute dehydration was a feature. Retrospective scrutiny of Keneba records some 10 to 15 years earlier,[16] and also of Marsden's data from a similar period,[5] indicates that this secondary peak is not just a recent phenomenon.

ETIOLOGICAL AGENTS

Pathogenic bacteria were sought in the stools of subjects with diarrhea (symptoms not more than 4 days) and healthy controls aged 6 to 36 months during the 1975 rainy-season epidemic. The list of pathogens sought in 1975 was notably deficient, including *Salmonella, Shigella,* and pathogenic *E. coli,* but failing to take account of toxin-producing *E. coli* and *Campylobacter* species. This may partly account for the remarkably low yield of pathogens obtained (5.6% of cases and 3.5% of controls) and the small difference in yield between the two groups.[3]

A resurvey in 1977 in children under 18 months of age confirmed the low isolation rate of these pathogens (unpublished data) but failed technically to shed more light on the pathogens omitted from the earlier protocol.

Rotavirus sought by immune electron microscopy was absent from the stools of cases and controls[17] in 1975, and we do not believe that the mainly rainy-season epidemic of diarrhea in Gambian children is due to this agent. However, it is clear from serological studies[15] that exposure to and/or disease from rotavirus is as common in these children as in other countries (86% in those aged 9 months to 2 years), and rotavirus has subsequently been found in the stools of children during the cool, dry season when the secondary epidemic occurs (unpublished results).

Of the parasitic diseases, only two organisms, both protozoa, were found with any degree of frequency, namely, *Giardia lamblia* and *Trichomonas hominis*, motile trophozoites of both being found in about 20% of children, particularly in association with protracted diarrhea. Screening for stool parasites was not sufficiently systematic to allow interpretation of this phenomenon, but some other information is relevant. In a small serosurvey of 17 children under 1 year of age, 7 had a positive *Giardia* fluorescent-antibody test,[18] a finding normally associated with malabsorption and suggestive of the presence of the parasite as a pathogen of importance. Of 27 village children between 12 and 20 months of age in whom small bowel flora was studied, 6 (22%) had *Giardia* in the jejunal aspirate.[3]

PATHOLOGY

The etiological information described above is clearly incomplete, but I wish to propose certain broad generalizations on the basis of it. First, rotavirus gastroenteritis is an important component of the secondary cool-season peak of disease with a relatively severe, acute, secretory diarrhea. The main rainy-season outbreak is in the first instance a largely bacterial phenomenon with giardiasis also important, perhaps in a synergistic capacity. Acute gastroenteritis at this time of the year, particularly in the older infant/toddler group, is frequently followed by intermittent, protracted symptoms compatible with the original description of weanling diarrhea. Jejunal aspirate studies, including measurement of total bile salt concentrations[3] (Table I), and the limited serological survey referred to above,[18] suggest that malabsorption may be a common phenomenon.

Concomitant food studies suggest that the degree of anorexia associated with diarrhea vis-à-vis other illness is not sufficient to explain the overriding importance of its effect on growth.[20] The postgastroenteritis complications may be primarily an infectious phenomenon, though detailed analysis of our evidence does not support this,[18] and the alternative or additional possibility of temporary food intolerance[21] deserves serious consideration. Our data do not permit us to determine whether

Table I.   Jejunal Intubation Findings in 37 Keneba Children Aged 6 to 20 Months

Jejunal aspirate	Mean value	"Abnormal" value	Percent abnormal
Log total bacterial count	5.0	>4.0	81
Giardia lamblia trophozoites	—	present	16
Total bile salt concentration (mm/liter)	2.3	<2	48
Ratio glycine:taurine conjugates	6.1	>3	74
Ratio dihydroxy:trihydroxy bile salt concentrations	0.4	<1.5	70

acute gastroenteritis due to any one particular agent is more or less likely to be followed by such complications, and this is an important area for future research. It may be that it is a particular sequence of events involving a series of acute infections with different pathogens, be they bacterial, viral, or parasitic, that determines the outcome.

THE ENVIRONMENT

Whatever the etiology or pathology of childhood diarrhea in The Gambia, the broad assumption will be made here that spread is via the fecal-oral route and environmental factors will be considered on this basis.

DOMESTIC WATER SUPPLIES AND SANITATION

Historically, shared water supplies have long been recognized as potential sources of major diarrheal epidemics. In Keneba, the needs of approximately 900 people are met by six wells within the village perimeter. These wells are major gathering points for women, not just when drawing water, but also for laundering. There is very little in the way of formal provision for sanitation within the village, and small children in particular commonly defecate within the main compound areas; nor are the well areas enclosed. The subsoil is porous laterite, allowing rapid leaching of surface material to deeper layers. The well water is polluted at all times, the pattern of organisms suggesting a mixture of human and animal fecal contamination, and there is a 10- or 100-fold increase in levels of fecal markers within 1 week of the onset of the rains. Specific pathogens such as *Salmonellae* have been found from time to time.[22] Water is stored in the homes in large earthenware pots, where the tendency is for the level of fecal organisms to fall off slightly.

Despite this rather alarming picture, small children do not in general consume large volumes of well water at any one time and thus may not commonly be exposed to infective doses of pathogens.[23] Against this we have to consider the effect of repeated subinfective doses in undernourished and sometimes otherwise immune-compromised children. Furthermore, the water is used for other domestic purposes, the most important of which in this context is food preparation.

WEANING FOODS

Detailed microbiological studies on weaning foods carried out at various stages of preparation have shown that well water is a major source of fecal contamination and that the organisms thereby introduced are reduced in number but certainly not eradicated by cooking.[24] Thus, excessively high contamination levels of freshly prepared foods[4] in the wet season are due in large part to the water supplies that, in turn, are affected by rainfall.[22] Other adverse factors come into play during the rains. It is a period of labor-intensive farming from which few able-bodied women are spared prolonged spells of heavy manual labor. From the age of 3 months, infants are increasingly left behind in the compounds in the care of nursemaids or other mother surrogates.[13]

In such cases, food is usually prepared for the child in the early morning and consumed in the course of the day, or even as late as 18 to 24 hours after. Not surprisingly, massive bacterial overgrowth occurs in these foods in the high ambient temperatures experienced (Table II).[25] Moreover, it is the lightly cooked cereal gruel or paps used to start weaning that are worse affected; the more adult-type boiled or steamed foods introduced at around 1 year are very much less contaminated when fresh, and sustain less rapid proliferation of organisms. The most polluted foodstuffs of all were those paps to which local cow's milk had been added, a commodity collected and stored in an extraordinarily unhygienic manner.[26,27]

Table II. Percentage of Weaning Foods
Hazardously Contaminated, by Season
(ICMSF, 1974)[a]

	Dry season	Wet season
Freshly cooked	6	35
After 8 hours	71	96

[a]From International Association of Microbiological Sciences[25]

Discussion

In most countries where strong seasonal climatic changes are observed there are equally clear-cut changes in the prevalence of childhood diarrhea. However, no uniform pattern is observed in this relationship; though diarrhea is probably related in most instances to wet seasons, it is a dry-season phenomenon in others. The Gambia shows both features. No explanation is offered here regarding the minor dry-season peak other than to say that it may in large part be due to rotavirus infection.[15] The upper respiratory symptoms that commonly accompany the early illness and the apparent susceptibility of the respiratory mucosa during hot, dry spells may hint at some explanation, but this is highly speculative.

The main rainy-season outbreak of diarrhea in The Gambia is a much less surprising phenomenon. Environmental hygiene deteriorates notably with the start of the rains. In explaining the tendency of increasing diarrheal prevalence to anticipate the onset of the rains, a number of explanations may be offered (Figure 2). First, at the end of the dry season, water availability, never good, is at absolute rock-bottom level. Women spend hours, often well into the night, drawing small quantities of muddy water from the drying wells. Mothers start to delegate child care and short-cut their food preparation just before the rains so that their farms will be ready for the earliest possible benefit when the rains arrive. Humidity rises and mean minimum–maximum temperatures also fall at this time, presumably permitting longer survival of fecal organisms in the environment. But the overall factor that appears to dominate the scene is the rain itself.

In low rainfall years, less diarrhea is seen than in years with high precipitation.[15] Monthly peaks in rainfall during any one season are usually accompanied by monthly peaks in diarrheal prevalence.[14] This can-

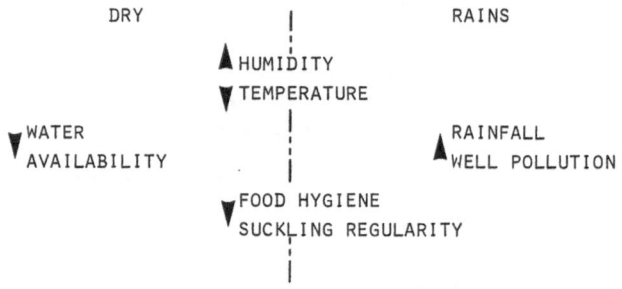

Figure 2. Weanling diarrhea: seasonality.

not be explained entirely on the basis of well pollution, as this tends to rise dramatically and be uniformly sustained throughout the rains.[22] The combination of enforced delegation of child care, the lack of a safe, traditional "convenience" weaning food, and poor environmental hygiene provides an almost insurmountable obstacle to the health planner, often constrained by limited financial and personnel resources, seeking single compromise intervention measures. The apparent ability of a small proportion of women to produce a milk that is so active in terms of antiinfective properties as to provide almost complete protection against diarrhea for 6 months or more[12] offers a useful lead when considering such solutions.

REFERENCES

1. Rowland, M. G. M., Cole, T. J., and Whitehead, R. G. A quantitative study into the role of infection in determining nutritional status in Gambian village children. *Br. J. Nutr.* **37**:441–450, 1977.
2. Cole, T. J., and Parkin, J. M. Infection and its effect on the growth of young children: A comparison of The Gambia and Uganda. *Trans. Roy. Soc. Trop. Med. Hyg.* **71**:196–198, 1977.
3. Rowland, M. G. M., and McCollum, J. P. K. Malnutrition and gastroenteritis in The Gambia. *Trans. Roy. Soc. Trop. Med. Hyg.* **71**:199–203, 1977.
4. Rowland, M. G. M., Barrell, R. A. E., and Whitehead, R. G. Bacterial contamination in traditional Gambian weaning foods. *Lancet* i:136–138, 1978.
5. Marsden, P. D. The Sukuta project: A longitudinal study of health in Gambian children from birth to 18 months of age. *Trans. Roy. Soc. Trop. Med. Hyg.* **58**:455–489, 1964.
6. Watkinson, M. Delayed onset of weanling diarrhea associated with high breast-milk intake, *Trans. Roy. Soc. Trop. Med. Hyg.* **75**:432–435, 1981.
7. Rowland, M. G. M., and Whitehead, R. G. The epidemiology of protein-energy malnutrition in a West African village community: A summary of the work of the Medical Research Council Dunn Nutrition Group 1974–1978. Medical Research Council, London, 1980.
8. Thompson, B. *Marriage, childbirth and early childhood in a Gambian village: A sociomedical study.* Unpublished doctoral dissertation Aberdeen University, 1965.
9. Whitehead, R. G., Rowland, M. G. M., Hutton, M. A., Prentice, A. M. Muller, E. M., and Paul, A. A. Factors influencing lactation performance in rural Gambian mothers. *Lancet* ii:178–181, 1978.
10. Gordon, J. E., Chitkara, I. D., and Wyon, J. B. Weanling diarrhea. *Am. J. Med. Sci.* **245**:345–377, 1963.
11. Dolby, J. M., Honour, P., Rowland, M. G. M., and Tully, M. Bacteriostasis of *Escherichia coli* V. The bacteriostatic properties of milk of West African mothers in The Gambia: *In vitro* studies. *J. Hyg. Camb.* **85**:347–358, 1980.
12. Rowland, M. G. M. Cole, T. J., Dolby, J. M., and Honour, P., 1980, Bacteriostasis of *Escherichia coli* VI. The *in vitro* bacteriostatic properties of Gambian mothers' breast-milk in relation to the *in vivo* protection of their infants against diarrhoeal disease, *J. Hyg. Camb.* **85**:405–413.

13. Rowland, M. G. M., and Paul, A. A. Factors affecting lactation capacity: Implications for developing countries. In: *Infant and Child Feeding*, J. T. Bond, L. J. Filer, Jr., G. A. Leveille, A. M. Thomson, and W. B. Weil (Eds.), Nutrition Foundation Monograph Series. pp. 63–75, Academic Press, London and New York, 1981.

14. Rowland, M. G. M., and Barrell, R. A. E. Ecological factors in gastroenteritis. In: *Disease and Urbanisation*, E. J. Clegg and J. P. Garlick (Eds.), *SSHB Symposia Proceedings*, 20:21–35. Taylor and Francis, London, 1980.

15. Rowland, M. G. M., Leung, T. S. M., and Marshall, W. C. Rotavirus infection in young Gambian village children. *Trans. Roy. Soc. Trop. Med. Hyg.* 74:663–665, 1980.

16. McGregor, I. A., Rahman, A. K., Thomson, A. M., Billewicz, W. Z., and Thompson, B. The health of young children in a West African (Gambian) village. *Trans. Roy. Soc. Trop. Med. Hyg.* 64:48–77, 1970.

17. Rowland, M. G. M., Davies, H., Patterson, S., Dourmashkin, R. R., Tyrell, D. A. J., Matthews, T. H. G., Parry, J., Hall, J., and Larson, H. E. Viruses and diarrhea in West Africa and London: A collaboratory study. *Trans. Roy. Soc. Trop. Med. Hyg.* 72:95–98, 1978.

18. Rowland, M. G. M., Cole, T. J., and McCollum, J. P. K. Weanling diarrhoea in The Gambia: Implications of a jejunal intubation study. *Trans. Roy. Soc. Trop. Med. Hyg.* 75:215–218, 1981.

19. Ridley, M. J., and Ridley, D. S. Serum antibodies and jejunal histology in giardiasis associated with malabsorption. *J. Clin. Pathol.* 29:30–34, 1976.

20. Rowland, M. G. M. Interactions between diarrhoea and malnutrition: Aetiological considerations. In: *Acute Enteric Infections in Children. New prospects for treatment and prevention* (Proceedings of Nobel Conference 3), T. Holme (Ed.), Amsterdam: Elsevier/North Holland, 1982.

21. Walker-Smith, J. A. Post-enteritis enteropathy. In: *Diseases of the Small Intestine in Childhood*, 2nd ed., pp. 245–246. Pitman Press, London, 1979.

22. Barrell, R. A. E., and Rowland, M. G. M. The relationship between rainfall and well-water pollution in a West African (Gambian) village. *J. Hyg. Camb.* 83:143–150, 1979.

23. Coward, W. A., Sawyer, M. B. Whitehead, R. G., Prentice, A. M., and Evans, J. New method for measuring milk intakes in breast-fed babies. *Lancet* ii:13–14, 1979.

24. Barrell, R. A. E., and Rowland, M. G. M. Commercial milk products and indigenous weaning foods in a rural West African environment: A bacteriological perspective. *J. Hyg. Camb.* 84:191–202, 1980.

25. International Commission on Biological Specifications for Foods of the International Association of Microbiological Sciences. *Microorganisms in Foods*, Vol. 2, *Sampling for Microbiological Analysis. Principles and specific applications.* University of Toronto Press, Toronto, 1974.

26. Barrell, R. A. E., and Rowland, M. G. M. Infant foods as a potential source of diarrhoeal illness in rural West Africa. *Trans. Roy. Soc. Trop. Med. Hyg.* 73:85–90, 1979.

27. Barrell, R. A. E., and Kelley, S. S. M. I., Cows' milk as a potential vehicle of diarrheal disease pathogens in a West African village. *J. Trop. Pediatr.* 28:48–52, 1982.

6

Malnutrition and Susceptibility to Diarrhea

With Special Reference to the Antiinfective Properties of Breast Milk

S. Sahni and R. K. Chandra

Introduction

Breast milk provides nearly optimum nutritional components for the growing infant. Its content of proteins, lipids, lactose, and minerals is ideally suited for the young infant. Moreover, it has several other advantages over formula, such as being readily available at proper temperature, being fresh and relatively sterile, and requiring no preparation, thereby reducing the potential risk of contamination. In addition, breast-feeding has psychological advantages for both the mother and the infant. It is satisfying to the mother because she is personally involved in nurturing her baby, and to the infant because of close contact and comfort from the mother. Another very important facet of breast-feeding that is being recognized and appreciated with increasing interest is its role in providing immunity to the newborn against infections. In the past 15 years or so, considerable work has focused on unraveling the biochemical and cellular bases of the antiinfectious properties of human milk, as well as on its role in preventing infections in the newborn and young infant and in prevention of allergic disorders; based on these data, breast-feeding is being strongly encouraged. This immunologic protective capacity of breast milk may indeed be a new frontier in infant nutrition.

S. Sahni • Janeway Child Health Center, St. John's, Newfoundland.   R. K. Chandra • Memorial University of Newfoundland, St. John's, Newfoundland.

IMMUNOLOGIC STATUS OF THE NEWBORN AND
YOUNG INFANT

Newborn infants have an increased susceptibility to infections, and morbidity and mortality from infections is higher than in older children and adults. This is attributed to the fact that specific, as well as nonspecific, immunologic mechanisms are both immature and antigenically inexperienced. Although the mechanism of antigen recognition and the resulting production of humoral antibodies and the ability to mount a cell-mediated immune response are present in fetal lymphoid cells by the end of the first trimester of pregnancy, their functional capability is suboptimal. Deficient cell-mediated immunity is reflected in diminished delayed cutaneous hypersensitivity reaction, impaired lymphoblast transformation on antigenic or mitogenic stimulation, decreased lymphokine production, and impaired cytotoxic reaction.

Humoral immune responses are also deficient in newborns. IgG is the only immunoglobulin present in significant amounts at birth. This is immunoglobulin of maternal origin that is actively transferred across the placenta, often against a concentration gradient. This transfer occurs late in pregnancy so that blood levels in preterm babies are even lower than in full-term infants. Serum half-life of IgG is 21 days, so that this maternal antibody gradually disappears from the circulation. Because of this decline in passively acquired immunity and the normal delay in acquiring active immunity after birth, there is a period of physiological hypoimmunoglobulinemia. Markedly low levels of IgG are associated with increased susceptibility to infection.

LOCAL IMMUNE STATUS OF THE NEONATAL
GASTROINTESTINAL TRACT

In newborn infants, the lymphoid follicles beneath the mucosal epithelium are infrequent and develop only after antigenic challenge. On antigenic stimulation, antigen-reactive lymphocytes present in these follicles proliferate and differentiate into IgA-secreting plasma cells. Secretory IgA is present in only trace amounts in the fetal intestine. The amounts, although higher in the newborn, are still very low and do not reach adult levels until several months after birth. Such maturation may be accelerated by repeated infections. This deficiency of the local immune mechanisms, which may be due in part to impaired cell-mediated immunity, is one of the factors making infants more susceptible to infections.

BREAST-FEEDING AND INFECTIONS

The practice of breast-feeding the newborn infant was quite prevalent until the close of the 19th century. With increasing socioeconomic status during the period 1930–1970, more infants were given artificial foods early in life. It was believed that feeding infants with hygienically prepared cow's-milk formula did not enchance the risk of infection and permitted optimal physical growth. This may largely be true for the developed countries. However, there are recent epidemiological data to suggest that these changes in feeding practices are responsible for increasing frequency of infections in nonindustrialized settings. This is particularly so in underprivileged populations, where the switch from the breast to the bottle invariably increases morbidity and even mortality.

The incidence of enteric bacterial and viral infections is lowest in breast-fed infants. Otitis media and respiratory infections are also fewer. Impure water supply and contamination of formula during preparation are important factors in predisposing infants to infections, especially in communities with low living standards, but they do not solely explain the higher incidence of, and increased mortality from, infections in artificially fed babies. This is supported by prospective studies in hospital nurseries, where it has been seen that breast-fed infants are almost completely protected from lethal infections like *Pseudomonas* septicemia and meningitis. A number of studies have looked into the relationship between feeding practices and the extent of gastrointestinal tract colonization with pathogenic organisms. Infants fed formula milks show increased colonization with enteropathogenic *Escherichia coli*, polio and rotaviruses, *Shigella*, *Salmonella*, and *Giardia lamblia*, and diarrheas caused by these organisms.

In prospective investigations carried out in India and Canada, the incidence of diarrheal disease in breast-fed infants was considerably lower than in cow's-milk-fed controls. In a study of 72,000 infants over a 1 year period, 253 cases of *Salmonella* infection in infants were observed. Only one of these infants was being breast-fed at the time of clinical infection, and there was a correlation between infection and age of the infant: 75% of the reported cases were less than 6 months of age. This report supports the concept that breast-feeding provides neonates and young infants with effective immunity against enteric infections. The study also highlights the fact that the younger the infant, the poorer the host defense response, and the higher the incidence of infection.

Human milk and colostrum have been used to prevent epidemics of *E. coli* diarrhea in the newborn and this is attributed to the presence in the milk of specific substances that neutralize or inactivate the toxins produced by these organisms. Some studies suggest a partial protective role of human milk in necrotizing enterocolitis; data in laboratory animals are more conclusive. Based on these observations, human milk banks are being proposed for preventing this disease in high-risk newborn infants.

Next in importance to its protection against gastrointestinal disease, breast milk protects against otitis media of bacterial, viral, or allergic origin. Retrospective as well as longitudinal prospective studies have clearly confirmed the preventive value of breast milk in this regard. Human milk also affords protection against respiratory tract infections according to both epidemiological surveys and hospital studies. This supports the concept that the high incidence of bacterial colonization and infection of the gastrointestinal tract in artifically fed babies is not solely because of contamination of formulas. Of 115 infants who presented for admission with respiratory syncytial virus infection, only 8 were being breast-fed compared to 46 of 167 healthy controls in the community. A recent study from northern New York State showed that significantly fewer infants hospitalized for infection were being exclusively breast-fed compared to the expected proportion being breast-fed in the community.

Human breast milk has been shown to have a significant beneficial effect in low-birth-weight infants. These infants, because of their immature immune system, are at high risk of developing infections. In a study of 70 high-risk, low-birth-weight infants, the incidence of infections was significantly higher (29 of 38) in artificially fed babies compared to those who received supplements of freshly expressed breast milk (9 of 32). On further analysis of those who did develop infection, serious infections like septicemia and meningitis were more common in the first group and their illnesses lasted longer. This further emphasizes the need for encouraging the use of breast milk for all newborn infants.

PROTECTIVE CONSTITUENTS OF HUMAN MILK

Human milk contains a variety of cellular and soluble factors that protect the newborn against infection. These include immunglobulins.

Cellular Components. Human colostrum and early milk contain up to 10 million cells per cubic millimeter. Macrophages constitute a major fraction of these cells after the first few days. Immunocompetent B and T lymphocytes, null cells, and neutrophils are the other cellular constituents of defense present in human milk. Although the cellular content of milk has been reported to vary widely, depending on factors like maternal hydration, emotional status, drug intake, and presence of mastitis, colostrum and early milk have a higher cellular content than found in mature milk (Table I).

Macrophages. Macrophages constitute the major fraction of the cellular components of human milk after the first few days of life, during which neutrophils predominate. These macrophages have been shown to be mobile and to exhibit phagocytic activity and adherence. This preponderance of macrophages in human milk and their activity suggest that these cells are important to the neonatal intestine. However, the mechanisms of the protection afforded by live, active macrophages are not clear. The macrophage is a scavenger cell known for its phagocytic activity, by virtue of which it can combat the uptake of microbial, environmental, and dietary antigens to which the infant is exposed immediately after birth. The protective role of macrophages against necrotizing enterocolitis in laboratory animals, and to some extent in human beings, has been documented. In addition to the phagocytic activity, it has a role in the production of some nonspecific factors of immunity, including lactoferrin, interferon, lysozyme, and complement components C3 and C4. Colostrum and milk macrophages have been shown by immunofluorescence techniques to possess surface and intracellular IgA and other immunglobulins, which suggests that they act as vehicles for the transient storage and transport of immunoglobulins. Finally, they are involved in antigen processing and regulation of production of antibody and T-cell-mediated immune response in the systemic and secretory sites.

T-Lymphocytes. Indirect immunofluorescence with anti-T-cell antibodies and rosetting techniques show approximately one-half of human colostral and milk lymphocytes to be thymic-derived. The source of these lymphocytes appears to be the gut- and bronchial-associated lymphoid tissue. On antigenic challenge, these lymphocytes are primed and appear in the milk via the enteromammary gland axis. This source of origin for these lymphocytes is based on the observation that proliferative response of milk lymphocytes from immune mothers is seen only to certain anti-

Table I. Average Cellular Content of
Human Milk

	1st day	7th day
Lymphocytes ($\times 10^6$/ml)	1.1	0.22
Macrophages ($\times 10^6$/ml)	2.5	0.68
Neutrophils ($\times 10^6$/ml)	6.24	0.48

gens like mumps, rubella, measles, and purified protein derivative (PPD), and not to others like *Candida albicans,* tetanus toxoid, or streptokinase. Furthermore, milk, and not the peripheral blood lymphocytes, shows blastoid response to K capsular antigen for *E. coli.*

Although it is by no means certain, T-lymphocytes may transfer delayed cell-mediated immunity to the infant during lactation. This is suggested by the studies of Orgra and co-workers (1979) on a small group of newborns. Cord blood was negative for PPD-reactive cells. After these infants were nursed by mothers who had PPD-reactive lymphocytes in blood and milk, the infants also showed the appearance of such cells in their circulation in 4 to 5 weeks. Whether this effect is through the passage of T-lymphocytes themselves, or to a T-cell-product-like transfer factor, is not clear. On the other hand, breast-fed infants of PPD-positive mothers and those with tuberculous disease rarely show a positive delayed cutaneous hypersensitivity response to tuberculin. Another point also unanswered is whether this tranfer of T-lymphocytes represents a major stimulus to the development of the newborn's cellular immune system.

T-cells are also responsible for the differentiation of IgA-bearing lymphocytes into IgA-secreting lymphocytes. This is suggested by the fact that in primary immunodeficiency states characterized by T-cell defect, there is increased incidence of IgA deficiency. Furthermore, a proportion of IgA-deficient individuals show T-cell dysfunction. The role of T-lymphocytes in proliferation of, and enhanced mucus secretion by, goblet cells of the gastrointestinal and bronchial mucous membranes has also been suggested. This provides another line of defense against invasion by microorganisms.

B-Lymphocytes. B-lymphocytes in human milk also appear to be derived from the enteromammary gland axis. This is suggested by laboratory *in vitro* studies showing that, of the 34% B-cell population of milk lymphocytes, only 3% bear the complement 3b (C3b) receptor, as compared to 11 of 15% B cells in the peripheral blood. These B-lymphocytes are the source of secretory IgA-producing plasma cells. Most of the B-lymphocytes in the mammary gland have surface IgA rather than other immunoglobulins.

Other Cells. Neutrophils constitute the major fraction of the cellular compartment of colostrum and milk for the first few days postpartum. Whether this is related to initial breast engorgement simulating an inflammatory response is not clear. Fluid-phase components promote chemotactic and opsonic properties, following which neutrophils phagocytose the foreign microorganisms and kill them. Although there are a number of reports in the literature comparing the chemotactic and phagocytic activities and intracellular killing by neutrophils from milk and blood, whether or not the former do protect the newborn against bacterial infection has not been established.

IMMUNOGLOBULINS AND ANTIBODIES

Human milk and colostrum are rich in immunoglobulins. These, by virtue of their antibody activity against microorganisms, provide antiinfective defense for the neonate. Antigen-sensitized precursor cells from gut, and probably bronchial-associated lymphoid tissue, home in on the mammary gland, where they initiate local synthesis of the antibody that appears in the colostrum and milk. Hormonal changes associated with pregnancy and lactation appear to be involved in induction of prolific immunoglobulin synthesis. A specific subclass of T-lymphocytes (T-helper cells) has a regulatory action in this process of antibody synthesis.

The dominant immunoglobulin in human milk is secretory IgA. Its concentration in colostrum and milk, on average, is 10 times higher than in serum. Early colostrum contains 20 to 40 mg per milliliter of IgA. After the first few days, the concentration in milk drops, but because of the increase in the total volume of milk produced, the total amount of IgA remains fairly constant in the first 2 to 3 months of lactation. Secretory IgA provides an antiinfective barrier at the mucosal surface. Secretory IgA production by the infant requires antigenic stimulation at the mucosal surfaces and does not reach adult levels before 2 years. Therefore, ingestion of this immunoglobulin by the neonate at a time when its own immune systems are immature helps to limit the colonization and replication of pathogenic organisms. Secretory IgA (sIgA) in the milk is adapted for a mucosal environment that is replete with proteolytic enzymes. sIgA in a dimeric form, in which two monomers of IgA are joined together by a J chain, is also produced by plasma cells. The presence of a secretory component synthesized by epithelial cells produces configurational changes in the IgA polymer so that the molecule becomes tightly packed and partially resistant to enzymatic degradation. sIgA, while in the neonatal intestine, is bound to the cysteine fraction of mucus and is thus not washed away by peristalsis. IgM is also present in appreciable amounts in human colostrum and milk and, as with sIgA, its concentration falls from an initial level of 27 to 30 mg/g of protein in the colostrum to 6 to 8 mg/g, again probably a dilutional phenomenon. Both these immunoglobulins contain antibodies against specific viruses and bacteria that cause maternal infection, and they provide specific protection to the neonate. IgG derived mainly from maternal blood is present in human milk in a concentration approximately one-third of serum levels and remains constant at these low levels in the milk. IgG is more easily inactivated by intestinal enzymes.

IMMUNOREGULATORY MEDIATORS

Complement. Colostrum contains quantities of complement component C3 and C4 in concentrations comparable to those in serum. After the first week, the concentration in human milk drops to 5 to 10% of the original. The source of these components appears to be macrophages in the milk. High concentrations of IgA in milk activates the complement system through the alternate pathway. C3 component thus activated helps in bacterial opsonization and phagocytic killing by macrophages and neutrophils.

Bifidus Factor. This is a nitrogen-containing polysaccharide present in appreciable quantities in human milk. While its concentration in cow's milk is very low, it promotes the growth of lactobacillus bifidus in the neonatal intestine.

Lipids. The antiviral properties of human milk lipids were first reported more than 30 years ago. This is attributed to the high lipase content of human milk. Lipase converts human milk lipids to free fatty acids and monoglycerides that have greater antiinfective activity than do triglycerides found in higher concentration in bovine and synthetic milks. Based on these facts, it has been suggested that when animal milks are used in synthetic formulas for infants, they should be fortified with monoglycerides rather than unsaturated vegetable oils.

Lactoferrin. Lactoferrin is a protein present in various exocrine secretions, including milk. Its concentration in human milk is about 7 mg/ml in colostrum and about 1 mg/ml in mature milk. It is a single polypeptide chain of molecular weight 75,000 to 90,000 daltons and binds two ferric ions. Lactoferrin is relatively resistant to degradation by gastric acidity or proteolytic activity. Whether this is because of low acid pepsin production in infants, the chemical nature of the protein itself, or the presence in the milk of inhibitors of proteolysis is not clear. The feature that is clear is the fact that the apolactoferrin (iron-free form) is most susceptible to proteolysis and loss of bacteriostatic property.

Considerable *in vitro* data are available to support the role of lactoferrin in protecting the neonate against gastrointestinal infections. However, no *in vivo* biological function of this protein has as yet been unequivocally established. Lactoferrin has been shown to inhibit the growth of certain microorganisms like enteropathogenic strains of *E. coli, Staphylococcus aureus* and *albus, Pseudomonas aeruginosa, Bacillum subtilis, Candida albicans,* and others. A bactericial effect on *V. cholerae* and *Strep-*

tococcus mutans has also been reported. The effects are synergistically enhanced in the presence of a specific antibody.

The bacteriostatic effect of lactoferrin is thought to be largely due to its high affinity for iron, thus making iron unavailable for bacterial growth. However, it may have direct bactericidal action.

Lysozyme. Lysozyme is a protein produced by macrophages. Its concentration in milk as measured directly or by the total stool content is higher in human breast milk than in artificial milk. By its property of clearing peptidoglycan of bacteria, it causes bacterial lysis. It may also act in conjunction with IgA immunoglobulin and complement, causing bacterial killing.

Epithelial Growth Factor. The newborn's intestinal epithelium, being immature, has a less effective protective function against the penetration of pathogens and macromolecules. Breast milk promotes and accelerates ontogenetic growth of gut mucosa.

IMMUNOLOGICAL PROTECTION AND DURATION OF BREAST-FEEDING

With the realization that breast milk is superior compared to artificial feeds with regard to nutritional, psychological, and immunological aspects, increasing numbers of educated mothers are breast-feeding their newborns. However, because of sociocultural stresses, they tend to stop early. In developing countries, this has disastrous effects on the child's health. There are some studies suggesting that there is a strong correlation between incidence of diarrhea and weaning, and mortality from this is proportional to the age of weaning. The factors contributing to this are removal of passive immunity afforded by maternal sIgA, more chances of exposure to pathogenic organisms via contaminated milk and other foods, and a compromise in nutritional status. The last two factors are not uncommon in the primitive conditions of the Third World. There are recent published data to suggest that exclusive breast-feeding may not provide adequate energy intake for a proportion of infants beyond 4 months of age. If this nutritional deficit alters immunocompetence, the frequency of infections may go up in such infants. This must obviously be balanced against the risk of infection resulting from ingestion of contaminated foods.

NUTRITIONAL DEFICIENCY, IMMUNOCOMPETENCE, AND SUSCEPTIBILITY TO INFECTION

Much of the information on the susceptibility of malnourished individuals to infection has been derived from clinical and epidemiological observations, further supported by controlled data collection in experimental laboratory animals. The most prominent effect of malnutrition is on the duration and severity of infectious illness. There is some evidence that the incidence and period of contagiousness of infection may also be increased, but the data on these aspects are inadequate. The results of many surveys support the common association of undernutrition, growth failure, infection, and diarrheal disease.

Prospective studies in the less developed countries indicate that among infants 6 to 24 months old, the duration of infectious episodes and incidence of complications correlate significantly with the presence of malnutrition. The Pan American Health Organization survey of childhood mortality patterns in the Americas showed that 57% of children under 5 years of age who died had signs of intrauterine and/or postnatal nutritional growth retardation as either the primary of associated cause of death. The severity of measles and diarrheal disease, as judged by mortality rates, is several-fold higher in the malnourished.

The pattern of microorganisms isolated from malnourished populations resembles the type seen in primary immunodeficiency states. These observations led to the investigation of the immunocompetence of undernourished subjects. Briefly, such studies have revealed consistent impairment of cell-mediated immunity, decreased levels of serum complement components C3 and Factor B and of secretory IgA, and reduced intracellular bactericidal activity. These changes are observed both in protein-energy malnutrition and in selected deficits of single nutrients such as zinc and iron. The topic has been extensively reviewed elsewhere (Chandra, 1980).

BIBLIOGRAPHY

Brock, J. H. Lactoferrin in human milk: Its role in iron absorption and protection against enteric infection in the newborn infant. *Arch. Dis. Child.* **55**:617–621, 1980.

Bullen, J. J., Rogers, H. J., and Leigh, L. Iron-binding protein in milk and resistance to *Escherichia coli* infection in infants. *Br. Med. J.* **1**:69–75, 1972.

Chandra, R. K., Mandeveille, R. P., and Dearlove, J. What's new in paediatric immunology? In: *Paediatric Problems in South East Asia,* I. S. Prasad (Ed.), pp. D1–16. Sanjivan Press, Patna, India, 1977.

Chandra, R. K. Immunological aspects of human milk. *Nutr. Rev.* **36**:265–272, 1978.

Chandra, R. K. Prospective studies of the effect of breast feeding on incidence of infection and allergy. *Acta Paediatr. Scan.* **68**:691–694, 1979.

Chandra, R. K. *Immunology of Nutritional Disorders.* Arnold, London, 1980.

Chandra, R. K. Breast feeding, growth and morbidity. *Nutr. Res.* **1**:35–41, 1981.

Cunningham, A. S. Morbidity in breast-fed and artificially fed infants. *J. Pediatr.* **90**:726–727, 1977.

Dowham, M. A. P. S., Scott, R., Simms, D. G., Webb, J. K. G., and Gardner, P. S. Breast feeding protects against respiratory syncytial virus. *Br. Med. J.* 3:274–276, 1976.

Fallot, M. E., Boyd, J. L., III, and Oski, F. A. Breast feeding reduces incidence of hospital admissions for infection in infants. *Pediatrics* 75:1121–1124, 1980.

France, G. L., Marmer, D. J., and Steele, R. W. Breast feeding and *Salmonella* infection. *Am. J. Dis. Child.* 134:147–152, 1980.

Gordon, J. E., Wyon, J. B., and Ascoli, W. The second year death rate in less developed countries. *Am. J. Med. Sci.* 254:357–380, 1967.

György, P. The uniqueness of human milk. Biochemical aspects. *Am. J. Clin. Nutr.* 29:970–975, 1971.

Hanson, L. A., and Winberg, J. Breast milk and defense against infections in the newborn. *Arch. Dis. Child.* 47:845–848, 1972.

Hanson, L. A., Carlsson, B., Ahlstedt, S., Svanborg, C., and Kaijser, B. Immune defense factors in human milk. *Mod. Probl. Pediatr.* 15:63–72, 1975.

Kabara, J. J. Lipids as host resistance factors of human milk. *Nutr. Rev.* 38:65–73, 1980.

Khan, A. J., Rosenfield, W., Vedapalli, M., Biagton, J., Khan, P., Huq, A., and Evans, H. E. Chemotaxis and random migration of human milk cells. *J. Pediatr.* 96:879–882, 1980.

Klaus, M. H., Jerauld, R., Kreger, N. C., McAlpine, W., Steffa, M., and Kennell, J. H. Maternal attachment. Importance of the first postpartum days. *N. Engl. J. Med.* 286:460–463, 1972.

Larsen, S. A., and Homer, D. R. Relation of breast vs. bottle feeding to hospitalization for gastroenteritis in a middle-class U.S. population. *J. Pediatr.* 92:417–418, 1978.

Masson, P. L, and Heremens, J. F. Lactoferrin in milk from different species. *Comp. Biochem. Physiol. (B)* 39:119–129, 1971.

Mata, L. J., and Urrutia, J. J. Intestinal colonization of breast-fed children in a rural area of low socio-economic level. *Ann. N.Y. Acad. Sci.* 176:93–109, 1971.

Mata, L. Breast-feeding: Main promoter of infant health. *Am. J. Clin. Nutr.* 31:2058–2071, 1978.

Miller, M. E. Host defenses in the human neonate. *Pediatr. Clin. North Am.* 24:413–423, 1977.

Narayanan, I., Parakash, K., Bala, S., Verma, S. K., and Gujaral, V. V. Partial supplementation with expressed breast milk for prevention of infection in low birth-weight infants. *Lancet* ii:561–563, 1980.

Nutrition Committee of the Canadian Paediatric Society and the Committee on Nutrition of the American Academy of Pediatrics. Breast feeding, a commentary on the international year of the child, 1979. *Pediatrics* 62:591–601, 1978.

Orgra, P. L., and Dayton, D. H. (Eds.). *Immunology of Breast Milk.* Raven Press, New York, 1979.

Pitt, J., Barlow, B., and Heird, W. C. Protection against necrotizing enterocolitis by maternal milk. 1. Role of milk leukocytes. *Pediatr. Res.* 11:906–909, 1977.

Pittard, W. B. Breast milk immunology. *Am. J. Dis. Child.* 133:83–87, 1979.

Robinson, J. E., Harvey, B. A. M., and Soothill, J. F. Phagocytosis and killing of bacteria and yeast by human milk cells after opsonization in aqueous phase of milk. *Br. Med. J.* 1:1443–1445, 1978.

Roitt, I. *Essential Immunology,* pp. 117–126. Blackwell Scientific Publications, London, 1974.

Winberg, J., and Wessner, G. Does breast milk protect against septicaemia in the newborn? *Lancet* i:1091–1093, 1971.

III

Mechanisms of Diarrhea and Malnutrition

7

Food Intake During and After Recovery from Diarrhea in Children

A. M. Molla, Ayesha Molla, S. A. Sarker, and
M. Mujibur Rahaman

Introduction

Published work suggests that the "nutritional status" of a child may represent as much the effect of infection as of dietary intake.[1,2] A study by Mata and co-workers[3] showed that the nutritional status of the children in rural Guatemala was more related to infections than to the availability of food. The same may be true for many other developing countries. That the nutritional consequences of diarrhea are protein-energy malnutrition and growth retardation has been established.[4,5] Several factors are involved in this process, among which partial anorexia or loss of appetite, cultural taboos, maternal behavior during diarrhea resulting in withholding of food as a measure to control it, and increased catabolic processes that compound direct loss due to malabsorption are important.

The purpose of this chapter is to review the available data on intake of food during diarrhea and the impact of diarrhea on the growth of children, and to present our recent study on the intake of food both during the acute stage and after recovery from diarrheas of different etiologies. Withdrawal or modification of food offered to reduce the stool volume and duration of diarrhea is widely practiced. Early investigators placed their reliance on the appearance, volume, and number of stools

A. M. Molla, Ayesha Molla, S. A. Sarker, and M. Mujibur Rahaman • International Centre for Diarrhoeal Disease Research, Dacca, Bangladesh.

as the criteria for success of treatment. This point of view was challenged in 1924 by Park,[6] who maintained that the child as a whole rather than stool volume and character should be taken as the criterion for evaluating therapy. This was scientifically examined for the first time by Chung and co-workers in 1948.[7]

They studied two groups of infants with diarrhea. The first group, younger than 6 months, was fed 100 to 120 kcal per kg of body weight per day, and those over 6 months old were given 80 kcal per kg per day. The older group received nothing p. o. for the first 48 hours, followed by oral feeding of 20 kcal/kg/day, which was increased at the rate of 20 kcal/kg per day. The mean intake of the group fed was 40.6 kcal greater during the first week than that of the group not fed for the first 48 hours. The duration of diarrhea in the group receiving food throughout was not significantly longer than in the younger group, but the weight gain was higher in infants and children given food, as shown in Figure 1. Chung further observed that the higher stool volume in the group receiving food was associated with greater absorption of nutrients.

Food intake is reduced in the acute phase of diarrhea. This has been amply demonstrated by different workers. According to FAO/WHO in 1973,[8] the daily recommended allowance for energy and protein was fixed at 100 kcal/kg and 1.25 g/kg, respectively, per day. Using this standard, Mata and co-workers[9] showed that Guatemalan village children consume diets deficient in calories but adequate in protein under normal conditions, as shown in Figure 2. This intake was affected by different kinds of illnesses, including diarrhea. The cause of infection lies in the nonnutritional factors, but malnourished children tend to harbor infections for longer periods and often have more severe clinical manifesta-

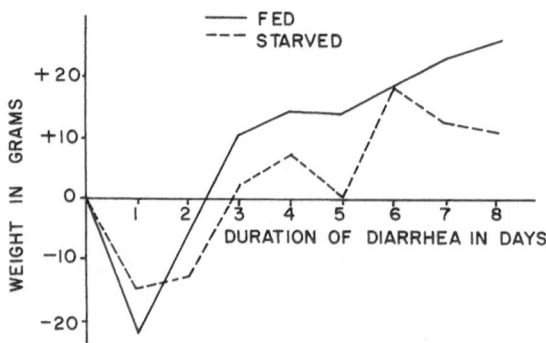

Figure 1. Weight curves showing algebraic sum of daily weight gains and losses in two groups of children (Chung *et al.*, 7).

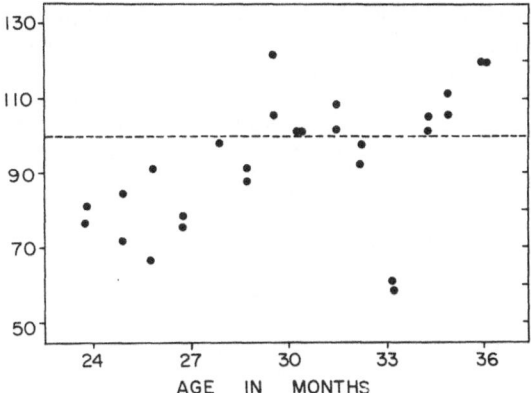

Figure 2. Estimates of percentage of recommended calories consumed by a child in Guatemala (Mata *et al.*, 9).

tions of disease.[10-13] Gyr and co-workers demonstrated that protein-deficient vervet monkeys exposed to cholera suffered more severe symptoms than monkeys eating their usual diets.[14]

Martorell and co-workers, in a longitudinal study in Guatemala[4] involving 477 preschool children, attempted to measure the effect of illnesses such as respiratory infections, diarrhea, and a group of selected common symptoms on food intake while the children were in their home environment. The authors found that, on average, the reduction of calorie and protein intake was 20%, which is equivalent to 175 kcal and 4.8 g protein per day. It became apparent that the effect of diarrhea on food intake was greater than that from respiratory infections.

Recently, at the International Centre for Diarrhoeal Disease Research, Bangladesh, studies were carried out to estimate the effect of diarrhoeal illness on food intake in the hospital and in the home. Hoyle *et al.*[15] studied the food intake in two groups of children with diarrhea admitted to a field hospital. The mothers of one group received intensive dietary education and the other group received routine hospital care. The authors compared the food intake of these two groups with that of a healthy group matched for age. The importance of this study lies in the fact that breast-feeding was continued for some children, and calorie intake from breast milk was measured separately. The results are presented in Table I.

Total calorie intake among children with diarrheas was 75 kcal/kg/day compared to 130 kcal/kg/day by healthy children. In other words, there was about a 40% reduction in intake during diarrhea. Most inter-

Table I.   Total Calorie Intake (kcal/kg per 24 hours) from Breast Milk, Oral Fluids, and Weaning Foods among Children with Diarrhea Compared to That of Health Controls (Mean ± SEM)[a]

Source of calories	Healthy controls (N = 11)	Children with diarrhea (N = 15)
Breast milk	53.6 ± 6.7	46.9 ± 5.5
Oral fluids	—	10.1 ± 2.0
Weaning foods	86.3 ± 21.1	33.3 ± 8.8
Total calories	129.9 ± 16.8	75.0 ± 8.3

[a]Source: reference 15.

estingly, calorie intake from breast milk did not decrease in children with diarrhea compared to calorie intake by healthy, breast-fed children. In this study, the intake of food was not studied in the same patients when they were healthy compared to intake when they had diarrhea. However, the study demonstrated that calorie intake from breast milk remains undisturbed even during diarrhea.

Another study carried out in a rural area in the southern part of Bangladesh (M. Rahaman, personal communication, 1978), which involved 65 children between the ages of 13 and 60 months, measured the food intake of these children in their homes during healthy periods as well as during diarrheal episodes. The investigators demonstrated that the intake of both calories and proteins was reduced by 70%, although environmental conditions remained unchanged. This severe reduction of calorie and protein intake may have been due to withdrawal of food in the home environment, which may be minimized in a hospital setting.

INTAKE OF FOOD IN THE ACUTE STAGE OF DIARRHEA AND AFTER RECOVERY

In the present study, intake of nutrients was measured among children below 5 years of age during the acute phase of diarrhea caused by *V. cholerae*, enterotoxigenic *Escherichia coli* (ETEC), rotavirus, and *Shigella*, and 2 and 8 weeks after recovery. The objectives of the study were to (1) make a quantitative estimation of nutrient intake during acute diarrhea of various etiologies in children and compare it with that after recovery, (2) study the pattern of intake of nutrients in acute and convalescent stages of diarrhea and after recovery, and (3) study the impact of food intake on stool volume during diarrhea.

PATIENTS AND METHODS

Sixty-three children below 5 years of age were involved in this study, of whom 29 had cholera, 15 rotavirus infection, 13 ETEC diarrhea, and 6 diarrhea due to *Shigella*. Patients with mild to moderate dehydration, whose diarrhea was of short duration and without any apparent complications, were selected from a diarrhea treatment center in Dacca, Bangladesh, for a food-intake study. The clinical information of the study patients is presented in Table II. Cholera patients were comparatively older and also lost more fluid. The patients in the other groups were comparable with respect to age, body weight, degree of dehydration, and purging rates. To correct dehyrdration and to maintain hydration, fluid was administered only by the intravenous route. Following rehydration, a charcoal marker was fed, and immediately after that, a familiar local diet was offered to the patients *ad libitum*. The composition of the diet is shown in Table III. The type of food was selected according to the choice

Table II. Clinical Summary of Study Patients (Mean ± SEM)

Particulars	Cholera (29)[b]	Rotavirus (15)[b]	ETEC (13)[b]	*Shigella* (6)[b]
Age (month)	43.8 ± 2.8	17.2 ± 3.9	33.1 ± 3.2	33.0 ± 7.6
Body weight (kg)	9.6 ± 0.3	9.1 ± 0.6	9.8 ± 0.5	9.4 ± 0.7
Hematocrit	35.4 ± 3.6	31.8 ± 0.9	32.8 ± 0.8	33.3 ± 2.0
Serum specific gravity	1.027 ± 0.001	1.026 ± 0.001	1.026 ± 0.001	1.026 ± 0.001
72-hour stool volume (ml/kg per 8 hr)	477 ± 63	142 ± 17	199 ± 23	247 ± 101
Total I.V. (liter)	5.75 ± 0.83	1.16 ± 0.21	1.16 ± 0.27	1.98 ± 0.46

[b]Figures in parentheses indicate number of subjects studied.

Table III. Composition of the Diet

Food item	kcal/g	Protein, g %
Boiled rice	1.2	2.12
Curry[a]	1.34	7.56
Banana	1.24	1.81
Khichuri[b]	0.94	2.57
Whole milk	0.77	2.37
Dessert/halua[c]	1.47	2.7
Bread	3.01	8.06

[a]Contained potato, oil, chicken, onion, and pumpkin.
[b]Contained rice, dal, oil, chicken, and potato.
[c]Contained milk, egg, semolina, oil, and sugar.

of the children in a prestudy trial. Actual amount of breast milk consumed was determined by test-weighing before and after nursing. The foods were offered at different times according to local customs, and special care was taken to keep the food habits of the children similar to those in the prediarrhea period.

After the appearance of the marker, the intake study was carried out for 72 hours. Same patients with diarrhea of each etiology were studied up to the seventh day after admission, which included a convalescent period. The appearance of the first formed stool was taken as the end of the acute stage and the beginning of the convalescent phase. Patients were discharged after clinical recovery and brought back 2 and 8 weeks after recovery. The intake study was repeated, employing the same procedures, during each of these two periods for 72 hours.

RESULTS

The mean intake of food in g/kg per day is shown in Table IV. Intake in the acute stage of *Shigella* was lowest compared to that in patients having diarrhea from all other etiologies. In the recovery stage, intake improved. Intake of patients with rotavirus was also low and they, too, showed less increase in food intake during the recovery stage compared to patients with diarrhea from other causes. The calorie intakes during acute diarrhea, and 2 and 8 weeks after recovery, are shown in Table V. The mean calorie intake in the acute stage was about 70 kcal/kg per day in patients with diarrhea of any type. However, 2 weeks after recovery, the calorie intake improved comparatively more for patients with diarrhea except for those with rotavirus, whose intakes became comparable only by 8 weeks after recovery.

The intake of fat, protein, and calories combined during different stages of diarrhea is shown in Figure 3, and the trend is the same as for calorie intake. The pattern of intake of calories showed a steady improvement day by day in cholera. It reached the FAO/WHO-recommended[8]

Table IV.   Intake of Food (g/kg per day) in Acute Stage and after Recovery from Diarrhea (Mean ± SEM)

Etiology	Acute	Recovery	% Reduced
Cholera	82 ± 8.5	110.4 ± 8.7	26
Rotavirus	87 ± 10.4	102.7 ± 11.1	15
ETEC	82.4 ± 7.87	106 ± 6.0	22
Shigella	73.2 ± 10.9	114.3 ± 8	36

Table V. Intake of Calories in Acute Stage (A), and 2 Weeks
(R₁) and 8 Weeks (R₂) after Recovery (Mean ± SD)

Etiology	A	R₁	R₂
Cholera	74.9 ± 36.20	111.1 ± 35.4	109.59 ± 31.7
Rotavirus	68.5 ± 22.6	87.2 ± 26.2	115.0 ± 20.2
ETEC	70.7 ± 37.9	90.97 ± 28.4	114.9 ± 19.0
Shigella	70.0 ± 28.2	100.5 ± 27.8	109.3 ± 18.8

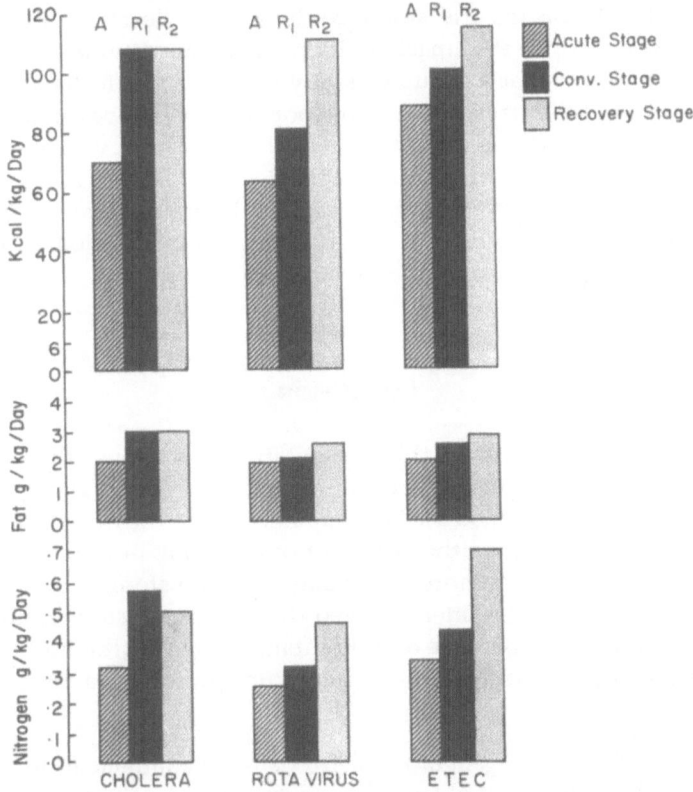

Figure 3. Nutrient intake in acute (A), convalescent (R₁), and recovery (R₂) stages of diarrhea.

intake of 100 kcal/kg per day on the fourth day in cholera and on the fifth day in ETEC and rotavirus infections. This coincided with the appearance of the first formed stool in all groups. The cholera patients showed an intake higher than the recommended allowances (120 kcal/ kg per day) on the seventh day, and it remained the same after recovery.

In ETEC patients, calorie intake was the highest (112 kcal/kg per day) on the seventh day and did not change in the recovery period. Rotavirus patients showed some differences. The highest calorie intake (115 kcal/ kg per day) was not reached until 8 weeks after recovery.

Table VI shows the percentage of estimated calorie requirements consumed in different stages of diarrheas of different etiologies—62.6, 44.7, 60, and 63.6 kcal/kg per day for cholera, rotavirus, ETEC, and *Shigella,* respectively. The calorie intake in the acute stage of rotavirus infection is comparatively less, but 2 weeks after recovery, substantial caloric intake was achieved in all groups.

For ethical reasons the study could not be designed properly to answer the question of impact of food on stool volume because this would have meant that a group of study children would have to fast to observe the impact of lack of food on stool volume. However, an attempt was made to measure the effect of food intake on stool volume for a 72-hour period in patients with diarrhea from all etiologies, as illustrated in Figure 4. The mean intake of food in each 24-hour study period is shown beside the mean stool volume in the same 24-hour period. No matter what the etiology, food intake steadily increased and stool volume decreased.

DISCUSSION

The literature review in this presentation has shown that diarrhea, like many other illnesses, affects the nutritional status and growth of children. Withholding food may or may not reduce the duration and volume of diarrhea or change the character of the stool. But the observation of Park, that the child is more important than the stool, is noteworthy.[6] Chung, over two decades later, showed that, although stool volume may increase in some cases because of food intake, it is nevertheless associated with higher nutrient absorption and does not prolong diarrhea.

Table VI.   Percent of Estimated Calorie Requirements in Different Stages of Diarrhea: Acute (A), and 2 Weeks (R_1) and 8 Weeks (R_2) after Recovery (Mean ± SD)

Etiology	A	R_1	R_2
Cholera	62.6 ± 35.0	99.1 ± 35.5	92.7 ± 47
Rotavirus	44.7 ± 22.6	76.9 ± 25.7	95.2 ± 23.2
ETEC	60 ± 32.1	76.3 ± 29.3	109.0 ± 9.1
Shigella	63.6 ± 23.0	80.9 ± 25.4	98.7 ± 14.4

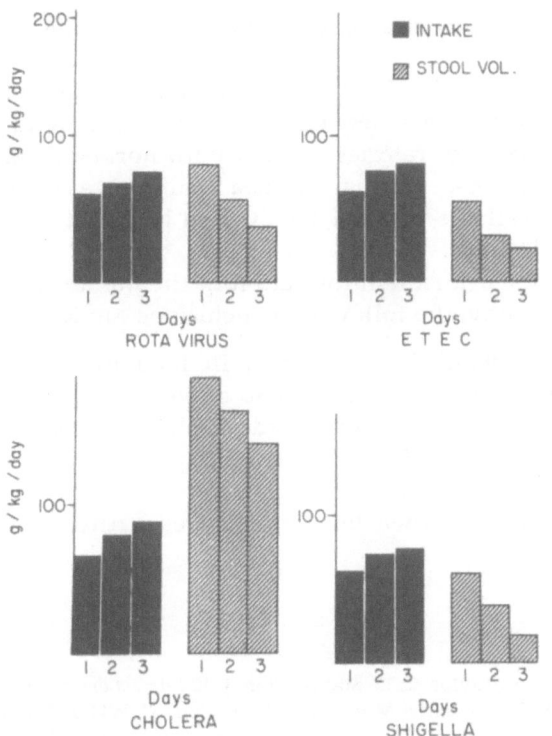

Figure 4. Relation between food intake and stool weight.

The virtue of breast milk has been elaborately studied, but the study of Hoyle *et al.*[15] showed that the anorexia of diarrhea mainly affects supplementary food intake, while the level of breast milk consumed remains unchanged. Thus, it provides a unique source of calories and much needed protein. Anorexia is a frequent consequence in diarrheal illnesses, and even dietary education for mothers may not alter this. However, this study shows that, if offered, there is substantial intake of food and calories by children suffering from diarrhea of different etiologies. The pathophysiology of the specific diarrhea is related to the amount of food consumed. In noninvasive diarrheas like cholera, calorie intake returns to the recommended amount by the fourth day, and during convalescent and recovery stages the intake even exceeds the recommended allowance. Patients with rotavirus, on the other hand, take a longer period to return to the same level of intake. This may be due to the pathology of rotavirus disease, selectively affecting the villous epithelial cells.[16]

In spite of anorexia, there was substantial calorie intake even in the acute stage of diarrhea when food was offered. If food had not been offered, the amount of calories necessary for normal metabolic activities and catabolic processes during diarrhea would have come from utilizing body fat and available protein. This would have put the child into further negative balance.

Based on the available information in the literature and on the data from our own study, the following conclusions can justifiably be drawn.

1. There is about 30% reduction in food intake during diarrhea among hospitalized patients no matter what the etiology.
2. Feeding, including breast-feeding, should be encouraged even in the acute phase of diarrhea from any cause.
3. There is no apparent deleterious effect of food on the volume or duration of diarrhea, but this requires further study.

REFERENCES

1. Scrimshaw, N. S., Taylor, C. E., and Gordon, J. E. *Interactions of Nutrition and Infection,* World Health Organization Monograph Series No. 57. WHO, Geneva, 1968.
2. Olson, R. E. (Ed.). *Protein-Calorie Malnutrition.* Academic Press, New York and London, 1975.
3. Mata, L. J., Urrutia, J. J., Albertazzi, C., Pellecer, O., and Arellano, E. Influence of recurrent infections on nutrition and growth of children in Guatemala. *Am. J. Clin. Nutr.* **25**:1267–1275, 1972.
4. Martorell, R., Yarbrough, C., Yarbrough, S., and Klein, R. F. The impact of ordinary illnesses on the dietary intakes of malnourished children. *Am. J. Clin. Nutr.* **33**:345–350, 1980.
5. Rowland, M. G., Cole, T. J., and Whitehead, R. G. A quantitative study into the role of infection in determining nutritional status in Gambian village children. *Br. J. Nutr.* **37**:441–450, 1977.
6. Park, E. A. Newer viewpoints in infant feeding. *Proc. Conn. State Med. Soc.* p. 190, 1924.
7. Chung, A. W., and Viščorová, B. The effect of early oral feeding versus early oral starvation on the course of infantile diarrhea. *J. Pediatr.* **33**:14, 1948.
8. *Energy and Protein Requirements, Report of a joint FAO/WHO ad hoc expert committee,* WHO Technical Report Series No. 522. World Health Organization, Geneva, Switzerland, 1973.
9. Mata, L. J., Kromal, R. A., Urrutia, J. J., and Garcia, B. Effect of infection on food intake and the nutritional state: Perspectives as viewed from the village. *Am. J. Clin. Nutr.* **30**:1215–1227, 1977.
10. Mata, L. J., Fernández, R., and Urrutia, J. J. Infección del intestino por bacterias enteropathogenas en niños de una aldea Guatemala, durante los tres primeros años de vida. *Rev. Latinoam. Microbiol.* **11**:103–110, 1969.

11. Schiefele, D. W., and Forbes, C. E. Prolonged giant cell excretion in severe African measles. *Pediatrics* **50**:867–873, 1972.

12. Hirschhorn, N., and Denny, K. M. Oral glucose electrolyte therapy for diarrhea: A means to maintain or improve nutrition. *Am. J. Clin. Nutr.* **28**:189–192, 1975.

13. Morley, D. C. Measles in the developing world. *Proc. Roy. Soc. Med.* **67**:1112–1115, 1974.

14. Gyr, K., Felsenfeld, O., and Zimmerlining, M. Effect of oral pancreatic enzymes on the course of cholera in protein-deficient vervet monkeys. *Gastroenterology* **74**:511–513, 1978.

15. Hoyle, B., Yunus, M., and Chen, L. C. Breast-feeding and food intake among children with acute diarrheal disease. *Am. J. Clin. Nutr.* **33**:2365–2371, 1980.

16. Davidson, G. P., Gall, D. G., Petric, M., Butler, D. G., and Hamilton, J. R. Human rotavirus enteritis induced in conventional piglets. *J. Clin. Invest.* **60**:1402–1409, 1977.

8

The Energy Cost of Diarrheal Diseases and Other Common Illnesses in Children

REYNALDO MARTORELL AND CHARLES YARBROUGH

INTRODUCTION

Diarrheal diseases and other common illnesses in children affect nutritional status by reducing appetite and by interfering with nutrient absorption and utilization.

The first objective of this paper is to estimate the effect of common illnesses on appetite by comparing the dietary intakes of children when they are healthy and when they are sick. The second objective is to compare common illnesses and food supplements in terms of their effects on physical growth. Both objectives seek to quantify the nutritional cost of diarrheal diseases and other illnesses. While the first objective involves a direct estimate of only one of the effects of illnesses (i.e., food-intake reduction), the second represents an indirect attempt to estimate their overall nutritional significance.

METHODOLOGY

POPULATION

The data come from a recently completed longitudinal study of malnutrition and mental development that took place in four small villages

REYNALDO MARTORELL • Food Research Institute, Stanford University, Stanford, California. CHARLES YARBROUGH • Computers for Marketing Corporation, San Francisco, California.

of Guatamala.* The initial sample included all mothers and all children 7 years old or younger at the time the study began in 1969. New cohorts of children were included until February 1973 and the study terminated in February 1977.

As in many areas of rural Guatemala, protein-energy malnutrition and respiratory and gastrointestinal illnesses were frequently observed. A vaccination and curative medical care program, staffed by paramedical personnel under the supervision of physicians, operated throughout the course of the study. A food supplementation program also functioned as described below. The study included measurements of supplement intake, growth, home dietary surveys, illness surveys, psychological test evaluations, and socioeconomic status.[1]

DATA COLLECTION PROCEDURES AND VARIABLES

Only those aspects of the data relevant to this study are briefly described.

Food Supplementation. The characteristics of the food supplementation design of the study reflect the emphasis in the late 1960s on the importance of adequacy of dietary protein. Two villages received a high-protein drink (11.5 g of protein per cup, 180 ml) called Atole, and two control villages, under identical conditions, a nonprotein drink called Fresco. The Atole contained 163 kcal per cup (180 ml), but the Fresco, with as little sugar and as few flavoring agents as necessary, contained only 59 kcal per cup. Both drinks contained vitamins and minerals, as detailed by Lechtig *et al.*[2] Both supplements were distributed daily in fixed locales. Individual intake was measured daily to the nearest 10 ml. Supplement ingestion was found to be unrelated to home food consumption.[3] Also, the effect of the food supplements on growth appear to have been caused by energy rather than protein.[3,4] Hence, for the purposes of this paper, supplement intake is expressed as calories.

Anthropometry. Anthropometric measurements were made at specific ages, following standardized techniques that did not vary during the course of the study. Supine length was measured on a standard measuring table and weight was measured on a beam balance.

Morbidity Survey. Mothers were interviewed every 2 weeks about the health of their children. Specifically, they were asked to recall any symp-

*The longitudinal study was carried out by the Division of Human Development, Institute of Nutrition of Central America and Panama (INCAP), Guatemala City, Guatemala. Support for data collection was by Contract PH 43-65-640 from the National Institute of Child Health and Human Development, National Institutes of Health, Bethesda, Maryland.

toms their preschool children might have had in the previous 2 weeks. The beginning and ending dates of each symptom were always noted. The quality control measures included periodic standardizations with a supervisor and routine inspections of the coded forms. The methodology is described in greater detail elsewhere.[5-7]

Information about 44 distinct items was collected. Four morbidity indicators were constructed from these data for the purposes of this study. Frequency of occurrence and likelihood of having an effect on diet were the criteria for selection.[7] The four indicators are described as follows: (a) *Respiratory infections.* This variable is defined by the presence of symptoms of upper respiratory infection (nasal discharge, sore throat) and/or lower respiratory infection (soreness of chest, shortness of breath). (b) *Diarrhea.* Any report of loose stools, whether or not accompanied by mucus and/or blood, and irrespective of the number of daily evacuations, was taken as evidence of diarrhea. (c) *Apathy.* A summary of reports of the child's not being "his usual self." Mothers might complain of the child's not wanting to eat (anorexia) or play as usual, or comment that he was a "cry-baby" or uncommonly irritable. These symptoms almost always occurred in conjunction with respiratory or gastrointestinal symptoms and other common complaints. (d) *Summary variable,* designated as SC (selected common) symptoms. This variable was designed to include common but important symptoms from the point of view of nutrition and health. It was defined by the presence of any of the following items: diarrhea, anorexia, fever, vomiting, signs of a rash, or any other indication of a communicable disease, and being so ill as to be confined to bed. The SC variable is largely a reflection of diarrhea and anorexia because the other symptoms were reported less frequently.

Dietary Survey. Dietary surveys were collected by the same workers responsible for the morbidity survey. Surveys were carried out on all children every 3 months, from 15 to 36 months of age and every 6 months thereafter, until they were 60 months old. The mother was asked to report all amounts of foods consumed by the child during the preceding day (24 hours). The information regarding cooking recipes and amounts consumed at every meal and between meals were recorded in precoded forms, and estimates of nutrients consumed were obtained by using the food composition tables developed for Central America. Two variables have been selected for the present study: energy and protein intake.

SAMPLE UTILIZED

The study began in 1969, but the morbidity methodology was not implemented in its final form until July 1970. The data for this study were collected between July 1970 and February 1977, when the study ended. Data subsets were used to address the issues of this paper, as detailed below.

Study of Effects on Appetite. Cases were identified that had both morbidity and dietary data for the same 24-hour period.* A total of 3,439 such "days" were identified. A total of 477 children were involved in this substudy, and each child was represented by an average of 7.2 observations. The prevalence of illness on the selected 3439 days did not differ significantly from that observed in the total sample.

COMPARISON OF EFFECTS OF SUPPLEMENT AND MORBIDITY ON GROWTH

Previous papers have dealt with the effects of the food supplementation program[3,4] and with the effects of the morbidity variables on growth.[5] These studies were carried out at different times in the life of the project and involved different samples. Ideally, a comparison of supplement and morbidity effects should be based on results from the same sample. Hence, for this study all available longitudinal data on morbidity, supplement, and growth rates available from 12 to 36 months of age were selected. This is a time when morbidity rates, particularly diarrheal diseases, are high and when the effects of both the supplement and the morbidity variable are marked.

RESULTS

EFFECTS ON APPETITE

The dietary intakes of children who were healthy were consistently greater than those of children who were sick. Figure 1 shows the percent reduction in calorie intake associated with having any of the selected common (SC) symptoms. Each bar represents a separate age group, starting at 15 months on the left and ending at 60 months on the right. The reduction in energy intakes as a percent of intakes in healthy children ranged from 12 to 28%. The average reduction across all ages was 19%.

---

*Because intake of the high-protein, high-calorie supplement (Atole) was substantial relative to home diets,[3] only data from the communities receiving the low-calorie supplement (Fresco) were used to test the hypothesis that illnesses reduce home dietary intakes. Interference from the food supplementation program was minimal because the average energy intake from the low-calorie drink was 28 kcal/day from 15 to 36 months of age and 63 kcal/day from 36 to 60 months of age. Moreover, home diet calories and supplement calories were unrelated.[3]

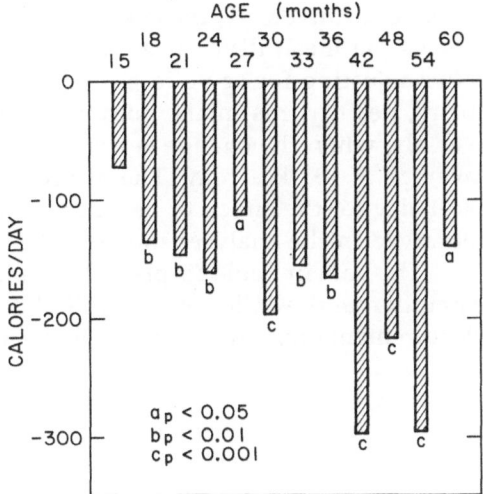

Figure 1. Caloric reduction associated with being sick (selected common symptoms).

The average reduction associated with SC symptoms is equivalent to 175 calories and 4.8 g of protein, as shown in Table I. Respiratory illnesses had the least effect of all variables: 67 calories and 1 g of protein. Diarrhea was associated with a reduction of 160 calories and 3 g of protein. Apathy had slightly higher effects: 175 calories and 5 g of protein.

It could be argued that the healthy children in Table I ate more because they came from different homes and not because they were healthy. To test this hypothesis, children with dietary data on two separate occasions were identified and two groups were selected for analyses: those who were sick with SC symptoms at first but were healthy

Table I. Average Reduction in Intake Associated with the Presence of Specific Symptoms[a]

Symptom	Energy (kcal/day) average		Protein (g/day) average	
	effect	p	effect	p
SC	−175	< .001	−4.8	< .001
Respiratory illness	−67	< .001	−1.0	.007
Diarrhea	−160	< .001	−3.0	< .001
Apathy	−175	< .001	−5.1	< .001

[a]Significance testing refers to an analysis of variance where the independent variables were age (11 groups) and presence or absence of the symptom. The dependent variable was either energy or protein. Degrees of freedom were 1/3438. The findings remained unchanged when dummy variables for either sex or village were added as independent variables.

later, and conversely, those who were well at first but sick later. Table II shows the mean differences, always the later minus the earlier period, after adjusting for age effects. When a child changes from being sick to being healthy, his intake goes up by an average of 139 kcal/day. Conversely, when the change is from healthy to sick, his intake drops by an average of 131 kcal/day. These results give a combined estimate of 124 kcal/day for the effects of being sick, a figure one-third smaller than that observed in the analyses shown in Figure 1 and Table I.

The data in Table III place the findings in perspective. Average consumption of the children studied fell below the 1973 FAO/WHO[8] energy requirements for their age and body weight by about 225 calories. The

Table II. Differences in Energy Intakes after Adjusting for Age Effects, Associated with Changes in Health (SC Symptoms in the Same Child)

	Age-adjusted changes[a]					
	Sick to well		Well to sick		Combined estimate $\Delta_2 - \Delta_1$	Average estimate (Figure 1)
Period Later–earlier (months)	N_1	Δ_1	N_2	Δ_2	$\dfrac{\Delta_2 - \Delta_1}{2}$	
18–15	40	87	34	−98	−93	−104
21–18	41	102	39	−164	−133	−141
24–21	44	93	25	−169	−131	−153
30–24	26	44	34	−205	−125	−179
36–30	47	116	27	−102	−109	−181
42–36	37	59	30	−241	−150	−231
42–48	27	313	25	−279	−296	−257
60–48	19	299	15	211	44	−178
Unweighted mean		139		−131	−124	−178

[a]Adjustments for age effects were made as follows. First, the increment observed in healthy children from one age to another was obtained from the data used in Figure 1. This number was then subtracted from the mean age change observed for both "sick to well" and "well to sick" children to obtain Δ. The sample size is denoted by N.

Table III. Significance of Findings

Energy gap in Guatemalan children	225 kcal/day
Average effect of SC symptoms	175 kcal/day
Average prevalence of SC symptoms	23%
Mean population effect	$-175 \times 0.23 = -40$ kcal/day
Percent of energy gap	$-40/-225 = 18\%$

average effects associated with the SC symptoms, −175 calories (Table I), are thus large relative to the energy gap and should have major biological significance for children who are frequently ill. The mean effect on the population as a whole, however, is dependent upon the percentage of children who are sick. In the population studied, 23% of the children were sick every day with one or more of the items included as SC symptoms. Therefore, the population mean effect is 40 calories per day (0.23 × −175), and illnesses called SC symptoms can be said to account for 18% (40/225) of the dietary energy deficiency.

MORBIDITY VARIABLES, SUPPLEMENT, AND GROWTH

The data in Table IV show the relationship between illness variables and weight gain for four different 6-month periods. Three types of values are shown: slopes, prevalences, and effects, the latter being the product of slopes times prevalences. The relationship between respiratory infections and growth rates in weight are not statistically significant. All analyses involving diarrheal diseases, apathy, and selected common symptoms are negative, and 11 out of 12 are statistically significant ($p <$ .05). The slope of the relationship between diarrhea and weight gain is larger than that for other symptoms (i.e., −3.5 g/day for diarrhea and −2.3 g/day for apathy and SC symptoms) but, because apathy and selected common symptoms have greater prevalences, their effects are greater than those of diarrheal diseases. Though the slopes in Table IV are small, it should be pointed out that at these ages children are only growing at the rate of about 6 g per day. It is likely that on days when children are sick, not only will growth cease but there might be weight loss in lean body mass and fat as well. Some catch-up growth during convalescence would be expected. As growth in this study was measured at 6-month intervals, the slopes shown in Table IV represent not what occurred on the actual days ill (i.e., instantaneous effect) but the residual, lasting impact of illnesses (i.e., permanent effect).

The effect of 100 daily calories from the supplements on 6-month weight gains is shown in the last column of Table IV. The relationship between supplement calories and weight gains are positive in all instances and statistically significant in all but one.* If home dietary intakes are not reduced appreciably, it would appear that most of the calories provided to these children went into physical activity and not growth.

---

*The strength and consistency of associations among supplement calories, morbidity variables, and growth rates have withstood rigorous testing in analyses that have taken into account a considerable number of confounding variables.[3−5]

Table IV. Effect of Morbidity Variables and of 100 kcal of Supplement on Growth Rates in Weight during 6-Month Periods[c]

Period	Sample size	Respiratory infections			Diarrhea			Apathy			Selected common symptoms			Effect of 100 daily supplement calories on 6-month weight gains E_c
		b_r	P_r	E_r	b_d	P_d	E_d	b_a	P_a	E_a	b_s	P_s	E_s	
12–18	308	0.5	73.0	37	−2.8[a]	23.1	−65	−3.3[b]	49.3	−163	−3.8[b]	36.9	−140	67[b]
18–24	366	1.0	70.7	71	−5.6[b]	14.4	−81	−2.3[b]	42.0	−97	−1.8[a]	33.3	−60	100[b]
24–30	391	0.1	76.1	8	−1.4	9.2	−13	−1.7[a]	30.9	−53	−2.1[a]	24.0	−50	43
30–36	447	−0.1	52.5	−5	−4.3[a]	6.5	−28	−1.7[a]	33.5	−57	−1.7[a]	32.6	−55	51[a]

[a] $p < 0.05$.
[b] $p < 0.01$.
[c] b (slope) = g of 6-month weight gain/day ill; P (prevalence) = days ill in 6-month period; E (effect) = b × P (g of 6-month weight gain).

Table V. Supplement Calorie Equivalent (kcal/day) of
Morbidity Effect[a]

Period (months)	Diarrhea	Apathy	Selected common symptoms
12–18	−97	−249	−209
18–24	−81	− 97	−60
24–30	−30	−123	−116
30–36	−55	−112	−108
Average value	−66	−145	−123

[a]The morbidity equivalent is calculated for each specific period and growth variable as $E_i/E_c \times 100$, where E_i is the morbidity effect and E_c the effect of 100 kcal of supplement (Table IV).

The supplement calorie equivalent of the effect of morbidity variables can now be estimated, as shown in Table V. The effect associated with each illness variable (E_i) was divided by the effect associated with 100 kcal/day from the supplements (E_c) and multiplied by 100. The results indicate that diarrheal diseases are equivalent to −66 supplement calories in terms of their effects on growth rates. That is, providing 66 kcal per day of the supplement would cause the same effect on growth rates as eliminating all diarrheal diseases. Apathy, and selected common symptoms, because of greater prevalences, have larger calorie equivalents, −145 and −123, respectively.

DISCUSSION

INFECTION AND FOOD INTAKES

Other authors also find that common illnesses have important effects on dietary intakes. Mata and co-workers[9] postulate that infections account for most of the energy deficits observed in children from developing countires. The results presented here do not seem to confirm this hypothesis in that common illnesses account for only 18% of the energy deficits in Guatemalan children.

There are reasons to suspect, however, that these effects are underestimates. Many infectious episodes are asymptomatic and many children reported as healthy may in reality be sick or in the convalescent phase. Many of the symptoms reported in the study communities were not included in the analyses. Also, the methodology used is known to underestimate the prevalence of symptoms, because mothers often fail to report them, either because they were not aware of the problem, or because they simply forgot about them.[5,6]

In fact, other authors find greater effects of diarrhea on dietary intakes. Hoyle, et al.[10] found that total calorie intakes in children with diarrhea were 40% lower than in healthy children. Molla and co-workers (chapter 7, this volume) report that diarrheal diseases reduce food intake by 30%. Combining all studies, diarrheal diseases, on average, lower food intakes by 20 to 40%. The mean effect on the population, as shown earlier in Table III, will depend upon the prevalence of illnesses. In this study, common illnesses reduced intakes by 40 kcal/day, which represents 18% of the energy deficit.

EFFECTS OF MORBIDITY ON GROWTH RATES

The results of studies of illness and physical growth are summarized in Table VI[11-18] for developed countries and in Table VII[19-29] for developing countries. The separation according to country of origin reveals contrasting results. While most of the studies from developed nations report no associations between illness and physical growth, those from developing nations report that common childhood ailments, in particular diarrheal diseases, are clearly associated with poor physical growth.

Differences in methodology may explain the results. The measurement of illness was more direct in developing countries, and greater reliance on the studies done in wealthier nations on school records and on lengthy recall interviews with parents may have obscured existing associations. However, it may be that the findings reflect contrasting ecological settings. The disease load experienced by children in developed countries is light in comparison to that of malnourished populations. Another obvious difference is the superior nutritional status of children from developed nations. Perhaps no associations were evident in the latter countries because such children, with ample nutritional resources, quickly made up the losses that the infrequent episodes of illness may have caused.

The magnitude of the impact of illness on physical growth can be estimated from the studies carried out in four rural Guatemalan villages.[3,26] Children who were relatively free from diarrhea from birth to 7 years of age grew significantly better than children not so fortunate. The differences in growth at 7 years of age between both groups were 3.5 cm in height and 1.5 kg in weight. These differences are of some magnitude if we consider that 7-year-old children from such communities differ from well-nourished children from the United States by about 13 cm in height and 5 kg in weight.

Table VI.   Illness and Physical Growth Indicators of Nutritional Status: Developed
Nations

Source	Illness variables	Growth variables	Conclusions
Evans[11]: 93 2.5- to 5-year-old children of high socioeconomic status (US)	Days absent from school; children were divided into 5 groups according to severity of illnesses	6-month increments in various measurements, including height and weight	The growth of all five groups was similar
Hardy[12]: 415 school children of all socioeconomic classes (US)	Incidence of ordinary diseases of childhood exclusive of minor colds and rickets as determined from a single interview of mothers (for history before age 8), and from yearly interviews of mothers and school records for absences due to illnesses (for history after age 8)	Annual growth rates in height from 8 to 12 years; various measurements of body size throughout childhood, middle childhood, and adulthood	No association was found between growth and disease; children in extreme categories of illness did not differ in terms of growth even when they were matched for national and social origins
Hewitt et al.[13]: 650 children followed from 2 to 5 years of age (UK)	Annual sickness records; the sample was divided into five diagnostic groups and into 3 categories according to severity of illness	Yearly height increments	The growth of all diagnostic groups was similar; however, the "severe" disease group grew less in height
Kubát et al.[14]: 333 middle-class children followed from birth to 6 years of age (Czechoslovakia)	The sample was divided into high and low groups according to disease-incidence data obtained from pediatric records	Height and weight at 6 years of age as well as increments from birth to 6 years of age	In all comparisons, the growth of frequently ill children was greater than that of the infrequently ill group. Only in the case of girls and with height increments did this reach statistical significance

Table VI. (*continued*)

Source[a]	Illness variables	Growth variables	Conclusions
Martens and Meredith[15]: 90 5- to 6-year-old children of high socioeconomic status	Days absent from school on account of illness	6-month increments and attained size of various measurements including height and weight	No association between absence from school on account of illness and physical growth
Meredith and Knott[16]: 35 elementary school children followed from 5 to 10 years of age (US)	Interviews of parents every 6 months; healthiest 20% compared to least healthy 20%; breakdown based on number of illnesses, severity, and duration	Various measurements of body size at 5 years; growth increments in height, weight, as well as in other measurements over a 5-year period	The growth of both groups was similar
Palmer[17]: 4,000 school children (US)	Days absent from school on account of illness	Attained height and weight	No associations were found
Turner et al.[18]: 120 school children 6 to 14 years of age (US)	School records and yearly recall interviews of parents and children by health center	60 children with poor weight gains were compared to 60 randomly chosen children of the same age and sex with above-average weight gains	Poor growers experienced more communicable, respiratory, and noncommunicable illnesses
Valvadian, Reed, Stuart, Burke, Pyle, and Cornoni: "Interrelationships between protein intake, illness, and growth as manifested by children from birth to 18 years." Unpublished manuscript (US)	Interviews at 3, 6, 9, and 12 months of age, every 6 months thereafter until 10 years, and every year from 10 to 18 years; complex score system used as the morbidity variable	Height and weight at various ages from birth to 17 years of age	The high-illness groups had the greater proportion of larger children at maturity; greater illness was associated with rapid growth in preschool children and to some extent also in adolescence

Table VII. Illness and Physical Growth Indicators of Nutritional Status: Developing Nations. All Samples Are from Rural Areas

Source[a]	Illness variables	Growth variables	Conclusions
Cole and Parkin[19]: 45 children followed from birth to 3 years of age (Uganda)	The children were examined routinely once a month and whenever they attended the clinic on account of illness; incidence per month was recorded for various symptoms	Monthly weight gains	The incidence of diarrhea, fever, and measles was significantly related to monthly weight gains; other illnesses, including respiratory infections, were not related to weight gains
London-Paoloni *et al.*[20]: 276 children studied from birth to 3 years of age (Mexico)	Illness histories collected every 2 weeks; the highest and lowest quartiles were identified for each of 3 variables: % of time ill with diarrhea, % with upper respiratory infections, and % with lower respiratory infections	Yearly increments in height and weight	Diarrheal diseases were significantly related to height but not to weight increments; respiratory infections were not related to growth in height or weight
Draper and Draper[21]: 88 infants (Tanzania)	Weekly clinic of irregular daily attendance	Two groups: 37 who lost more than 1 pound in a month and 51 who lost only 0.5 to 1 pound in a month	The group who lost more weight had more diarrhea but less respiratory infection and fever
Guzmán et al.[22]: Indian children studied from birth to 2 years of age (Guatemala)	Illness histories collected every 2 weeks; information obtained about diarrhea, respiratory problems, and all other causes of disease	Growth rates in height and weight	No association between terciles of growth and frequency or extent of illness; No significant relationship between days of illness and growth
Mata et al.[23]: 43 Indian children followed from 0.5 to 3 years (Guatemala)	Weekly interviews with mothers; incidence of various illnesses was recorded	Weight increments over a 2½-year period	There was no association between number of illnesses and growth rates in weight; the 10 best growers had significantly more dysentery but not more overall diarrhea than the 10 worst growers
Mata et al.[24]: 45 Indian children followed from birth to 6 months of age (Guatemala)	Weekly laboratory cultures; the sample was divided into high and low groups according to their enterovirus attack rates	Height and weight at 6 months of age	At 6 months, high and low groups were similar in height, but different in weight by 140 g (low group heavier)

Table VII. (*continued*)

Source[a]	Illness variables	Growth variables	Conclusions
Mardsen[25]: 95 children followed from birth to 18 months (The Gambia)	Regular weekly and daily clinic; more reliance on examination than on interview with mother	Faltering in weight (a gain of less than ½ pound in 3 months	63% of attacks of diarrhea and 14% of lower respiratory infections associated with weight faltering
Martorell et al.[5,26]: 716 Ladino children under 7 years old studied for 23 months (Guatemala)	Illness histories collected every 2 weeks; Data were expressed as % of time ill per semester per year	Semester and yearly increments in height and weight	Diarrheal diseases were related to weight and height gains; this finding was independent of potentially confounding factors; no relationship with fever and respiratory illness
Morley et al.[27]: 232 children (Nigeria)	Clinical diagnosis of whooping cough from an "under 5" clinic and hospital admissions	Weight gains	Whooping cough resulted in weight loss; nearly 20% lost between 5 to 10% of their weight, while 26% took more than 2, and 15% more than 3 months to recover their weight
Morley et al.[28]: 104 children studied from birth to 12 months (Nigeria)	Regular monthly clinic and "under 5," irregular attendance clinic	Two groups: 52 children had weights below the 10th percentile at 6, 9, or 12 mos. (Group A), and 52 children were always above the 50th percentile (Group B)	From 0 to 6 incidence of diarrhea was greater in Group A; From 6 to 12, whooping cough and measles greater in Group A; no difference in respiratory infections
Rowland et al.[29]: 152 children 0.6 to 3 years old, studied for 19 months (The Gambia)	The children were examined approximately once a month and whenever they attended the clinic because of illness; data were expressed as % of time ill with each of 9 disease categories	Weight and height gains per month	Diarrhea was negatively related to growth in height and weight. Malaria was related to growth in weight but not in height. All other symptoms, including fever and respiratory infections, were not.

[a]The Guatemalan samples studied by Guzmán et al.,[22] Mata et al.,[23,24] and Martorell et al.[5,26] were independent studies carried out in separate communities.

In conclusion, the common childhood illnesses in developing nations, in particular those syndromes that involve diarrheal symptoms, have a negative impact on nutritional status. The vulnerability of malnourished children to infection is best illustrated by the fact that immunizations with live agents (BCG, smallpox, polio, DPT + polio), which are innocuous experiences for most well-nourished children, can lead to substantial weight loss, particularly in children less than 6 months of age, or with a poor initial status.[30]

SUMMARY

Public health officials concerned with problems of malnutrition can implement programs oriented to increasing food intake, decreasing the prevalence of infections, or both. In choosing among alternatives, the literature offers little guidance. In this paper, a simple analysis is proposed that would allow comparisons of various types of interventions. The only requirement is that the effects of the diverse interventions be expressed in terms of common units. In this paper, the effects of a calorie supplementation and of a number of morbidity variables were expressed in terms of common units, i.e., grams of weight gain. It was found that providing 66 kcal/day of the supplement was similar, in order of magnitude, to eliminating all diarrheal diseases in children from 12 to 36 months of age. Eliminating two other variables, apathy and selected common symptoms, was equivalent to providing 145 and 123 kcal/day, respectively. The numbers can be taken as rough and preliminary estimates of the total energy cost of common morbidity problems.

There is no question that infectious diseases, and in particular diarrheal diseases, are a major cause of poor dietary intakes, and through this and other mechanisms, of malnutrition.

REFERENCES

1. División de Desarrollo Humano. Nutrición, crecimiento y desarrollo. *Bol. Of. Sanit. Panam.* **78**:38–51, 1975.
2. Lechtig, A., Habicht, J-P., Delgado, H., Klein, R. E., Yarbrough, C., and Martorell, R. Effect of food supplementation during pregnancy on birth weight. *Pediatrics* **56**:508–520, 1975.
3. Martorell, R., Klein, R. E., and Delgado, H. Improved nutrition and its effects on anthropometric indicators of nutritional status. *Nutr. Rep. Int.* **21**:219–230, 1980.
4. Martorell, R., and Klein, R. E. Food supplementation and growth rates in preschool children. *Nutr. Rep. Int.* **21**:447–454, 1980.

5. Martorell, R., Habicht, J-P., Yarbrough, C., Lechtig, A., Klein, R. E., and Western, K. A. Acute morbidity and physical growth in rural Guatemalan children. *Am. J. Dis. Child.* **129**:1296-3101, 1975.

6. Martorell, R., Habicht, J-P., Yarbrough, C., Lechtig, A., and Klein, R. E. Underreporting in fortnightly recall morbidity surveys. *J. Trop. Pediatr.* **22**:129-134, 1976.

7. Martorell, R., Yarbough, C., Yarborough, S., and Klein, R. E. The impact of ordinary illnesses on the dietary intakes of malnourished children. *Am. J. Clin. Nutr.* **33**:345-350, 1980.

8. *Energy and Protein Requirements,* Report of a joint FAO/WHO ad hoc expert committee, WHO Technical Report Series No. 522. World Health Organization, Geneva, Switzerland, 1973.

9. Mata, L. J., Kromal, R. A., Urrutia, J. J., and Garcia, B. Effect of infection on food intake and the nutritional state: Perspectives as viewed from the village. *Am. J. Clin. Nutr.* **30**:1215-1227, 1977.

10. Hoyle, B., Yunus, M., and Chen, L. C. Breast feeding and food intake among children with acute diarrheal disease. *Am. J. Clin. Nutr.* **33**:2365-2371, 1980.

11. Evans, M. E. Illness history and physical growth. II. A comparative study of the rate of growth of preschool children of five health classes. *Am. J. Dis. Child.* **68**:390-394, 1944.

12. Hardy, M. C. Frequent illness in childhood, physical growth and final size. *Am. J. Phys. Anthropol.* **23**:241-246, 1938.

13. Hewitt, D., Westropp, D. K., and Acheson, R. M. Oxford child health survey: Effect of childish ailments on skeletal development. *Br. J. Prev. Soc. Med.* **9**:179-186, 1955.

14. Kubát, K., Kourim, J., Nováhová, M., Moderová, M., and Stloukalová, M. The relation of acute morbidity in preschool age to the weight and height in six years old children. *Cesk. Pediatr.* **26**:105-106, 1971.

15. Martens, E. J., and Meredith, H. V. Illness history and physical growth. I. Correlation in junior primary children followed from fall to spring. *Am. J. Dis. Child.* **64**:618-630, 1942.

16. Meredith, H. V., and Knott, V. B. Illness history and physical growth. III. Comparative anatomic status and rate of change for schoolchildren in different long-term health categories. *Am. J. Dis. Child.* **103**:146-151, 1962.

17. Palmer, C. E. The relation of body build to sickness in elementary school children. *Am. J. Phys. Anthropol.* **21 (Suppl)**:7-8, 1936.

18. Turner, C. E., Longee, W. W., Saravia, K., and Fuller, R. P. Rate of growth as a health index. *Res. Q.* **6**:29-40, 1935.

19. Cole, T. J., and Parkin, J. M. Infection and its effect on the growth of young children: A comparison of The Gambia and Uganda. *Trans. Roy. Soc. Trop. Med. Hyg.* **71**:196-198, 1977.

20. Condon-Paoloni, D., Cravioto, J., Johnston, F. E., de Licardie, E. R., and Scholl, T. O. Morbidity and growth of infants and young children in a rural Mexican village. *Am. J. Public Health* **67**:651-656, 1977.

21. Draper, K. C., and Draper, C. C. Observations on the growth of African infants: With special reference to the effects of malaria control. *J. Trop. Med. Hyg.* **63**:165-171, 1960.

22. Guzmán, M. A., Scrimshaw, N. S., Bruch, H. A., and Gordon, J. E. Nutrition and infection field study in Guatemalan villages, 1959-1964. VII. Physical growth and development of preschool children. *Arch. Environ. Health* **17**:107-118, 1968.

23. Mata, L. J., Urrutia, J. J., and Lechtig, A. Infection and nutrition of children of a low socioeconomic rural community. *Am. J. Clin. Nutr.* **24**:249-259, 1971.

24. Mata, L. J., Urrutia, J. J., Albertazzi, C., Pellecer, O., and Arellano, E. Influence of

recurrent infections on nutrition and growth of children in Guatemala. *Am. J. Clin. Nutr.* **25**:1267–1275, 1972.

25. Mardsen, P. D. The Sukuta project. A longitudinal study of health in Gambian children from birth to 18 months of age. *Trans. Roy. Soc. Trop. Med. Hyg.* **58**:455–489, 1964.
26. Martorell, R., Yarbrough, C., Lechtig, A., Habicht, J-P., and Klein, R. E. Diarrheal diseases and growth retardation in preschool Guatemalan children. *Am. J. Phys. Anthropol.* **43**:341–346, 1975.
27. Morley, D., Woodland, M., and Martin, W. J. Whooping cough in Nigerian children. *Trop. Geogr. Med.* **18**:169–182, 1966.
28. Morley, D., Bicknell, J., and Woodland, M. Factors influencing the growth and nutritional status of infants and young children in a Nigerian village. *Trans. Roy. Soc. Trop. Med. Hyg.* **62**:164–195, 1968.
29. Rowland, M. G. M., Cole, T. J., and Whitehead, R. G. A Quantitative study into the role of infection in determining nutritional status in Gambian village children. *Br. J. Nutr.* **37**:441–450, 1977.
30. Kielmann, A. A. Weight fluctuations after immunization in a rural preschool child community. *Am. J. Clin. Nutr.* **30**:592–598, 1977.

9

Effects of Acute Diarrhea on Absorption of Macronutrients During Disease and After Recovery

Ayesha Molla, A. M. Molla, S. A. Sarker, M. Khatoon, and M. Mujibur Rahaman

Introduction

Nutritional consequences of diarrhea are thought to be due to several factors: (a) decreased intake of food resulting from loss of appetite or withholding of food as practiced in communities as a measure to control diarrhea, (b) loss of major nutrients as well as vitamins and minerals in the feces because of rapid transit or malabsorption, and (c) increased catabolism in response to infection.

The main purpose of this presentation is to report our current research on absorption of macronutrients during and after acute diarrheal attacks. To cite some information from previous work, we will summarize the results reported earlier on loss of enzymatic activity in the gut secondary to cholera[1,2] and then review the work of Chung and Chung and Viščorová[3,4] on net absorption of nutrients and the effect of oral feeding and starvation during pediatric diarrhea.

Two kinds of mucosal enzymes, namely, adenosine triphosphatase and disaccharidase, in acute cholera and other diarrheal diseases were studied by Hirschhorn and co-workers.[1,2] Sodium-potassium-stimulated

Ayesha Molla, A. M. Molla, S. A. Sarker, M. Khatoon, and M. Mujibur Rahaman • International Centre for Diarrhoeal Disease Research, Dacca, Bangladesh. This study was partially funded by a United Nations University research grant.

adenosine triphosphatase (Na-K-ATPase), an enzyme implicated in active sodium transport, was demonstrated in homogenates of human jejunal and ileal mucosa. They found that in cholera, acute nonspecific gastroenteritis, and bacterial enteritis there was a significant loss of Na-K-ATPase activity during the acute phase of the disease compared to the convalescent period. Loss of Na-K-ATPase in cholera and other enteric diseases probably contributes to a worsening of, if not the initiation of, intestinal fluid loss.

The significance of depressed Na-K-ATPase in acute diarrhea is uncertain. Diarrhea, however, may directly influence membrane enzyme activity, possibly contributing to the loss of absorptive capacity in the gut. Sucrase, maltase, and palatinase activities were low during the acute disease in the studies of Hirschhorn et al., and lactase activity was low during both the acute and convalescent periods compared to that in healthy North Americans. Enzymatic activities were estimated in serial jejunal and ileal biopsies on patients. The authors concluded that diarrhea probably was responsible for the changes in enzymatic activity. However, the significance of the loss of disaccharidase activities is not clearly understood. Further research is necessary to correlate these findings with studies related to nutrient malabsorption in acute diarrhea.

Net absorption of nutrients in acute diarrhea was first studied by Chung and Chung and Viščorová in 1948.[3,4] The important results are summarized in Tables I and II. Table I presents the data obtained from a study on four infants who were fed three diets successively: low-, medium-, and high-calorie in the first, second, and third 24-hour periods, respectively. The results showed that the absorption of nitrogen and fat was approximately proportional to the amount of intake. Table II presents results obtained from a study on two infants treated first with a high-calorie diet and then with complete starvation (maintaining electrolyte balance with continuous I.V. drip). Results showed that in acute

Table I. Percentage of Absorption of Nitrogen and Fat at Different Levels of Calorie Intake during Acute Diarrhea[a]

Case No.	Low (30–45)		Moderate (60–69)		High (100–137)	
	N$_2$	Fat	N$_2$	Fat	N$_2$	Fat
12	40	72	50	67	63	60
26	27	48	40	39	74	59
22	38	−27	—	—	60	30
23	—	—	63	70	60	49

[a]Source: reference 3.

Table II. Percentage of Absorption of Nitrogen and Fat
during a Period of High Calorie Intake and of Starvation in
Acute Diarrhea[a]

| Case No. | High (100–106) | | Starvation | |
	N_2	Fat	N_2	Fat
27	75	68	−0.30	−2.22
28	65	46	−0.15	−0.51

[a]Source: reference 4.

diarrhea, a substantial absorption of nitrogen and fat did occur if food was ingested, while no positive absorption occurred during the period of starvation. In a separate report, Chung and Viščorová[4] studied 153 patients with diarrhea, 50 treated by starvation and 53 by feeding. They observed that duration of diarrhea was comparatively longer in the starved group, though the statistical difference between the starved and the fed group was not significant. The observations are listed in Table III.

Since the work of Chung and Viščorová, no attempt has been made to demonstrate the importance of continuing feeding during acute diarrhea. Cholera, rotavirus, *Shigella,* and enterotoxigenic *Escherichia coli* (ETEC) are the major causes of diarrheal illness among the under-5 population in most developing countries.[5,6] Rotavirus continues to be one of the important causative organisms responsible for childhood diarrhea even in developed countries.[7] The aim of the present study was to determine the effect of diarrhea caused by rotavirus, *Shigella,* and ETEC on net absorption of fat, calories, nitrogen, and carbohydrate during acute diarrhea, and 2 weeks after discharge. The absorption study was repeated 8 weeks after discharge to see if there was any difference in the absorption of nutrients between the two periods of recovery. The absorption data

Table III. Mean Observations on 50 Patients with Diarrhea
Treated by Starvation and 53 Treated by Feeding[a]

Observations	Starvation	Feeding
Age (months)	7.9	7.3
Initial weight (kg)	5.97	5.56
Weight gain at discharge	Lesser gain	Greater gain
Duration of diarrhea (days)	7.8	6.1

[a]Source: reference 4.

obtained from the above study were analyzed to determine whether the absorption pattern varied in patients with diarrhea caused by rotavirus, *Shigella*, and ETEC.

However, before going into detail about the Dacca study, we would like to point out the important differences between the studies of Chung and Viščorová and the present research (Table IV). In the current research, specific etiologic agents were identified and their relation to nutrient absorption was studied. Previous work dealt only with nonspecific diarrheas.

PATIENTS AND METHODS

Twenty-nine male children under 5 years of age with a history of acute, watery diarrhea and moderate to severe dehydration were selected at random for study. Patients with any obvious complication were excluded from the study. Informed consent was obtained from the parents or guardians of the patients. Out of a total of 29 patients, 13 had rotavirus infection diagnosed by the enzyme-linked immunosorbent assay (ELISA),[8] and 10 had *E. coli;* the colonies were tested for toxigenicity by infant mouse assay for heat-stable toxin (ST) and adrenal cell assay[9] for heat-labile toxin (LT), and 6 had *Shigella*, isolated by standard methods.[10] The patients were rehydrated intravenously with the Dacca solution* and maintained on it for 18 to 24 hours. After an overnight fast, the patients were fed 5 grams of D-xylose in 100 ml of water. One hour

Table IV.   Differences between the Study of Chung and the Present Research[a]

Chung	Molla *et al.*
Subjects: infants, age 12 to 70 days	Subjects: children, age 1 to 4 years
Sample size: 6	Sample size: 29
Causative organisms: not isolated	Causative organisms: isolated from the stool
A liquid formula diet commonly employed for this age group was used	Familiar semisolid and solid diet was used
Three different calorie levels of formula fed: low, medium, or full	No restriction applied
Study period: 24 hours' duration, with each formula level	Study period: 72 hours' duration using same foods

[a]Source: reference 3.

*Composition: Na$^+$ 133 mmol/L; K$^+$ = 13 mmol/L; Cl = 99 mmol/L; and HCO$^-$3 (as acetate) = 48 mmol/L.

after ingestion, 1 ml of venous blood was drawn for the estimation of xylose.

Charcoal tablets were fed as markers for collection of stool. The time taken by the charcoal to makes its appearance in the stool was considered the transit time. Four meals were offered daily *ad libitum* to each patient at regular intervals during the study period. Two types of diets were used in this study. A semisolid cooked meal containing rice, chicken, lentils, and oil was offered to the patients for lunch and supper. Another cooked meal, consisting of a mixture of rice, egg, milk, butter, and sugar was given to the patients for breakfast. Banana, cow's milk, and bread were given to them at specified intervals during the period of the study. Each item of food was weighed before being offered to the patients, and any left over was weighed again to quantify the actual amount of intake.

Test weighing was done before and after each breast-feeding to measure the amount of milk consumed. Samples of all types of food consumed were saved for analysis of fat, nitrogen, and calories. Breast milk was collected from the mothers and analyzed for calories, fat, and nitrogen. Collection of stool was started after the first appearance of the marker and it was continued until the appearance of the second marker, fed at 72 hours. The stool samples collected between markers were pooled and homogenized in a blender. Aliquots from the stool specimens were saved for analysis of fat, nitrogen, and calories. Vomitus collected from the patients during the study was analyzed and subtracted. No antibiotics were administered during the study. Patients went home after diarrhea had stopped. All 29 patients were studied 2 weeks after discharge, and 18 were also studied 8 weeks after discharge (8 rotavirus, 6 ETEC, 4 Shigella). These two recovery stages will be termed, respectively, R_1 and R_2 in the text.

Serum xylose estimation was done by the method of Roe and Rice.[11] Fat estimation was done by the Van de Kamer procedure,[12] and total nitrogen content was measured according to the micro-Kjeldahl procedure.[13] Calorie estimation from all samples was performed by using an adiabatic bomb calorimeter, with benzoic acid as the standard.

Coefficients of absorption of nutrients both in the acute stage and at the recovery period was calculated using the following expression: (Intake − Output) × 100/Intake.

RESULTS

Clinical features of the study patients are presented in Table V. Rotavirus patients were comparatively younger than those with ETEC and

Table V.   Characteristics of the Study Patients (Mean $\pm$ 1 *SD*)

Particulars	Rotavirus		ETEC		Shigella	
N studied	13		10		6	
Age (months)	23	$\pm$ 14.2	36.3	$\pm$ 10.6	34.1	$\pm$ 8.8
Admission body weight (kg)	8.7	$\pm$ 1.8	9.2	$\pm$ 2	9.4	$\pm$ 1.7
Body weight at recovery 1	9.1	$\pm$ 1.9	9.8	$\pm$ 2	9.9	$\pm$ 2.2
Body weight at recovery 2[a]	10.2	$\pm$ 2.2	10.0	$\pm$ 1.8	10.9	$\pm$ 2.4
Serum hematocrit admission	31.2	$\pm$ 3.8	32.6	$\pm$ 2.5	33.3	$\pm$ 4.9
First 24-hour stool volume (liters)	0.70	$\pm$ 0.31	0.68	$\pm$ 0.55	0.93	$\pm$ 0.57

[a]The number of patients available for the study at stage 2 were 8, 6, and 4 for rotavirus, ETEC, and *Shigella*, respectively.

Shigella. Body weight increased from acute to recovery stages 1 and 2 in all groups. All of the patients were anemic.

The coefficient of absorption of nitrogen was compared in patients experiencing diarrhea of the three different etiologies (Table VI). During the acute stage, absorption of nitrogen was significantly less ($p < 0.01$) in rotavirus than in ETEC. At recovery stage 1, absorption of nitrogen did not differ significantly among the patients with the three different diarrheas. However, even after 8 weeks of recovery, absorption of nitrogen was comparatively less in the rotavirus group than in the others. Coefficients of absorption of fat, calories, and carbohydrates are shown in Tables VII, VIII, and IX, respectively. During the acute stage, absorption of fat and calories was significantly less ($p < 0.01$) in rotavirus patients compared to ETEC patients. There was no statistical difference in the absorption of both fat and calories between rotavirus and *Shigella* patients during the acute stage. In patients with diarrhea from any of the three etiologies, absorption of carbohydrate was least affected, even during

Table VI.   Coefficient of Absorption ($\pm$ 1 *SD*) of Nitrogen during Acute (A) Diarrhea and after Recovery Stages (R_1 and R_2)[a]

Etiology	Coefficient of absorption		
	A	R_1	R_2
Rotavirus (13)[b]	43.3 $\pm$ 22.3[A]	68.5 $\pm$ 13.0[B]	59.9 $\pm$ 28.2[C]
ETEC (10)	58.3 $\pm$ 13.9[D]	54.0 $\pm$ 33.3[E]	72.8 $\pm$ 9.3[F]
Shigella (6)	41.3 $\pm$ 45.6[G]	73.6 $\pm$ 4.8[H]	72.3 $\pm$ 9.7[I]

[a]Student's *t* test: A vs. D:significant.
[b]Figures in parentheses indicate number of patients.

Table VII. Coefficient of Absorption ($\pm$ 1 SD) of Fat during Acute (A) Diarrhea and after Recovery Stages (R_1, R_2)[a]

Etiology	Coefficient of absorption		
	A	R_1	R_2
Rotavirus (13)[b]	42.3 ± 27.6^A	79.0 ± 20.0^B	81.3 ± 10.1^C (8)
ETEC (10)	78 ± 14.2^D	80.4 ± 15.3^E	88.4 ± 8.3^F (6)
Shigella (6)	61.8 ± 34.8^G	88.8 ± 3.6^H	93.8 ± 2.1^I (4)

[a]Student's t test: A vs. D:S, C vs. I:S, F vs. I:S.
[b]Figures in parentheses indicate number of patients.
S = significant

Table VIII. Coefficient of Absorption ($\pm$ 1 SD) of Calories during Acute (A) Diarrhea and after Recovery Stages (R_1, R_2)[a]

Etiology	Coefficient of absorption		
	A	R_1	R_2
Rotavirus (13)[b]	55.4 ± 23.7^A	91.1 ± 4.6^B	81.2 ± 10.1^C (8)
ETEC (10)	86.7 ± 7.7^D	82.2 ± 10.9^E	88.7 ± 6.5^F (6)
Shigella (6)	68.1 ± 32.0^G	79.7 ± 13.9^H	90.4 ± 2.5^I (4)

[a]Student's t test: A vs. D:S, B vs. E:S, C vs. I:S.
[b]Figures in parentheses indicate number of patients.
S = significant

Table IX. Coefficient of Absorption ($\pm$ 1 SD) of Carbohydrate during Acute (A) Diarrhea and after Recovery Stages (R_1 and R_2)[a]

Etiology	Coefficient of absorption		
	A	R_1	R_2
Rotavirus (13)[b]	73.8 ± 26.0^A	88.8 ± 5.8^B	84.1 ± 11.6^C
ETEC (10)	91.7 ± 5.2^D	86.8 ± 9.8^E	91.0 ± 6.3^F
Shigella (6)	77.0 ± 31.7^G	78.3 ± 20.8^H	$91.6 \pm. 3.7^I$

[a]Student's t test: A vs. D:significant.
[b]Figures in parentheses indicate number of patients.

acute diarrhea (Table IX). In ETEC cases, absorption of all the nutrients was comparatively better in the acute stage compared to recovery stage 1. However, in recovery stage 2, absorption of nutrients in ETEC patients increased compared to absorption in stage 1.

Serum xylose levels were measured during the acute stage and after recovery (Table X). Patients absorbing less than 20 mg% of xylose were defined as xylose-malabsorbers. On average, 75% of patients were found to be xylose-malabsorbers in the acute stage, which fell to 10% at recovery stage 1. An attempt was made to see the relationship between xylose absorption and the absorption of nutrients during acute and recovery stages (R_1 and R_2) in diarrhea. Figure 1 shows that in rotavirus infection, when xylose absorption was poor, carbohydrate absorption was as high as 74%, even during acute diarrhea. However, results were not similar for the *Shigella* group. Results in Figure 2 indicate that in *Shigella*, though xylose absorption remained unaffected (39 mg%) in acute diarrhea, carbohydrate absorption (77%) was not significantly higher than in the rotavirus group (74%).

Stool weight was taken every 24 hours during the acute and early recovery stages. Table XI shows the mean percent change in stool weight in the first and second 24-hour period during acute diarrhea. A general tendency of gradually decreasing stool weight was noticed from the first to the second 24-hour period of acute diarrhea.

DISCUSSION

The results of the present research indicate several differences with regard to the absorption of nutrients during acute and recovery stages of diarrhea, depending on etiology.

Table X. Mean 1-Hour Serum Xylose Level ($\pm$ 1 *SD*) during Acute (A) and Recovery Stages (R_1,R_2) in Patients with Diarrhea of Different Etiologies

Etiology	Serum xylose level (mg%)		
	A	R_1	R_2
Rotavirus (13)[a]	13.9 $\pm$ 6	26.3 $\pm$ 7	33.7 $\pm$ 10
ETEC (10)	15.2 $\pm$ 6	26.7 $\pm$ 8	24.3 $\pm$ 5
Shigella (6)	38.6 $\pm$ 4	28.6 $\pm$ 5	32.1 $\pm$ 14

[a]Figures in parentheses indicate number of patients.

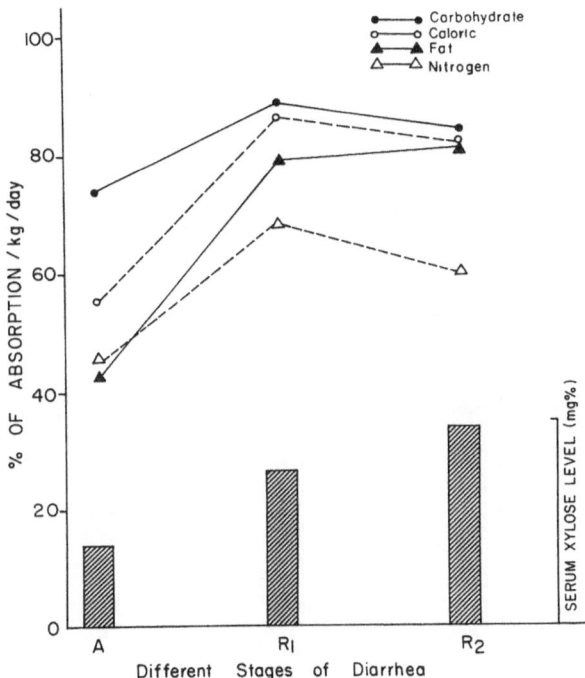

Figure 1. Relation Between Xylose Absorption and Percentage of Nutrient Absorption During Acute (A) and Recovery Stages (R₁ and R₂) of Diarrhea Caused by Rotavirus.

In the acute stage of rotavirus, absorption of all the nutrients was significantly lower compared to the absorption in patients with ETEC diarrhea. Absorption of nitrogen in rotavirus did not improve even after 8 weeks of recovery, suggesting a period of prolonged malabsorption. This observation might be explained by the fact that, in rotavirus infection, villous epithelial cells are specifically affected[14] and that the stool in rotavirus diarrhea contains a large amount of reducing substance compared to the stool in cholera.[15,16] However, in this study we observed that as much as 74% of ingested carbohydrate was absorbed in the acute stage of rotavirus infection compared to 92% absorption in ETEC and 77% in *Shigella* diarrheas.

During the acute stage of ETEC diarrhea, absorption of all nutrients was comparatively better than in diarrhea of other etiologies but failed to show improvement after 2 weeks of recovery. After 8 weeks of recovery, increased absorption of nutrients was clearly evident. The mechanism of mucosal damage by the ST toxin is not yet wholly understood.

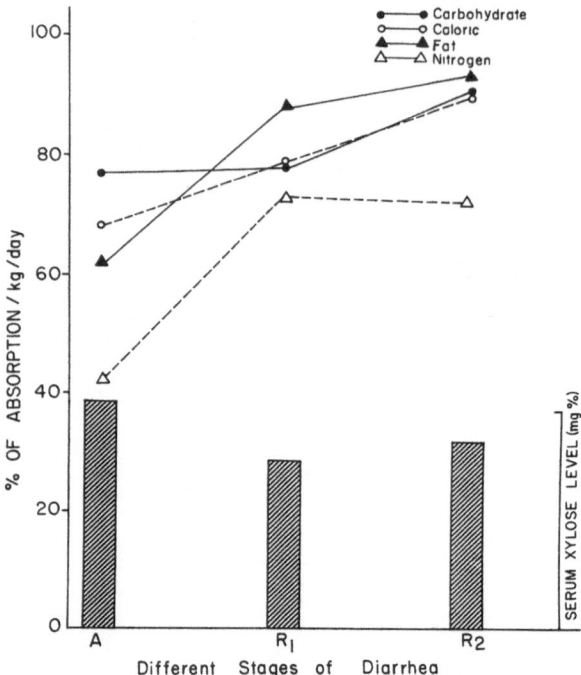

Figure 2. Relation Between Xylose Absorption and Percentage of Nutrient Absorption and Percentage of Nutrient Absorption During Acute (A) and Recovery Stages (R₁ and R₂) of Diarrhea Caused by *Shigella.*

Table XI.   Mean Percent Change (Decrease) in Stool Weight in First and Second 24-Hour Periods of Acute Diarrhea

		\% change in stool weight	
Etiology	N	First 24 hr.	Second 24 hr.
Rotavirus	13	19	26
ETEC	10	56	33
Shigella	6	47	69

In the present group of ETEC patients, we had four with pure ST, two with pure LT, and four with a mixture of ST and LT. The combined presence of ST and LT toxins on the epithelial cells might have adversely affected absorption of nutrients after 2 weeks of recovery, but it improved thereafter.

During the acute stage of *Shigella*-induced diarrhea, absorption of nitrogen was minimum (41%) compared to the absorption of other nutrients, which was in the range of 62 to 77%. *Shigella* is a disease of the lower bowel, and absorption of nitrogen may have been caused by direct loss of protein from the gut rather than failure of intestinal absorption. Absorption of all nutrients was significantly higher after 2 weeks of recovery.

Similarly, serum xylose level in the acute stage of rotavirus diarrhea and ETEC diarrhea was below 20 mg%, but in *Shigella* it was 37 mg%. In spite of the lower xylose level, absorption of carbohydrate was 74% in rotavirus and 92% in ETEC. During the acute stage of *Shigella* diarrhea it was 77%, though serum xylose level was much higher. This discrepancy between xylose and carbohydrate absorption indicates that xylose absorption is not a valid reflection of the absorption of a natural carbohydrate and other macronutrients.

Early feeding of those patients with diarrhea did not seem to increase stool volume. However, Chung and Chung and Viščorová[3,4] showed that in some of their patients, feeding during diarrhea was associated with increased stool volume, though absorption of nutrients was not affected.

Finally, the following conclusions can be derived from this study. Despite reduced absorption of nutrients, feeding of children should be encouraged because substantial absorption does take place even in acute diarrheal infection. This might help in the prevention of more seriously compromised nutritional status. This observation has profound practical implications, especially in developing countries where diarrhea is endemic.

References

1. Hirschhorn, N., and Rosenberg, I. H. Sodium-potassium stimulated adenosine triphosphatase of the small intestine of man: Studies in cholera and other diarrhea diseases. *J. Lab. Clin. Med.* **72**:28–39, 1968.
2. Hirschhorn, N., and Molla, A. Reversible jejunal disaccharidase deficiency in cholera and other acute diarrheal diseases. *Johns Hopkins Med. J.* **125**:291–300, 1969.
3. Chung, A. W. The effect of oral feeding at different levels on the absorption of foodstuffs in infantile diarrhea. *J. Pediatr.* **33**:1–13, 1948.

4. Chung, A. W., and Viščorova, B. The effect of early oral feeding versus early oral starvation on the course of infantile diarrhea. *J. Pediatr.* **33**:14–22, 1948.
5. Mosley, W. H., Bart, K. H., and Sommer, A. An epidemiological assessment of a cholera control programme in rural East Pakistan. *Int. J. Epidemiol.* **1**:5–11, 1972.
6. Black, R. E., Merson, M. H., Huq, I., Alim, A. R. M. A., and Yunus, M. Incidence and severity of rotavirus and *Escherichia coli* diarrhoea in rural Bangladesh. Implications of vaccine development. *Lancet* **i**:141–143, 1981.
7. Estes, M. K., and Graham, D. Y. Epidemic viral gastroenteritis. *Am. J. Med.* **66**:1001–1007, 1979.
8. Yolken, R. H., and Kim, H. W., Clem, T., Wyatt, R. G., Chanock, R. M., Kalica, A. R., and Kapikian, A. Z. Enzyme-linked immunosorbent assay (ELISA) for detection of human reovirus-like agent of infantile gastroenteritis. *Lancet* **ii**:263–266, 1977.
9. Merson, M. H., Sack, R. B., Kibriya, A. K. M. G., Al Mahmood, A., Ahmed, Q. S., and Huq, I. The use of colony pools for diagnosis of enterotoxigenic *Escherichia coli* diarrhea. *J. Clin. Microbiol.* **9**:493–497, 1979.
10. Edwards, P. R., and Ewin, W. H. *Identification of Enterobacteriaceae.* Burgess, Minneapolis, 1972.
11. Roe, J. H., and Rice, E. W. Photometric method for determination of free pentoses in animal tissues. *J. Biol. Chem.* **173**:507–512, 1948.
12. Van de Kamer, J. H., Ten Bokkel Huinink, H., and Weyers, H. A. Rapid method for determination of fat in feces. *J. Biol. Chem.* **177**:347–355, 1949.
13. Henry, R. J. *Clinical Chemistry: Principles and Technics.* Harper & Row, New York, 1964.
14. Davidson, G. P., Gall, D. G., Petric, M., Butler, D. G., and Hamilton, J. R. Human rotavirus enteritis induced in conventional piglets. *J. Clin. Invest.* **66**:1402–1409, 1977.
15. Sack, D. A., Chowdhury, A. M. A. K., Eusof, A., Ali, M. A., Merson, M. H., Islam, S., Black, R. E., and Brown, K. H. Oral hydration in rotavirus diarrhoea: A double-blind comparison of sucrose with glucose electrolyte solution. *Lancet* **ii**:280–283, 1978.
16. Sack, D. A., Islam, S., Brown, K. H., Islam, A., Kabir, A. K. M. I., Chowdhury, A. M. A. K., and Ali, M. A. Oral therapy in children with cholera: A comparison of sucrose and glucose electrolyte solutions. *J. Pediatr.* **96**:20–25, 1980.

10

Direct Nutrient Loss and Diarrhea

M. Mujibur Rahaman and M. A. Wahed

Introduction

The pathogenesis of malnutrition in diarrheal diseases is the principal
theme of this volume. A meeting held in 1976 summarized the literature
and drew renewed attention to the infection–nutrition relationship.[1]
New information on the specific interactions of diarrhea and nutrition is
presented in this volume. Reduced dietary intake resulting from partial
loss of appetite, lower digestive and absorptive capacity of the gastrointestinal tract caused by enzymatic deficiencies, short transit-time, and
morphological changes in the intestinal villi, induced by repeated attacks
of diarrheal diseases, are considered to be some of the main causes of
malnutrition in tropical developing countries. Catabolic breakdown of
body protein because of inflammation also contributes to malnutrition in
some invasive diarrheas. There is, however, another cause of malnutrition, brought about by direct loss of nutrients into the gut, that has not
so far been investigated adequately, mainly because of technical difficulties involved in its measurement. Loss of protein or other nutrients into
the gut in a healthy individual is extremely small; whatever is secreted
into the intestine undergoes breakdown and reabsorption. The major
protein in the feces is in mucous secretions, undigested food material,
and bacteria. Loss from the gastrointestinal tract becomes obvious when
the quantity secreted exceeds the capacity of the intestine to reabsorb.

Protein-losing enteropathy (PLE) has been extensively investigated
in many diseases of children and adults since the early 1960s.[2] Excessive

M. Mujibur Rahaman and M. A. Wahed • International Centre for Diarrhoeal Research,
Dacca, Bangladesh.

loss of protein has been documented in children suffering from celiac disease,[3] measles,[4] and kwashiorkor,[5] all of which may cause considerable loss of body mass and severe malnutrition. The dysenteries, particularly those caused by *Shigella dysenteriae* type 1 and *S. flexneri,* also cause extreme hypoproteinemia, which has been documented in our center.[6] The mechanism of loss of protein was easy to explain on the basis of extensive ulceration of the large bowel and exudation of serum protein; it was, however, not simple to quantify the loss. This paper describes the methodology developed to estimate the quantitative loss of protein in diarrheal diseases, particularly in shigellosis, and attempts to explain the pathogenesis of this loss.

METHODOLOGICAL CONSIDERATIONS

The nitrogen content of the feces is easily estimated by the standard Kjeldahl method, but it is difficult to determine its source(s), as protein entering the gut also undergoes breakdown and reabsorption during its passage through the intestinal tract. The time-honored method employed to measure such loss involved the use of radioisotopes such as [131]albumin, [131]polyvinylprolidone (PVP), ^{59}Fe-dextran, or [51]Cr. Feces had to be collected for several consecutive days after administration of the isotope.[2] Despite the difficulty and cost involved, the method was not considered to be very precise. Also, it was not easy to observe the day-to-day changes in loss of serum protein during recovery.

A recently introduced technique obviates the necessity of using radioisotopes and allows a more precise estimation, over a shorter period of time, of loss of serum protein into the gut. The method is based on estimation of alpha 1-antitrypsin, an inhibitor of proteolytic enzymes found in measurable quantities in serum.[7,8] This method, being specific for alpha 1-antitrypsin alone, ignores other sources of protein. Once secreted into the gut, alpha 1-antitrypsin is resistant to further breakdown and its quantity can be measured by the radial immunodiffusion technique using hyperimmune sera against purified alpha 1-antitrypsin. By measuring its concentration simultaneously in feces and serum and calculating the ratio between the two, quantitative loss of protein into the gut can be estimated. The ratio has been found to be consistently low, i.e., < 1, in all healthy subjects and in many states not involving protein-losing enteropathy.[8]

Measuring the volume of stool collected over a 24-hour period permits assessment of the amount of serum lost into the gut. The distinctive advantages of the method are not only its low cost, simplicity, and avoidance of handling hazardous radioisotopes; it also allows day-to-day estimation of protein loss into the gut. This was not possible with isotope techniques that required a long period to establish the so-called steady state.

RESULTS

The method of estimating alpha 1-antitrypsin in feces was found to be very useful in our investigation of protein loss in patients with diarrhea. An earlier analysis indicated that almost all patients with dysenteric symptoms, including pus and red blood cells in the stool, had a high stool:serum ratio. Nearly two-thirds of patients with enterotoxigenic *Escherichia coli* (ETEC) and 40% of those with rotavirus diarrhea also showed excessive loss of protein in the feces (Figure 1).

Figure 2 shows the mean value and the distribution of the alpha 1-antitrypsin ratio according to microscopic examination of the stool. The mean and standard errors, respectively, were 2.19 ± 0.47, 1.52 ± 0.36, and 0.58 ± 0.15, for patients with both white blood cells (WBC) and red blood cells (RBC), for those with only WBC, and for those without either in their stools. Protein loss was seen in 88% of patients with both WBC and RBC in their stools and in 63% of those with WBC only. Twenty-two percent of patients showing neither WBC nor RBC in their stools were positive for PLE.

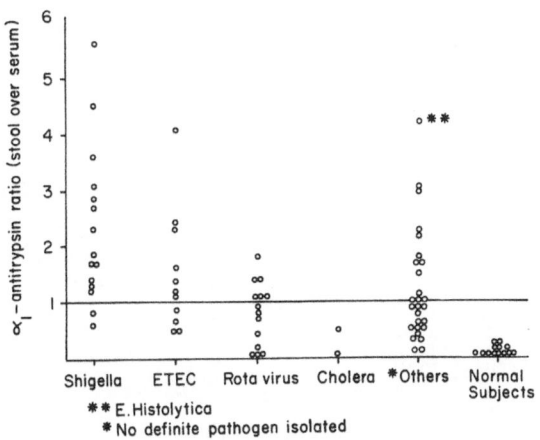

Figure 1. Distribution of alpha$_1$–antitrypsin ratios according to etiology.

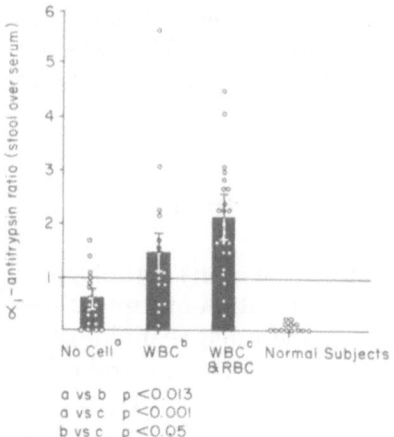

Figure 2. Mean and distribution of alpha$_1$-antitrypsin ratios according to presence of red blood cells and white blood cells in stool.

When the data were recalculated, it became apparent that, on admission, patients with shigellosis were losing between 100 to 500 ml of serum in feces each day. It was also shown that antibiotic therapy during hospitalization progressively reduced such losses (Figure 3). A new study is under way that will attempt to measure the loss of protein in the gut from the onset of disease through convalescence and recovery.

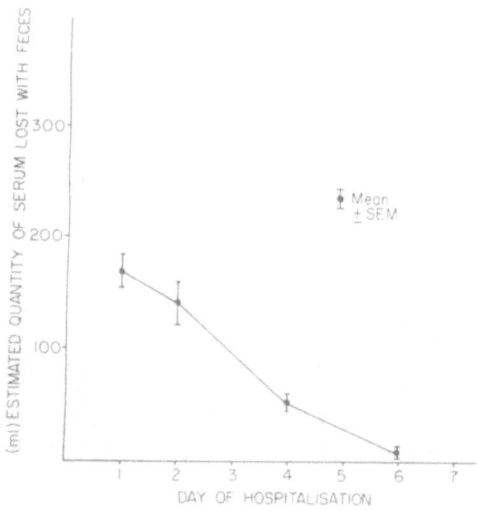

Figure 3. Calculated amounts of serum lost in the feces of a *Shigella* patient on each day of hospitalization.

DISCUSSION

Alpha 1-antitrypsin has been found to be a simple and useful quantitative marker for estimating the loss of protein into the gut in diarrheal diseases. The method also provides a reasonably satisfactory answer to some of the theoretical objections raised in carrying out studies involving estimation of protein loss. The pathogenesis of serum protein losses through the ulcerated and inflamed colonic mucosa in shigellosis is not difficult to explain. A number of additional factors may help precipitate the quick development of hypoproteinemia in patients with dysentery. Endotoxemia is a frequent feature of severe shigellosis[9] that may interfere with hepatic function. The liver is responsible for synthesis of the bulk of plasma protein, mainly albumin. Reduced intake of food following diarrheal attacks and increased catabolism during the inflammatory process also help to explain hypoproteinemia in dysenteric illnesses.

The presence of protein-losing enteropathy in rotavirus diarrhea was another important finding. Rotavirus is perhaps the main cause of diarrhea in the weaning period, i.e., between 6 months and 2 years of age. This disease causes patchy mucosal damage in the upper intestine,[10] which may take a number of days, perhaps weeks, to recover its full digestive and absorptive capacity. This pathological process may contribute to the pathogenesis of protein loss into the gut, not only through possible exudation but perhaps through shedding of the mucosal epithelium.

It has been estimated that under normal circumstances 250 g of cells containing 25 g of protein are desquamated each day, but most of the protein is reabsorbed in healthy individuals. In rotavirus infection, partial destruction of epithelial cells has been established as one of the principal pathological changes, and the quantitative loss of protein could therefore be many times higher. Loss of protein into the gut in rotavirus patients is manifested only when secretion exceeds the absorptive capacity of the intestine. Shorter transit-time in diarrhea and low levels of proteolytic enzymes may also hinder reabsorption of protein.

The mechanism of action of enterotoxigenic *E. coli* bacterias, particularly ST or heat-stable toxin, on the small intestine has yet to be fully understood. Heat-labile (LT) toxin is supposed to behave like cholera enterotoxin. Although it has been repeatedly confirmed that loss of protein in cholera stools is minimal, it is difficult to explain the finding that nearly two-thirds of patients with ETEC diarrhea showed an excessive loss of protein in the diarrheal stool. Could there be epithelial damage like that seen in rotavirus infection? Since the large majority of the ETEC strains in Bangladesh produce ST and ST/LT toxins, the loss of significantly high quantities of protein in ETEC diarrhea may be associated only with ST toxin. This interesting speculation gains some credence from the fact that intestinal absorptive capacity is not fully recovered in ETEC diarrhea even after 2 weeks of apparent clinical recovery (A. M. Molla *et al.*, unpublished data).

CONCLUSION

Use of alpha-1 antitrypsin as a marker protein derived from serum offers both theoretical and practical advantages over the time-honored radioisotope methods in diagnosing protein-losing enteropathy and measuring protein loss in diarrheal diseases. This method, when combined with longitudinal studies of intraluminal and cellular enzymes in the gut, correlated with the histologic appearance of the gastrointestinal tract, should reveal the pathogenesis of malnutrition in a large proportion of patients with diarrheal disease. It might be useful to encourage a multicenter study to confirm these findings.

REFERENCES

1. Proceedings of a symposium: Impact of infection on nutritional status of the host. *Am. J. Clin. Nutr.* 30: 1203–1369, 1977.
2. Waldman, T. A. Protein-losing enteropathy. In: *Modern Trends in Gastroenterology*, W. I. Card and B. Creamer (Eds.), pp. 125–142, Butterworths, London, 1970.
3. Rotem, Y, and Czerniak, P. Gastrointestinal protein leakage in celiac disease as studied by labeled PVP. *Am. J. Dis. Child.* 107:58–66, 1964.
4. Axton, J. H. M. Measles: A protein-losing enteropathy. *Br. Med. J.* 3:79–80, 1975.
5. Cohen, H., Metz, J., and Hart. D. Protein-losing gastroenteropathy in kwashiorkor. *Lancet* i:52, 1962.
6. Rahaman, M. M., Alam, A. K. M. J., and Islam, M. R. Leukaemoid reaction, haemolytic anaemia, and hypoproteinaemia in severe *Shigella dysenteriae* type-1 infection. *Lancet* i:1004, 1974.
7. Crossley, J. R., and Elliott, R. B. Simple method for diagnosing protein-losing enteropathies. *Br. Med. J.* 1:428–429, 1977.
8. Bernier, J. J., Florent, C., Desmazures, C., Aymes, C., and L'Hirondel, C. Diagnosis of protein-losing enteropathy by gastrointestinal clearance of alpha 1-antitrypsin. *Lancet* ii:763–764, 1978.
9. Koster, F., Levin, J., Walker, L., Tung, K. S. K., Gilman, R. H., Rahaman, M. M., Majid, M. A., Islam S., and Williams, R. C., Jr. Hemolytic-uremic syndrome after shigellosis. *N. Engl. J. Med.* 298:927–933, 1978.
10. Davidson, G. P., Gall, D. G., Petric, M., Butler, D. G., and Hamilton, J. R. Human rotavirus enteritis induced in conventional piglets: Intestinal structure and transport. *J. Clin. Invest.* 60:1402–1409, 1977.

11

Diarrhea and Nutrient Requirements

ELIZABETH D. MOYER AND MICHAEL C. POWANDA

Any discussion of protein and energy requirements arising from the occurrence of diarrhea is complicated by a number of factors, not the least of which is an incomplete understanding of these requirements in healthy individuals.[1-8] Protein and energy requirements vary considerably as a function of age, sex, size of frame, rate of growth, activity, and genetic makeup.[8] The variation in requirements is likely to increase considerably when the effects of disease, injury, and/or prior malnutrition become factors in the equation.[9-12] Thus, it may not be possible, based on available knowledge, to establish absolutely the protein and energy requirements occasioned by diarrhea. However, it may still be feasible to develop operational guidelines for assessing the relative nitrogen and energy depletion in various forms of diarrhea as well as for judging the success of nutrient repletion.

Diarrhea is a symptom of a diverse series of diseases of widely disparate etiologies. It can occur as a result of bacterial and parasitic infections, chronic inflammatory bowel disease, malabsorption syndrome, pancreatic insufficiency, and genetic disorders as well as after jejunoileal resection. This list is by no means inclusive, but it does indicate the variety of conditions in which diarrhea may be a component. The nutrient loss occasioned by diarrhea may depend upon the region or regions of

ELIZABETH D. MOYER • Research Division, Cutter Laboratories, Berkeley, California. MICHAEL C. POWANDA • Department of the Army, Letterman Army Institute of Research, Presidio of San Francisco, California. This work was partially supported by Grant No. NIAMDD/AM1820. The views of the authors do not purport to reflect the position of the Department of the Army or the Department of Defense.

the gastrointestinal tract affected as well as on whether the pathologic process involves the presence of abnormally large quantities of osmotically active substances, intestinal secretions, and derangements of active transport systems, or alterations in intestinal motility.

Transient, mild diarrhea in an otherwise healthy adult may be more of a social inconvenience than a nutritional liability. In contrast, repeated bouts of infection-associated diarrhea in infants and young children, or persistent diarrhea in children with inflammatory bowel disease, retard growth and development [13-15] and may increase susceptibility to infection. Chronic diarrhea has such potentially severe consequences in infants and young children, in part because their protein and energy resources are quite limited,[16] but mostly as a result of their high protein and energy requirements[3-8] related to growth processes. Although growth is not a concern in adults with diarrhea caused by inflammatory bowel disease or gastrointestinal tract resection, nutrient losses can be significant [17,18] and may result in considerable tissue wasting and impairment in healing. Since recurrent diarrhea may profoundly affect the growth and development of infants and young children, much of this chapter will be devoted to developing an assessment of the protein and energy costs of diarrhea in this age group. However, the application of this approach for assessing protein and energy requirements in adolescents and adults with persistent diarrhea caused by various forms of inflammatory stress will be discussed *pari passu.*

A rather extensive review of the literature regarding protein and energy demands of diarrheal diseases failed to reveal any comprehensive study that (a) assessed nutrient intake *and* (b) measured total nutrient excretion *and* (c) determined the efficiency of nutrient utilization *and* (d) quantified alterations in lean body mass as well as growth and body weight *and* (e) encompassed the entire period of illness and convalescence to ensure that the cumulative negative nutrient balances engendered by the disease that caused the diarrhea were totally recompensed. All of these measurements are necessary to allow a quantitative assessment of the protein and energy requirements occasioned by diarrheal diseases.

However, there are a number of reports that do give some indication of reduction in food intake or efficiency of a given nutrient's absorption, the loss of nonfood protein, or the diminution in growth rate associated with diarrheal diseases. Thus, in order to estimate protein and energy requirements, we are forced to make a number of assumptions and assemble the evidence from a number of studies, not all of which are in agreement with one another. We have therefore chosen to present our assessment of protein and energy requirements in a best case/worst case

Table I.   Assumptions Used in Estimating Protein and Energy Requirements
Engendered by Diarrheal Diseases

Best case	Worst case
The 1973 FAO/WHO protein allowances are correct	The 1973 FAO/WHO protein allowances are insufficient
There is a constant relationship between protein and energy needs	The relationship between protein and energy needs varies
Nutrient intake during diarrhea is reduced by about 20%	Nutrient intake during diarrhea is reduced by about 50%
Protein absorption 90% of intake; normal loss of body protein	Protein absorption 40–80% of intake; increased loss of body protein
Fat absorption 90% of intake	Fat absorption 50–80% of intake
Carbohydrate absorption 98% of intake	Carbohydrate absorption 75% of intake
There is no additional metabolic cost other than directly related to diarrhea	The underlying disease increases metabolic requirements from 20 to 50%
Efficiency of metabolism during health and illness is comparable	Efficiency of metabolism during illness is less than in health
There is little or no damage to gastrointestinal tract	Damage to the intestinal tract is appreciable (surgery may be required)

format. The assumptions behind each of these factors are shown in Table I. The following summarizes the evidence underlying the assumptions.

With regard to the 1973 FAO/WHO allowance for protein for young adults, Scrimshaw has assembled data indicating that nitrogen balance at this level of intake was achieved only when caloric intake was considerably in excess of recommended energy allowances.[1] Moreover, a recent study of obligatory nitrogen losses in adults gave evidence that the FAO/WHO-recommended safe intake of protein appears to be but marginally adequate.[19] The FAO/WHO-recommended protein intake for adults (0.57 g/kg/day) was based on ingestion of a high-quality protein such as egg. However, if a wheat-soy-milk mixture was used instead of egg protein, then even 0.8 g/kg/day was insufficient to maintain positive nitrogen balance in five of eight young adults (23 to 39 years) and in three of seven older subjects (60 to 73 years) when they were provided with a caloric intake of 40 kcal/kg/day.[20]

There is also some disagreement on accepted levels of protein intake sufficient to promote growth in infants and young children,[4,5] arising in part from the choice of units used to express the requirement, e.g., g/kg versus g/100 kcal,[21] as well as the source of protein, e.g., breast milk versus unprocessed cow's milk.[4,22] Since the presence of infection and/or injury increases nitrogen utilization,[9,10] levels of protein intake that are marginally adequate for healthy individuals are likely to become inadequate during inflammatory stress.

Although a constant relationship between protein and energy needs would simplify calculations, this assumption is useful only in providing a lower limit, because there is evidence that protein utilization is affected by caloric intake,[1,11] just as energy utilization is affected by the quality and quantity of protein.[23] Thus, fat deposition and accumulation of lean body mass can occur to some degree independently of one another[11,12,23] in patients recovering from nutrient depletion.

Diarrheal diseases appeared to have reduced nutrient intake by approximately 20% in preschool children in Guatemala,[24] while preschool children with diarrhea in Bangladesh had a nutrient intake 50 to 70% that of controls of similar age[25] (see also A. M. Molla et al., chapter 7, this volume). In studies designed to assess the effect of early oral feeding versus early oral starvation on the course of diarrhea in infants, a greater than 60% decrease in nutrient intake was observed in children less than 2 years old for the first day after hospitalization; however, by the second day the children were ingesting more than 90% of expected normal intake.[26]

Protein absorption in healthy, young American adults eating an American diet appears to be 91 to 92% of intake.[27] Approximately 0.7 to 2% of the protein ingested is excreted in the feces.[28] Consumption of a typical Indian diet by young adults appears to result in less efficient nitrogen absorption (approximately 80% of intake), with a greater proportion of the nitrogen appearing in the feces.[27] In infants, severe diarrhea has been reported to cause a 25% loss of ingested protein via the stool as compared to an 8% loss in children without diarrhea.[29] The authors of this last study[29] felt that not all of the fecal protein loss during severe diarrhea was derived from food, and they suggested that a portion of the protein loss might arise from intestinal secretions.

Indeed, recent evidence indicates that a portion of the protein found in fecal samples from children with certain forms of diarrheal diseases, especially shigellosis, may be the result of the enteric loss of serum proteins (see Rahaman and Wahed, chapter 10, this volume). If the loss of serum proteins via the gastrointestinal tract is appreciable during certain forms of diarrhea, then estimates of the efficiency of absorption of protein would be spuriously low. Ayesha Molla and co-workers (see chapter 9, this volume) indicate that children 1 to 4 years old with diarrhea caused by rotavirus or Shigella have a severely reduced efficiency of nitrogen absorption (approximately 40% of intake) during the acute stages of the illness. Although the estimate of efficiency of nitrogen absorption may have been affected by intestinal serum protein leakage in those patients with shigellosis, the estimate is likely to be reasonable in children infected with rotavirus, because there appears to be little secretion of serum proteins in these patients (see Rahaman and Wahed, chapter 10, this volume).

Fat absorption in healthy children and young adults eating an American diet,[27,28,30-32] and in Indian adults[27] and young children (3 to 7 years old) eating an Indian diet,[31] averages 93 to 97% of intake even when the children are infected with *Ascaris lumbricoides.*[33] However, the coefficient of fat absorption in children 1 to 4 years old decreases significantly during diarrhea caused by rotavirus or *Shigella*, but less so in the case of diarrhea caused by enterotoxigenic *Escherichia coli* (see Ayesha Molla et al., chapter 9, this volume).

In contrast to children and young adults, infants less than 6 months of age excrete 6 to 14% of their fat intake.[34] Mild diarrhea increases fat excretion to about 28%.[34] These data are consistent with the values for fecal fat obtained by Holt et al.[29] Healthy infants 4 to 13 months of age excreted 12.4% of fat intake, while mild diarrhea increased the fecal fat content to 23.1% and severe diarrhea raised it to 40.5%. Chronic, severe malnutrition (presumably accompanied by infection and diarrhea) also reduces the efficiency of fat absorption in children to about 50% of intake; upon recovery, the efficiency of fat absorption rises to about 80%.[35]

Carbohydrate absorption ranges from 97 to 99% in young adults whether consuming an American or an Indian diet.[27] The presence of *Ascaris* in Bangladeshi children 3 to 7 years old did not significantly alter the efficacy of their carbohydrate absorption, which amounted to 94 to 95%.[33] Children with diarrhea caused by rotavirus or *Shigella* had reduced absorption of carbohydrate—73 to 77% of intake (see Ayesha Molla et al., chapter 9, this volume). However, diarrhea induced by toxigenic *E. coli* did not reduce carbohydrate absorption in these subjects.

In the case of diarrhea caused by a microorganism generally thought to be noninvasive, such as *Vibrio cholerae*,[36] conceivably the only additional metabolic cost to the host, other than the loss of nutrients caused by decreased intake and vomiting[37] (see also D. Mahalanabis, chapter 14, this volume), would be that occasioned by the activation of the Na-K-dependent ATPase-linked sodium pump (see R. L. Guerrant, chapter 2, this volume). When the diarrhea is the result of an invasive infection, such as typhoid fever,[38] or a consequence of inflammatory bowel disease, there will be increased energy requirements related to altered metabolism and redistribution of nutrients as well as to fever.[39-42] During a severe case of typhoid, the caloric expenditure of patients may increase by as much as 50%,[39] and protein loss may average 500 to 800 grams.[39,41]

Even milder diseases such as sandfly fever, which is self-limiting and transient, or experimentally induced, promptly treated tularemia and Q fever engender significant caloric demands and protein losses.[39]

Based on weight losses of 1.5, 2.1, and 2.7 kg, the caloric cost of sandfly fever, Q fever, and tularemia would be, respectively, 11,500, 16,170, and 20,790 kcal; based on excess nitrogen excretion, protein losses would amount to 94, 220, and 312 g, respectively. In other words, even mild infections can cause cumulative losses of protein and calories equivalent to 2 to 8 days and 3.5 to 7 days, respectively, of the recommended allowances for a healthy, mildly active 70-kg adult. Thus, it is not surprising that the nutrient deficits generated by even mild infections persist for weeks after the acute phase of the illness.[40]

With regard to infants, diarrhea in conjunction with various infections can easily cause a weight deficit or loss in a 1-year-old child of 2.5 kg,[13] i.e., equal to that occasioned by experimentally induced tularemia in an adult. Though the weight loss is similar, it represents a longer period of inadequate nourishment equivalent to an 11-day loss of protein and a 20-day deficit in calories. A 4- to 5-kg weight deficit such as observed in the infants studied by MacLean et al.[43] would be tantamount to a 17- to 23-day absence of protein and a 31- to 38-day lack of calories, which is consistent with the 5- to 6-weeks period these authors suggest as the minimum effective treatment period for these patients.

It would appear from much of the foregoing discussion that the efficiency of metabolism during illness would be less than that in health, especially considering the decrements in efficiency of absorption and the metabolic demands of invasive and/or inflammatory diseases; and indeed, during the acute phase of illness and even early into the recovery period this may be so.[44,45] However, in terms of energy expended for the deposition of new tissue, infants 12 months of age appear to be quite efficient, requiring but 4,400 kcal/kg of new tissue.[44] This value is lower or comparable to that measured by other investigators under similar conditions,[44] and less than the average caloric intake required for new tissue deposition in patients recovering from anorexia nervosa.[46]

Spady et al. predicted that the composition of the new tissue accumulated by infants was 31% fat and 14% protein.[44] Based on data from animal studies, the cost of depositing new tissue with this composition would be about 5700 kcal/kg.[47] The apparent inefficiency in weight gain in infants noted by some authors may be explained, at least in part, in terms of the criteria used in estimating caloric needs. For example, in the absence of disease and/or malnutrition, a 1-year-old child should weigh about 10 to 11 kg and require 100 kcal/kg per day to cover basal metabolism, activity, losses of energy via excreta, and growth.[7,48] However, a 1-year-old child who is severely malnourished may weigh only 5 to 6 kg.[43] If, after determining that a weight deficit based on age and/or height does indeed exist, one looks at charts of the estimated caloric requirements of a child of that weight, not age, then it becomes apparent that such a child would require at least 120 kcal/kg, per day[7,48] a value closer to the observed needs of these infants.[43]

In a noninvasive diarrhea-inducing infection such as cholera, there is little or no gastrointestinal tract damage[36] and little loss of nutrients other than that caused by diminished intake[37] (see also D. Mahalanabis, chapter 14, this volume). Moreover, cholera-induced diarrhea leaves the glucose and amino acid transport mechanisms intact (see R. L. Guerrant, chapter 2, this volume), which makes possible the rapid replenishment of depleted patients[37] (see also D. Mahalanabis, chapter 14, this volume.

In contrast, *Shigella*-induced diarrhea is associated with inflammation and ulceration of the lower bowel leading to the exudation of serum proteins (see Rahaman and Wahed, chapter 10, this volume). If the alpha$_1$-antitrypsin marker used by Rahaman and Wahed reflects losses of serum proteins of molecular weight (MW) less than, or equal to, 100,000 daltons, then the 100 to 500 ml of serum that they report may be lost in the feces of patients with shigellosis increases the daily protein deficit by 4 to 20 grams. If appreciable amounts of the larger MW serum proteins, such as the immunoglobulins, are also lost, the daily exudation of serum proteins into the gut may range from 7 to 35 grams.

Crohn's disease, an inflammatory condition of the intestinal tract, results in a loss of serum proteins via feces.[49] The nutritional consequences of Crohn's disease may be sufficient to retard growth in children and adolescents.[14,15,50] Although there may be intestinal loss of serum proteins, the major deficit in these patients appears to be in calories rather than protein,[15,50] because their protein intake generally appears to exceed the recommended daily allowance for their age, whereas their caloric intake ranges from 45 to 100% of expected. However, this too may be an instance of using the wrong criterion for judging the extent of requirements.

If the intestinal tract inflammation is of sufficient magnitude and hazard to the patient to require surgery, or if other conditions require intestinal resection,[51,52] there is a high likelihood of diarrhea occurring for months or maybe years after the surgery,[18,51,52] and selective decrements in nutrient absorption may persist for years.[51] The occurrence of diarrhea appears to be related to perturbations of the colon rather than of the ileum.

Studies of transit time of a meal in normal subjects showed that stool weight was a function of whole gut transit time but not small intestinal transit time, thus implicating the colon as being the key in the rate of normal stool production and osmotically induced diarrhea.[53] These data complement the findings from patients who had undergone intestinal resection, namely, that though the severity of diarrhea was a function of both the amount of colon and the centimeters of ileum removed, the extent of missing colon had an effect three times that of the excised ileum.[54] Though rapid transit of ingested food such as occurs during diarrhea certainly would have a deleterious effect on the efficiency of nutrient absorption, the actual loss of jejunum and ileum would also impose a defect in nutrient absorption even if there were no diarrhea. Unfortunately, it is difficult to assess just how much of a loss in the ability to absorb nutrients is caused by such surgery.

Some of the pitfalls associated with evaluating the protein and energy requirements occasioned by diarrhea resulting from infection, inflammation, and/or malnutrition have been presented. It remains to ascertain whether any reasonable estimate of these requirements can be made from the available data. Starting with the simplest case, patients, especially children, with cholera-induced diarrhea, it would appear that the protein and energy losses are primarily the result of decreased intake with little other metabolic cost and seemingly no defect in the absorptive capacity of the intestinal tract[37] (see also D. Mahalanabis, chapter 14, this volume). Thus, once the diarrhea is successfully treated, it should be merely a matter of providing protein and calories in excess of the recommended daily allowance until the deficit—the difference between the RDA and actual intake during the diarrheal episode times the number of days of illness—is abolished.

In the case of an invasive infection that causes fever and considerable alterations in systemic metabolism as well as diarrhea, the metabolic alterations appear to produce the greatest deficit, especially in protein.[55] In adults, the protein losses may reach 0.9 g/kg per day (greater than 100% of the RDA) during illness, and the caloric requirements may increase by 50%. If there is a loss of serum proteins into the feces, as in shigellosis, the protein loss may range from 1.0 to 1.4 g/kg per day.

Considering these consequential losses and the fact that there may be residual defects in nutrient absorption for some weeks after the acute phase of the illness, it should be readily apparent why it takes so long to make up the deficits induced by such infections. It also would seem reasonable that the protein-to-energy ratio would have to increase during the repletion period. A 30% increase in calories and a 100% increase in protein has been recommended by Whitehead to optimize repletion in young children depleted by infection.[56] Whitehead's estimate of caloric requirements for catch-up growth (approximately 143 kcal/kg per day) are at the upper range of energy needs specified in the RDA for children in the 6- to 7-kg weight range[7] and found to be required by MacLean *et al.* in their treatment of malnourished infants.[43] Whitehead's estimate of protein requirements (approximately 4 g/kg per day), though high by present standards (approximately 2 g/kg per day), coincides with the observed protein intake of children reported by Holt and Fales.[22]

All of the preceding cases have dealt with situations in which the diarrhea and its underlying cause is transient and thus one needs only to replenish what has been momentarily lost. However, in the case of inflammatory bowel disease or intestinal resection, the diarrhea and increased metabolic cost may be a chronic condition requiring a longer-term dietary adjustment to provide adequate protein and energy. As stated earlier, in the case of Crohn's disease, especially in patients who have not undergone extensive intestinal tract resection, the primary deficit appears to be in calories, and by increasing the caloric intake so it exceeds the presumed caloric needs of these patients, adequate growth is achieved.[50] Unfortunately, protein requirement is also increased.

In the case of intestinal resection, there appears to be a direct relationship between the extent of the resection and the percentage of protein and fat intake lost in the stool as long as the ileocecal valve is left intact.[18] If indeed this is a consistent finding, then by knowing the extent of excision, an adjustment can be made so that the intake of protein and energy will be sufficient to prevent wasting. However, there are other studies suggesting that nitrogen absorption does not vary appreciably with the extent of excision.[51]

The foregoing provides a guide to, rather than standards for, the protein and energy costs of diarrhea in a somewhat limited set of cases. This seems appropriate, considering the incomplete state of our knowledge of protein and calorie requirements in healthy populations and the anticipated greater variation in these requirements in diseased and/or malnourished populations. In order to establish the extent of protein and energy needs occasioned by diarrhea, more complete balance studies are needed encompassing the entire period of illness and recovery. But it is not sufficient to measure intake and output; we must also learn how the nitrogen and calories are being used during the illness, injury, or inflammation[57,58] that precipitates the diarrhea as well as afterward, to promote repletion and the deposition of new tissue.[58,59] We require more information about the cost of tissue deposition in infants, children, and adults, whether it differs in efficiency with age, and how it is influenced by the protein-to-energy ratio of the diet. We need to know the composition of the tissue deposited and to what extent the composition of the new tissue is affected by the ratio and amounts of protein and energy supplied. We need to have a simple, accurate measure of the accumulation of lean body mass. In this regard, perhaps the nomogram used to predict lean body mass in men[60] could be extended to and validated for women and children.

REFERENCES

1. Scrimshaw, N. S. Shattuck lecture—Strengths and weaknesses of the committee approach. An analysis of past and present recommended dietary allowances for protein in health and disease. *N. Engl. J. Med.* **294**:136–142; 198–203, 1976.

2. Rand, W. M., Scrimshaw, N. S., and Young, V. R. Determination of protein allowances in human adults from nitrogen balance studies. *Am. J. Clin. Nutr.* **30**:1129, 1977.

3. Ghadimi, A., and Tejani, A. Protein and amino acid requirements. In: *Total Parenteral Nutrition: Premises and Promises*, A. Ghadimi (Ed.). pp. 213–230 John Wiley, New York, 1975.

4. Irwin, M. I., and Hegsted, D. M. A conspectus of research on protein requirements of man. *J. Nutr.* **101**:385, 1971.

5. Swaminathan, M., and Parpia, H. A. B. Human protein requirements. *Nutr. Rep. Int.* **3**:39, 1971.

6. Gentz, J., and Persson, B. Energy metabolism. In: *Total Parenteral Nutrition: Premises and Promises*, A. Ghadimi (Ed.), pp. 9–22 John Wiley, New York, 1975.

7. Food and Nutrition Board. *Recommended Dietary Allowances*, 9th ed., pp. 16—29. National Academy of Sciences/National Research Council, Washington, D.C., 1980.

8. Young, V. R., and Scrimshaw, N. S. Genetic and biological variability in human nutrient requirements. *Am. J. Clin. Nutr.* **32**:486, 1979.

9. Wilmore, D. W. *The Metabolic Management of the Critically Ill*. Plenum Medical, New York, 1977.

10. Wilmore, D. W., and Kinney, J. M. Panel report on nutritional support of patients with trauma or infection. *Am. J. Clin. Nutr.* **34**:1213, 1981.

11. Elwyn, D. H., Gump, F. E., Munro, H. N., Iles, M., and Kinney, J. M. Changes in nitrogen balance of depleted patients with increasing infusions of glucose. *Am. J. Clin. Nutr.* **32**:1597, 1979.

12. MacLean, W. C., Jr., and Graham, C. G. The effect of energy intake on nitrogen content of weight gained by recovering malnourished infants. *Am. J. Clin. Nutr.* **33**:903, 1980.

13. Mata, L. J., Kromal, R. A., Urrutia, J. J., and Garcia, B. Effect of infection on food intake and the nutritional state: Perspectives as viewed from the village. *Am. J. Clin. Nutr.* **30**:1215, 1977.

14. McCaffery, T. D., Nasr, K., Lawrence, A. M., and Kirsner, J. B. Severe growth retardation in children with inflammatory bowel disease. *Pediatrics* **45**:386, 1970.

15. Werlin, S. L. Growth failure in Crohn's disease: An approach to treatment. *JPEN* **5**:250, 1981.

16. Heird, W. C., and Greene, H. L. Panel report on nutritional support of pediatric patients. *Am. J. Clin. Nutr.* **34**:1223, 1981.

17. Colin, R., Hecketsweiler, P., Galmiche, J-P, Le Bihan, M., and Geffroy, Y. Etude de l'absorption intestinale dans la maladie de Crohn. *Gastroenterol. Clin. Biol.* **2**:705, 1978.

18. Chen, K. M. Massive resection of the small intestine. *Surgery* **65**:931, 1969.

19. Bodwell, C. E., Schuster, E. M., Kyle, E., Brooks, B., Womack, M., Steele, P., and Ahrens, R. Obligatory urinary and fecal nitrogen losses in young women, older men

and young men and the factorial estimation of adult human protein requirements. *Am. J. Clin. Nutr.* **32**:2450, 1979.

20. Cheng, A. H. R., Gomez, A., Bergan, J. G., Lee, T. C., Monckeberg, F., and Chichester, C. O. Comparative nitrogen balance study between young and aged adults using three levels of protein intake from a combination wheat-soy-milk mixture. *Am. J. Clin. Nutr.* **31**:12, 1978.

21. Fomon, S. J., Thomas, L. N., Filer, L. J., Anderson, T. A., and Bergmann, K. E. Requirements for protein and essential amimo acids in early infancy. *Acta Paediatr. Scand.* **62**:33, 1973.

22. Holt, E., and Fales, H. L. The food requirements of children. II. Protein requirements. *Am. J. Dis. Child.* **22**:371, 1921.

23. MacLean, W. C., Jr., and Graham, G. G. The effect of level of protein intake in isoenergetic diets on energy utilization. *Am. J. Clin. Nutr.* **32**:1381, 1979.

24. Martorell, R., Yarbrough, C., Yarbrough, S., and Klein, R. E. The impact of ordinary illnesses on dietary intakes of malnourished children. *Am. J. Clin. Nutr.* **33**:345, 1980.

25. Hoyle, B., Yunus, M., and Chen, L. C. Breast-feeding and food intake among children with acute diarrheal diseases. *Am. J. Clin. Nutr.* **33**:2365, 1980.

26. Chung, A. W., and Viščorová, B. The effect of early oral feeding versus early oral starvation on the course of infantile diarrhea. *J. Pediatr.* **33**:14, 1948.

27. Briscoe, J. The quantitative effect of infection on the use of food by young children in poor countries. *Am. J. Clin. Nutr.* **32**:648, 1979.

28. Wollaeger, E. E., Comfort, M. W., and Osterberg, A. E. Total solids, fat and nitrogen in the feces. III. A study of normal persons taking a test diet containing a moderate amount of fat; comparison with results obtained with normal persons taking a test diet containing a large amount of fat. *Gastroenterology* **9**:272, 1948.

29. Holt, L. E., Courtney, A. M., and Fales, H. L. The chemical composition of diarrheal as compared with normal stools in infants. *Am. J. Dis. Child.* **9**:213, 1915.

30. Wollaeger, E. E., Comfort, M. W., Weir, J. F., and Osterberg, A. E. The total solids, fat and nitrogen in the feces. I. A study of normal persons and of patients with duodenal ulcer on a test diet containing large amounts of fat. *Gastroenterology* **6**:83, 1946.

31. Willimas, H. H., Endicott, E. N., Shepherd, M. L., Galbraith, H., and Macy, T. G. Fat excretion by normal children. *J. Nutr.* **25**:379, 1943.

32. Stier, L. B., Taylor, D. D., Pace, J. K., and Eisen, J. N. Metabolic patterns in preadolescent children. IV. Fat intake and excretion. *J. Nutr.* **73**:347, 1961.

33. Brown, K. H., Gilman, R. H., Khatun, M., and Ahmed, M. G. Absorption of macronutrients from a rice-vegetable diet before and after treatment of ascaris in children. *Am. J. Clin. Nutr.* **3**:1975, 1980.

34. MacLean, W. C., Klein, G. L., de Romana, G. L., Massa, E., and Graham, G. G. Transient steatorrhea following episodes of mild diarrhea in early infancy. *J. Pediatr.* **92**:562, 1978.

35. Gomez, F., Galván, R. R., Cravioto, J., Frenk, S., Santaella, J. V., and De La Pena, C. Fat absorption in chronic severe malnutrition in children. *Lancet* **ii**:121, 1956.

36. Carpenter, C. C. J. Cholera (Asiatic cholera). In: *Cecil Textbook of Medicine*, 15th ed., P. B. Beeson, W. McDermott, and J. B. Wyngaarden (Eds.), pp. 460–462, W. B. Saunders, Philadelphia, 1979.

37. Mahalanabis, D. Nitrogen balance during recovery from secretory diarrhea of cholera in children. *Am. J. Clin. Nutr.* **24**:1548, 1981.

38. Gorbach, S. L. Typhoid fever. In: *Cecil Textbook of Medicine*, 15th ed., P. B. Beeson, W. McDermott, and J. B. Wyngaarden (Eds.), pp. 446–449, W. B. Saunders Co., Philadelphia, 1979.

39. Coleman, W., and DuBois, E. F. Clinical calorimetry. VII. Calorimetric observations on the metabolism of typhoid patients with and without food. *Arch. Intern. Med.* **15**:887, 1915.

40. Beisel, W. R., Sawyer, W. D., Ryll, E. D., and Crozier, D. Metabolic effects of intracellular infections in man. *Ann. Intern. Med.* **67**:744, 1967.

41. Powanda, M. C. Changes in body balances of nitrogen and other key nutrients: Description and underlying mechanisms. *Am. J. Clin. Nutr.* **30**:1254, 1977.

42. Beisel, W. R. Infectious diseases: Effect on food intake and nutrient requirements. In: *Nutrition: Metabolic and Clinical Applications,* R. E. Hodges (Ed.), pp. 329–346, Plenum, New York, 1979.

43. MacLean, W. C., Jr., de Romana, G. L., Massa, E., and Graham, C. G. Nutritional management of chronic diarrhea and malnutrition: Primary reliance on oral feeding. *J. Pediatr.* **97**:316, 1980.

44. Spady, D. W., Payne, P. R., Picou, D., and Waterlow, J. C. Energy balance during recovery from malnutrition. *Am. J. Clin. Nutr.* **29**:1073, 1976.

45. Powanda, M. C., and Beisel, W. R., Hypothesis: Leukocyte endogenous mediator/endogenous/pyrogen/lymphocyte-activating factor modulates the development of nonspecific immunity and specific immunity and affects nutritional status. *Amer. J. Clin. Nutr.* **35**:762, 1982.

46. Walker, J., Roberts, S. L., Halmi, K. A., and Goldberg, S. C. Caloric requirements for weight gain in anorexia nervosa. *Am. J. Clin. Nutr.* **32**:3196, 1979.

47. Pullar, J. D., and Webster, A. J. F. The energy cost of fat and protein deposition in the rat. *Br. J. Nutr.* **27**:355, 1977.

48. Holt, E., and Fales, H. L. The food requirements of children. I. Total caloric requirements. *Am. J. Dis. Child.* **21**:1, 1921.

49. Jensen, K. B., Golterman, N., Jarnum, S., Weeke, B., and Westergaard, H. IgM turnover in Crohn's disease. *Gut* **11**:223, 1970.

50. Kelts, D. G., Grand, R. J., Shen, G., Watkins, J. B., Werlin, S. L., and Boehme, C. Nutritional basis of growth failure in children and adolescents with Crohn's disease. *Gastroenterology* **76**:720, 1979.

51. Ladefoged, K., Nicolaidou, P., and Jarnum, S. Calcium, phosphorus, magnesium, zinc and nitrogen balance in patients with severe short bowel syndrome. *Am. J. Clin. Nutr.* **33**:2137, 1980.

52. Aly, A., Barany, F., Kollberg, B., Monsen, U., Wisen, O., and Johansson, C. Effect of an H_2-receptor blocking agent on diarrhoeas after extensive small bowel resection in Crohn's disease. *Acta Med. Scand.* **207**:119, 1980.

53. Read, N. W., Miles, C. A., Fisher, D., Holgate, A. M., Kime, N. D., Mitchell, M. A., Reeve, A. M., Roche, T. B., and Walker, M. Transit of a meal through the stomach, small intestine and colon in normal subjects and its role in the pathogenesis of diarrhea. *Gastroenterology* **79**:1276, 1980.

54. Mitchell, J. E., Breuer, R. I., Zuckerman, L., Berlin, J., Schilli, R., and Dunn, J. K. The colon influences ileal resection diarrhea. *Dig. Dis. Sci.* **25**:33, 1980.

55. Scrimshaw, N. S. Effect of infection on nutrient requirements. *Am. J. Clin. Nutr.* **30**:1536, 1977.

56. Whitehead, R. G. Protein and energy requirements of young children living in the developing countries to allow for catch-up growth after infections. *Am. J. Clin. Nutr.* **30**:1545, 1977.

57. Wilmore, D. W., Goodwin, C. W., Aulick, L. H., Powanda, M. C., Mason, A. D., Jr., and Pruitt, B. A., Jr. Effect of injury and infection on visceral metabolism and circulation. *Ann. Surg.* **192**:491, 1980.

58. Powanda, M. C., and Moyer, E. D. Plasma protein alterations during infection: Potential significance of these changes to host defense and repair systems. In: *Infection: The Physiologic and Metabolic Responses of the Host*, M. C. Powanda and P. G. Canonico (Eds.). Elsevier/North Holland, Amsterdam , 1981, pp. 271–296

59. Powanda, M. C., and Moyer, E. D. Plasma proteins and wound healing. *Surg. Gynecol. Obstet.* **153**:749–755, 1981.

60. Fuchs, R. J., Theis, C. F., and Lancaster, M. C. A nomogram to predict lean body mass in men. *Am. J. Clin. Nutr.* **31**:673, 1978.

Interventions against Diarrhea and Malnutrition

Promotion of Breast-Feeding, Health, and Growth among Hospital-Born Neonates, and among Infants of a Rural Area of Costa Rica

LEONARDO MATA, MARÍA A. ALLEN, PATRICIA JIMÉNEZ,
MARIA E. GARCÍA, WILLIAM VARGAS, MARÍA E.
RODRÍGUEZ, AND CARLOS VALERIN

INTRODUCTION

A decline in the incidence of breast-feeding in many developing nations has been recorded in recent years, often in conjunction with (a) rapid changes in way of life, (b) migration from rural to urban centers, (c) incorporation of women into the labor force (especially in industry), and (d) increase in stress, anxiety, and violence in transitional and modern societies. The marked decline in incidence and duration of breast-feeding throughout the world is a matter of international concern. The importance of breast-feeding, particularly in developing societies, stems from its health-promoting effect, as it provides the best food known for infants, protects the child against a variety of debilitating infectious

LEONARDO MATA, MARIA A. ALLEN, PATRICIA JIMENEZ, MARIA E. GARCIA, WILLIAM VARGAS, MARIA E. RODRIGUEZ, and CARLOS VALERIN • Instituto de Investigaciones en Salud, Universidad de Costa Rica, San Pedro, Costa Rica.

processes, and encourages attachment between mother and infant.[1-6] Furthermore, successful breast-feeding indirectly reduces the ills of bottle-feeding, especially in developing nations, as epidemiological observation in many countries has revealed that early weaning is often associated with severe infant malnutrition, neglect, child abuse, abandonment, and premature death.[7-9]

Latin American countries in transition from traditional to modern societies have experienced a rapid decline in breast-feeding according to surveys conducted in the period 1975 to 1978 (Table I).[10-15] The causes for the decline have not been investigated thoroughly, but they are expected to be similar to those detected in other societies where the same phenomenon has been recorded.[7] However, in nations like Costa Rica, where the trend toward hospital childbirth has occurred so rapidly, separation of mothers and infants after delivery may play a more important role than currently realized. If this proves to be the case, a new approach different from that emphasizing routine educational aspects must be tried to promote breast-feeding.

A survey conducted in Costa Rica in 1978 showed that as many as 24% of infants from the rural areas were not breast-fed or were weaned in the first days of life; by 3 to 6 months, approximately one-half had been weaned onto cow's and formula milks. Furthermore, breast-fed infants were given supplements (mainly cow's milk) at an early age and only 19% were exclusively at the breast by age 4 months (Table II).[16]

Such a situation undoubtedly resulted from a combination of factors in our transitional society, such as (a) many years of practicing drastic separation of mothers and infants immediately after delivery, and formula-feeding in hospitals and clinics, (b) many years of intense promotion of processed cow's milk for infants by the medical and commercial establishments, (c) a powdered milk distribution program by the govern-

Table I.   Percentage of Women Who
Nursed Last Child, 1976–1979[a]

	Urban	Rural
Honduras (East)	97	96
Peru	87	95
Colombia	88	92
Panama	70	88
Nicaragua	72	85
Costa Rica	60	76

[a]Source: references 10–14, 16.

Table II. Prevalence of Breast-Feeding, Costa Rica 1978 and Puriscal 1979–1981

| | % Prevalence | | | |
| | | Puriscal subcohorts | | |
Age (months)	Costa Rica $N = 286$	1.1 $N = 114$	1.2 $N = 219$	1.3 $N = 218$
1	76	95	95	86
3	52	82	79	71
6	57	66	59	46
9	31	62	47	36
Total breast-fed[a]	74	95	98	95

[a]One week or longer.

ment to all new mothers in effect for several years, and (d) cultural distortion of the role of the breasts and breast-feeding.

Although no account of the sequence of events leading to the situation uncovered by the surveys was available, the decline in breast-feeding probably began several decades ago. Early weaning was already common in the 1950s and probably contributed to the exceedingly high rates of diarrheal disease, malnutrition, infant death, and demographic change recorded in that decade. In spite of this, a sustained emphasis by governments on social development and improved nutrition and health resulted in consistent reduction in infant deaths, particularly in the 1970s.[17]

While Costa Rica coped with some of the ill effects of an increasing rate of premature weaning, incidence and duration of breast-feeding continued their decline. By the middle of the 1970s, measures intended to promote breast-feeding emanated from the Social Security and the Ministry of Health, with collaboration of the Costa Rican Association of Demography. They promoted educational programs through the radio, television, and press, but, according to the 1978 nutrition survey, the effect of such programs on breast-feeding was judged to be limited, as no significant changes were detected in the years since the preceding surveys (Table II). In fact, a further decline in breast-feeding was noted in 1978 compared to 1975.[10,16]

The present paper is a preliminary report of a collaborative study permitting implementation of certain hospital and field interventions and an assessment of their possible impact on maternal behavior, the practice of breast-feeding, and infant nutrition and health. The report summarizes findings of interventions affecting neonates at the San Juan de Dios Hospital in San José, as well as results of a long-term, prospective field observation of mothers in Puriscal, most of whom deliver their infants in that hospital. The municipal seat of Puriscal, Santiago, is just 45 kilometers by paved road from San José, the capital of Costa Rica, but the study region extends to the Pacific Coast, comprising about 800 square kilometers, with approximately 24,000 inhabitants in eight districts containing about 170 localities of a very sparsely distributed rural population (Figure 1). The region is in rapid transition and its population enjoys a better standard of living than most traditional societies in Latin America. Most children have access to schools and health services, and

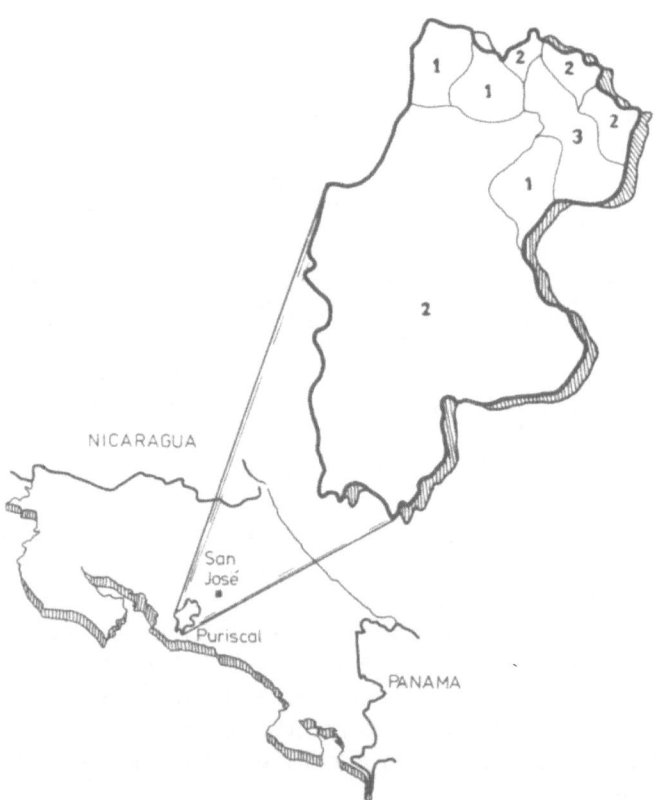

Figure 1. Region of Puriscal in the Republic of Costa Rica. Numerals 1 represent, from left to right, districts of Grifo Alto, Barbacoas, and Candelarita, or subcohort 1.1; numerals 2 are, from left to right, districts of Mercedes Sur, Desamparaditos, San Antonio, and San Rafael, or subcohort 1.2; and numeral 3 is the central district of Santiago, or subcohort 1.3 (see Table III).

about 70% of the homes are connected to piped water supplies. The population lives mainly on agricultural production and sales of food crops, complemented with cash crops such as tobacco.

The Puriscal study was planned simultaneously with several interventions in the Gynecology and Obstetrics Service of the San Juan de Dios Hospital. While planning began in 1976, hospital interventions started in September 1977, and the recruitment of mothers and infants for the study was initiated in September 1979.[15,18]

HOSPITAL INTERVENTIONS

The San Juan de Dios Hospital is the oldest and one of the largest and most prestigious institutions in the country. Up to August 1977, the norm in the hospital obstetrics facility (total births: 7,500 to 9,000 per year) was to separate mothers and infants completely for the whole period of hospitalization (Table III). After delivery, neonates were examined, bathed, clothed, and placed in the neonatal ward, where they were fed glucose solution and formula milk; mothers and infants were reunited upon hospital discharge, usually 1 to 2 days after delivery.

In 1977 a series of innovations were initiated, as indicated in Table III. A partial rooming-in system was progressively developed after September 1977, with an ensuing increase in breast-feeding. The measure consisted of leaving the approximately 95% of normal infants with their mothers during the day (Figure 2). Infants born at night stay apart from their mothers until a neonatologist examines them. If they are found normal, they stay with their mothers during the day for the remainder of the hospitalization. Preterm, high-risk, and other very ill neonates (about 5%) are separated from their mothers and kept in an adjoining ward under supervision.

A milk bank was established in December 1977 and January 1978 adjacent to the rooming-in ward. Mothers and staff are very appreciative of the Syster Majas and Schuco breast pumps (Figure 3). The machines often serve to demonstrate the obvious to mothers: that they do produce colostrum and milk. Since most women do not undergo nipple massage before delivery, the pump may be of help in nipple formation and lactation stimulation. We believe the pumps have been important in assuring certain mothers of their capacity to lactate.[18] Donation of colostrum is carried out before or after the mother has breast-fed her own infant for the first time. However, emphasis is on suction of colostrum by the infant itself, and this often occurs on the delivery table, or soon after rooming-in is effected. The program has also encouraged feeding hos-

Table III. Interventions in the Gynecology and Obstetrics Service, San Juan De Dios Hospital, 1977–1980

Intervention	Date of onset	Description	Approximate percent of population exposed
A. Mother–infant separation; formula-feeding	1969–1976	a. Brief visual contact at delivery; total separation during hospitalization b. Infants fed glucose solution and milk formulae	100%
B. Rooming-in	September 1977	a. Infants stayed with mothers for about 8 hours per day; infants separated at night	66% (in 1977) 95% (in 1978+)
C. Colostrum; promotion of breast-feeding	January 1978	a. Colostrum and milk given to preterm and high-risk neonates b. Education of nurses and mothers on lactation practices	50% (mid-1978) 95% (in 1979+)
D. Early stimulation	July 1979	a. Skin-to-skin contact b. Suction of nipple shortly after birth c. Physical contact of mothers and preterm and high-risk neonates	50% (end 1979) 75% (in 1980+)

pitalized infants their own mother's milk; nursing mothers from the hospital staff use the pumps to extract their own milk during working hours. Some of these women have donated milk and some have breast-fed infants other than their own under special circumstances. This intervention has been very successful. Mothers transfer breast-feeding techniques to newcomers; the hospital environment has improved, and a relaxed and optimistic atmosphere prevails.

In 1978 a colostrum program for all neonates was initiated. For high-risk neonates who had hyaline membrane disease (HMD), congenital abnormalities, birth trauma, infections, or other pathology, and remained in the hospital for varying lengths of time, pooled fresh colostrum and milk were obtained by breast-pump extraction from donating postpartum women and mothers of hospitalized infants and fed to neonates in varying amounts of about 5 ml per kg of body weight per day.

Colostrum is administered by tube or bottle as soon as 4 hours after birth; some very ill infants may receive colostrum at a later time. Normal neonates (about 95% of the total population) suckle colostrum from their own mothers, a situation favored by the partial rooming-in system established the preceding year and availability of breast-pumps. By the middle of 1978, breast-feeding in this hospital had become almost universal.

A program of early stimulation of mother–infant bonding was started in 1979 and covered about one-half of the mother–infant pairs by the end of the year. Newborns are given to their mothers in the delivery room, although in many instances the infants are already clothed. Eye-to-eye contact, and stimulation of the infant's mouth and maternal nipple are emphasized by nurses attending in the delivery room, but this is not universally practiced. The program has not been wholly successful due, in great part, to the firmly established tradition of separation of mother and infant immediately after delivery, lack of knowledge on the importance of mother–infant interaction, alleged limitations to space and time by the nursing staff, and similar reasons. In 1979 a professional member from INISA commenced interviews of mothers and provided assistance

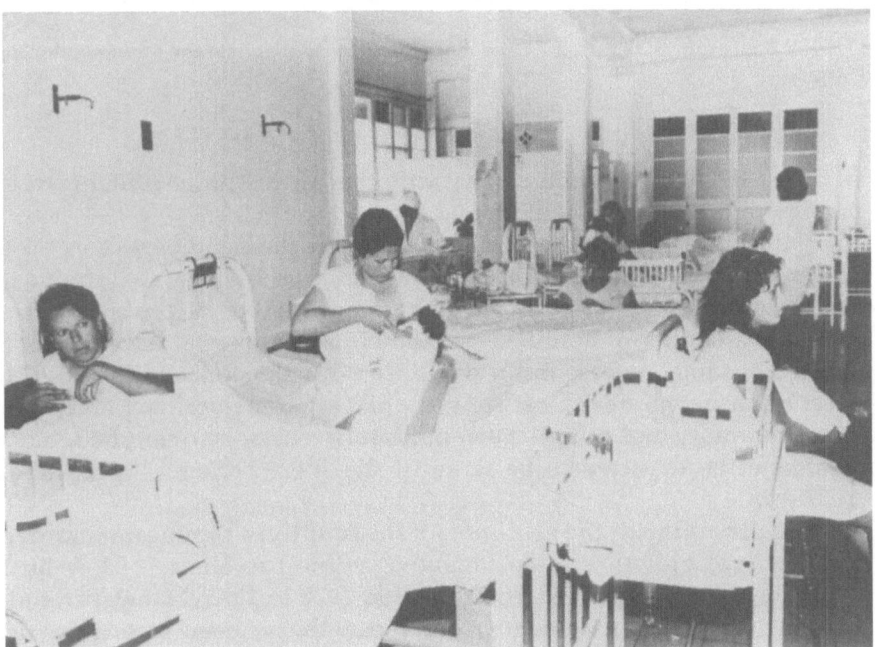

Figure 2. Rooming-in at the San Juan de Dios Hospital.

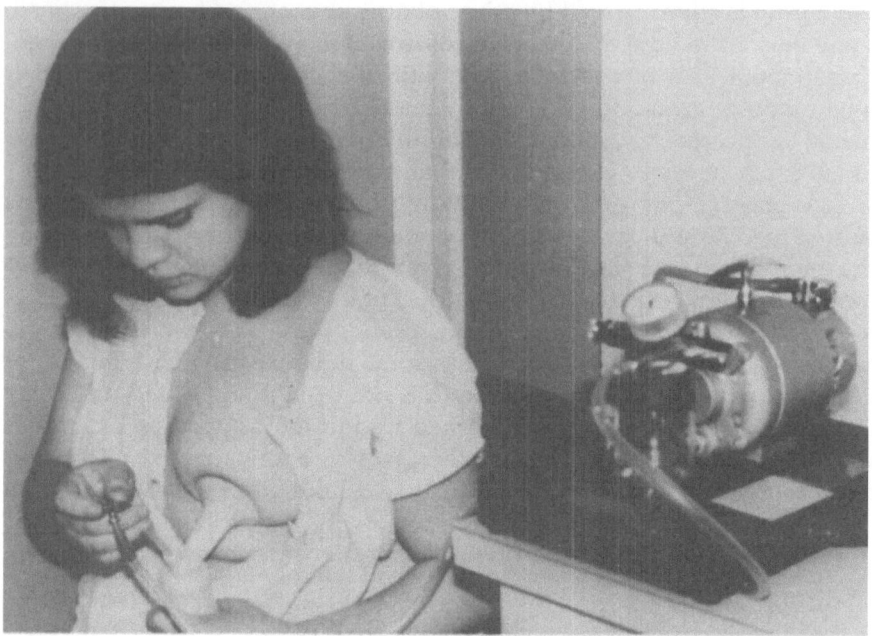

Figure 3. Colostrum is extracted with a mechanical breast pump at the San Juan de Dios Hospital.

in breast-feeding techniques. The activities of this professional focused mainly on the mothers of Puriscal.

Other interventions were effected during the same period, as Costa Rica is a country in rapid transition and continuously tries to improve its health care delivery system. An increasing number of physicians and greater availability of qualified personnel in the hospital have probably resulted in some increase in survival for high-risk neonates. The possible effect of improved health care and sophisticated medical technology on infant mortality and other health indicators cannot be quantified, but it would not be expected to be large in the short period of observation (1977–1981).

Concordant with the evolution of the country, a significant improvement in fetal growth was documented, as the prevalence of low birth weight fell from 9.2 to 7.5% in the period 1970 to 1975.[19] However, only a slight further improvement in fetal growth has been recorded since then (unpublished data).

THE PURISCAL STUDY

The planning of the study began in 1976; recruitment of cases in the hospital and in the field began in September 1979 and paralleled and inspired some of the hospital interventions mentioned above. The Puriscal study is a long-term, prospective observation of mothers and infants predominantly of Spanish and, to a lesser extent, Spanish-Amerindian descent. The population lives partly in the district centers, partly dispersed in valleys and hills surrounding the centers. The localities are "rural dispersed" if they have fewer than 500 people, or "rural concentrated" if they have 500 to 2000 people. The population yields from 600 to 650 newborns per year, and the aim of the study is to include at least two complete yearly cohorts. Although traditionalism and ruralism are still prevalent, the social development of Puriscal and most of rural Costa Rica is significantly high if compared with populations where long-term studies have also been conducted—i.e., in Tezonteopan and Tláltizapán, Mexico,[20,21] Santa María Cauqué, Guatemala,[22] Khanna and Narangwal in India,[23,24] and Matlab, in Bangladesh.[25] However, ruralism in Puriscal is more marked than in the Guatemalan and Mexican villages, and distances between houses may require several hours of walking through forests and fields, while some houses may be more than 2 km from the nearest school.

Many Puriscal mothers are included in the study through prenatal clinics; others are included in connection with delivery; a few are entered at a later date. About 84% of deliveries occur in the San Juan de Dios Hospital, 13% occur in other maternity units and clinics in San José, and 3% occur in the home, a situation contrasting with that of traditional villages in which most births occur at home.

Adequate coordination between our office at the hospital and other hospitals and clinics allows the staff of the field station to know about most deliveries in Puriscal. Inevitably, our personnel at the hospital pay more attention to these women, and stimulation of mothers and infants by a neonatologist, a social scientist, and a nurse should favor bonding and breast-feeding.

Because Puriscal women are harder to reach in their widely dispersed homes, mothers are interviewed while in the hospital. This contact also serves to further stimulate mothers to breast-feed. The base of operations for the medical officer, nurses, health workers, dietary technicians, and other staff is the INISA Field Station in Santiago de Puriscal. Coordination with health workers from the Ministry of Health for coverage of the highly scattered population has been required. Rural motor

Table IV. Subcohorts of the Puriscal Study, 1979–1981

Subcohort districts[b]		Type of population	Field intervention[c]
1.1 (114)[a]	Grifo Alto Barbacoas Candelarita	Rural dispersed	a. Visit by INISA's field worker within 10 days postpartum b. Contact with INISA's physician c. Monthly visits by INISA's field workers
1.2 (308)	Mercedes Sur Desamparaditos San Antonio San Rafael	Rural dispersed	a. Monthly visits by health workers from Ministry of Health b. Occasional contact with INISA's physician
1.3 (190)	Santiago	Rural concentrated, rural dispersed	a. Occasional contact with health personnel from Social Security, Ministry of Health, and INISA

[a]Number of infants born into subcohort.
[b]See text and Figure 1.
[c]Infants in all subcohorts were equally stimulated in the hospital (see text).

vehicles, motorcycles, and horses are used, but surveillance still includes foot travel in each instance.

The cohort comprised 612 infants 1 year after the study began, distributed in three subcohorts according to the type and intensity of intervention and prospective observation (Table IV and Figure 1). All mother–infant pairs were similarly treated in the hospital (Table III). Those of the rural dispersed districts of Grifo Alto, Barbacoas, and Candelarita (subcohort 1.1) were visited within the first 10 days postpartum and then were studied by the physician and health nurses through monthly consultations. Visits served to collect data on physical growth, breast-feeding, food intake, and morbidity.

Mother–infant pairs of four other districts (Mercedes Sur, Desamparaditos, San Antonio, and San Rafael, constituting subcohort 1.2), equally rural and dispersed, were visited monthly by the staff of the Ministry of Health, coordinated by INISA, to collect information on breast-feeding and physical growth. Contact with INISA's physician and field staff was less than for subcohort 1.1. Mother–infant pairs of Santiago, the central district of Puriscal (subcohort 1.3), both rural dispersed and concentrated, attended the health services of the locality and had more access to resources of the region and the capital city. They could consult with INISA's personnel, but monthly visits were primarily coordinated through the staffs of the Social Security and Ministry of Health.

Standard forms and procedures were used to collect data in all districts within the epidemiologic framework of a long-term prospective study.

Results

Incidence of Breast-Feeding in the Hospital. Prior to the interventions at the San Juan de Dios Hospital, most infants did not receive colostrum and were not breast-fed while in the hospital. About 20 to 30% of infants did not breast-feed, a figure in accord with the 24% of rural infants who were not breast-fed at all in Costa Rica in 1978 (Table II). This apparently resulted from the drastic separation of mother and infant and the lack of support of the mother during hospitalization. The current interventions resulted in about 95% of infants being given the breast to receive colostrum soon after birth, in agreement with the theory of bonding and lactation induction.[2,4,7]

Postpartum Breast-Feeding in Puriscal. Rates of breast-feeding after hospital discharge were computed for the population of Puriscal newborns delivered in the San Juan de Dios Hospital. Extreme differences in the rate of breast-feeding in all Puriscal subcohorts, as compared with rural Costa Rica in 1978, became evident (Table II and Figure 4). The Puriscal data in Figure 4 represent prevalences of monthly observations for all

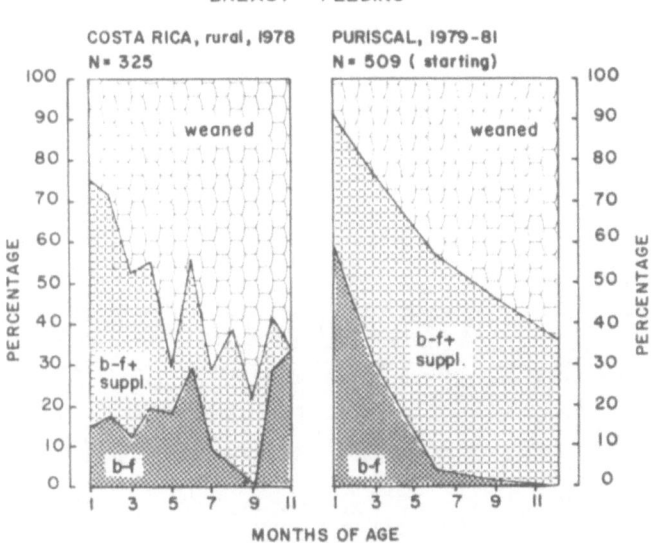

BREAST - FEEDING

Figure 4. At left is the prevalence of breast-feeding in rural Costa Rica, 1978. Data from the national nutrition survey[16] were derived from a representative sample that included the region of Puriscal. At the right is the cumulative prevalence of breast-feeding among the subcohorts of the Puriscal study.

infants of the three subcohorts combined, consisting of 509 newborns 1 month old, 513 3 months old, 454 6 months old, 294 9 months old, and 86 infants 1 year old—a natural attrition because the subcohorts were growing older. In the first months of life, breast-fed infants in Puriscal may receive small amounts of orange juice and fluid and semisolid foods, and this could account for the low rate of exclusive breast-feeding, as illustrated in Figure 4. Significant food supplementation (ablactation) begins at 3 to 4 months for many infants. This also includes cow's milk or other formula milks. Our criteria to define exclusive breast-feeding are more stringent than those used in the 1978 survey. The important consideration is that only 9% of infants did not breast-feed as compared with a 24% weaning rate in rural Costa Rica in 1978 (Figure 4).

A contrast is noted when the prevalence of breast-feeding in rural Costa Rica in 1978 is compared with that of subcohort 1.1 (stimulated by INISA's personnel, as indicated above). Only 7% of infants in this subcohort were weaned by 1 month of age, while at 6 months, more than 60% were still at the breast (Figure 5). The prevalence of exclusive breast-feeding was also greater in subcohort 1.1 than in the others.

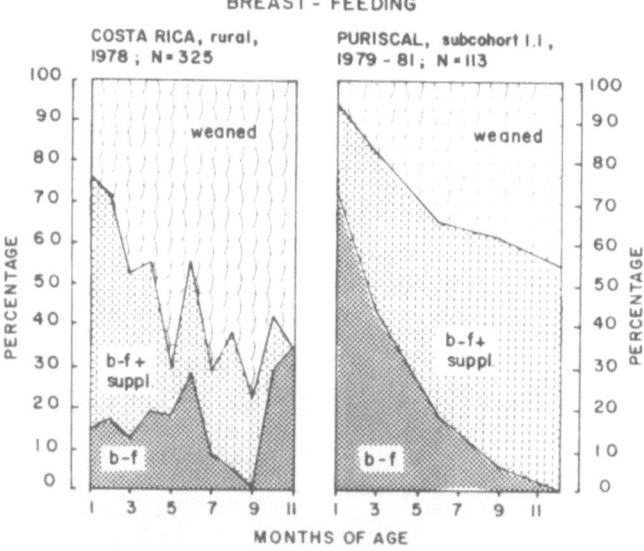

Figure 5. At left is the prevalence of breast-feeding in rural Costa Rica, 1978, as in Figure 4. At right is the prevalence of breast-feeding in subcohort 1.1, where a postpartum prospective observation is made by INISA's field workers. Note that a significantly greater number of infants were breast-fed in this subcohort as compared with the total cohort population (see Figure 4).

Although there should not have been any reason for the Puriscal population to adopt improved lactation practices before our intervention began compared to the rest of the rural Costa Rican area, a retrospective survey of the siblings of cohort infants was undertaken. The survey included siblings under 6 years of age, and therefore the data correspond to the period 1975 to 1979, that is, before the Puriscal study was established. The prevalence of breast-feeding in all subcohorts (data corresponding to 1, 3, 6, 9, and 12 months were used for all children who were at least 1 year old) was significantly greater than that of their siblings (Figure 6). A more stringent criterion of defining exclusive breast-feeding in the current study may have accounted for the lower prevalence in the cohort infants than in the siblings.

Since subcohort 1.1 exhibited the greatest prevalence of breast-feeding, a comparison was made with the siblings of infants in this group (Figure 7). All siblings of subcohort 1.1 infants were surveyed. Again, the prevalence was significantly greater for cohort infants than for the corresponding siblings.

Subcohort 1.3 is the least rural of the three and received less stimu-

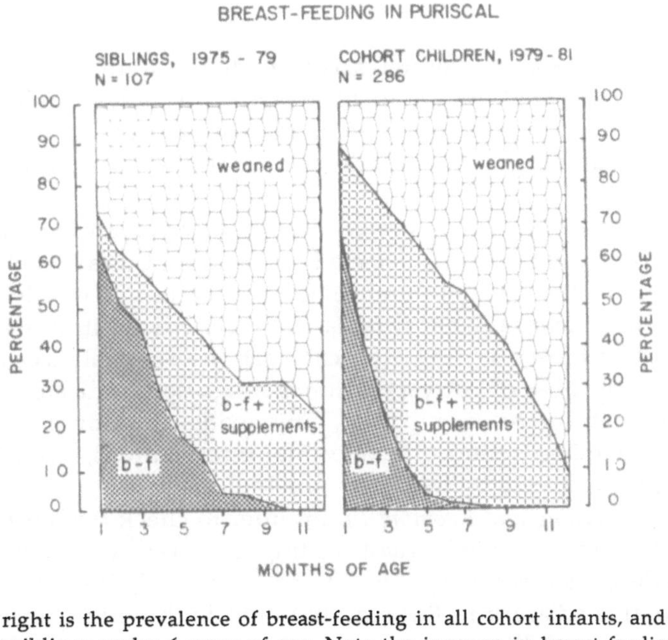

BREAST-FEEDING IN PURISCAL

SIBLINGS, 1975 - 79
N = 107

COHORT CHILDREN, 1979 - 81
N = 286

MONTHS OF AGE

Figure 6. At right is the prevalence of breast-feeding in all cohort infants, and at left is that of their siblings under 6 years of age. Note the increase in breast-feeding among infants of the Puriscal study.

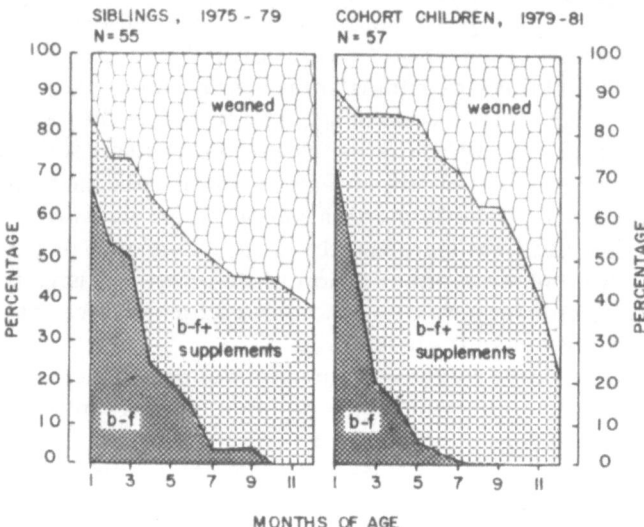

BREAST-FEEDING, SUBCOHORT I.I

Figure 7. At right is the prevalence of breast-feeding for infants of subcohort 1.1 only, and at left is the prevalence in the corresponding siblings under 6 years of age.

lation from INISA's personnel, according to the study design. The prevalence of breast-feeding in this subcohort again showed an improved situation in the current study population compared with the siblings (Figure 8), although the difference was less than that in the other subcohorts.

It is evident that there is significantly more breast-feeding in Puriscal now compared to levels detected for the rural Costa Rican population as a whole in 1978. The difference becomes more noteworthy for subcohort 1.1, which was further stimulated by periodic visits of field workers interested in breast-feeding. The comparison of prevalences in the subcohorts with those of corresponding siblings does indicate an improvement over the preceding period. This evidence strongly suggests an effect of rooming-in and other hospital interventions, strengthened by periodic surveillance by field personnel.[2,3,7]

Breast-Feeding and Rooming-In. In order to check further the relation of bonding to improved breast-feeding practices, a prevalence survey was made in two rural regions similar to Puriscal. One (Acosta, Aserri, and Mora) is adjacent to Puriscal, but outside the influence of the field intervention of INISA; most women of this region deliver at the San Juan de Dios Hospital, and therefore mothers and infants are affected by the

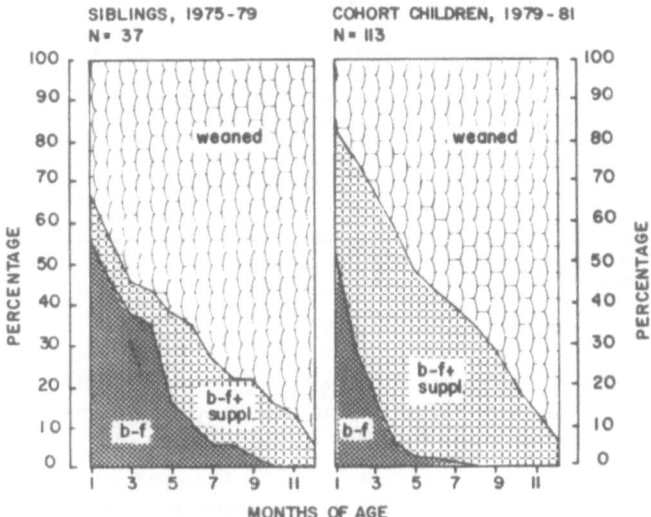

Figure 8. At right is the prevalence of breast-feeding for infants of subcohort 1.3 only, and at left is that of their siblings under 6 years of age.

ongoing interventions. The other (Moravia, Santo Domingo) is about 60 kilometers from Puriscal and is not influenced by INISA's field intervention either; women of this region deliver at the Calderón Guardia Hospital, where separation of mothers and infants and formula feeding of neonates is the norm.[18] The community survey results in Table V clearly show a high rate of early weaning among all infants separated from their mothers soon after birth. Furthermore, most infants had been completely weaned by 9 months of age. This finding is in support of observations on the effect of bonding on breast-feeding.[9,26]

Neonatal Morbidity. A significant reduction in neonatal morbidity of infectious origin was recorded in the population of live-borns during the observation period (Table VI).[27] Data were from clinical records corresponding to the first few days of life and covered all newborns at the San Juan de Dios Hospital, including those of Puriscal. The decline in morbidity was more striking for diarrheal disease and meningitis. Such a reduction was probably not influenced by improved medical attention, but rather by the colostrum program and promotion of bonding, as shown by Larguía's group in Argentina.[28,29]

A decline in the incidence of hyaline membrane disease (HMD) was also noted (Table VII). HMD appeared at a rate similar to that reported

Table V. Breast-Feeding by Hospital Practice, Two Rural Areas of Costa Rica, 1980

Age (months)	Acosta-Aserrí-Mora (incomplete rooming-in[a])		Moravia-Sto. Domingo (no rooming-in[b])	
	Number	% at breast	Number	% at breast
0–3	43	86	31	77
4–7	40	78	49	35
8–11	25	52	40	10

[a]San Juan de Dios Hospital and Carit Institute.
[b]Dr. Calderón Guardia Hospital.

in the medical literature and in accord with the 7.7% rate of prematurity (less than 37 weeks of gestation) before the hospital interventions began. While the frequency of prematurity had declined to 5.1% (a 34% reduction from 1976 to 1979), this does not seem to explain the 56% decrease in the incidence of HMD in the period. Administration of cortisol to high-risk pregnant women is not practiced for all women; it would not have accounted for the total reduction recorded. It appears possible that colostrum has a maturing effect on preterm infants that may help prevent HMD. Colostrum and breast milk might promote or support maturation phenomena, especially because the newborn is an immature, exterogestate fetus.[1] This possibility, currently under investigation, would help explain excess rates of HMD where newborns are customarily deprived of colostrum.

Table VI. Neonatal Morbidity Attributed to Infection, San Juan de Dios Hospital

Year	Intervention[a]	Number of live births	Cases per 1000 live births			
			Diarrheal disease	Sepsis	Lower respiratory infection	Meningitis
1976	A	7629	135(17.7)	41(5.4)	32(4.2)	10(1.3)
1977	B	8582	71(8.3)	52(6.1)	35(4.1)	5(0.6)
1978	B + C	8931	62(6.9)	29(3.2)	27(3.0)	12(1.3)
1979	B + C + D	8638	55(6.4)	28(3.2)	18(4.9)	0
1980	B + C + D	8963	14(1.6)	NA[b]	22(2.4)	1(0.1)
% reduction in rates 1976–1979			91		43	92

[a]See Table III and text.
[b]NA = not yet available

Table VII. Hyaline Membrane Disease (HMD), San Juan de Dios Hospital

| | | | Number (%) of | Hyaline membrane disease | | |
| | | Number of live | infants < 37-week | Observed | Observed | Observed minus expected case rates |
Year[a]	Intervention[b]	births	gestation	cases (%)	deaths (%)	as %[d]
1976	A	7629	589(7.7)	154(2.0)[c]-	47(0.62)[c]	0
1977	B	8582	618(7.2)	161(1.9)	37(0.43)	−5.0
1978	B + C	8931	597(6.7)	133(1.5)	32(0.36)	−25.0
1979	B + C + D	8638	437(5.1)	85(1.0)	31(0.36)	−50.0
% reduction in rates 1976–1979						
			33.8	50.0	41.9	

[a]In 1978 most moderate and severe cases were transferred to the National Children's Hospital; they are excluded from these statistics.
[b]See Table III and test for description and timing of interventions.
[c]In parentheses, percent cases or deaths among total infants.
[d]Arbitrarily, the 1976 rate (2.0%) was assumed to be the expected value for the following years.

Neonatal Mortality. Expectedly, a decrease in neonatal mortality of infectious origin should also have occurred (Table VIII). This was computed only from deaths in the hospital. Most neonatal deaths occur in the first few hours or days of life, and since many high-risk and preterm babies remain hospitalized, the figures should be close to accurate.[27] No deaths from diarrhea, lower respiratory tract infection, or meningitis have been recorded since 1979, in accord with the known antiinfectious protection afforded by colostrum.[1,3,5–7,28–30]

Other causes of neonatal death remained relatively unaltered, as

Table VIII. Neonatal Mortality Attributed to Infection, San Juan de Dios Hospital

Year	Intervention[a]	Diarrheal disease	Sepsis	Lower respiratory infection	Meningitis	Total
1976	A	3(3.9)[b]	7(9.2)	4(5.2)	2(2.6)	16(20.9)
1977	B	1(1.2)	9(10.5)	6(7.0)	2(2.3)	18(20.9)
1978	B + C	0	4(4.5)	1(1.1)	4(4.5)	9(10.1)
1979	B + C + D	0	4(4.6)	0	0	4(4.6)
1980	B + C + D	0	4(4.5)	0	0	4(4.5)
% reduction in rates						
1976–1980		100	51	100	100	78

[a]See Table III and text.
[b]Deaths (rate per 10,000 live births), number of live-borns as in Table VI.

shown in Table IX for congenital defects. Deaths associated with immaturity decreased by 38%, in accord with the gradual reduction in the incidence of low-birth-weight infants in the country.[19] In this regard, the
percent incidence of HMD decreased as a cause of death by 71%, in agreement with the 50% reduction in incidence of HMD (see above). Since
better systems to cope with the high-risk mother and with the disease
would not likely be solely responsible for this marked decline, other
explanations must be sought; for instance, the possibility that colostrum
has a maturing capacity that prevents HMD in some infants and ameliorates it in others.

Infant Mortality in Puriscal. The evolution of infant mortality in Puriscal is shown in Table X, next to the interventions that might have
affected it, and in comparison with the national figures. Only two deaths
of cohort infants, both occurring in the first week of life, were recorded.
Monitoring survival was by monthly visits of all cohort infants. Furthermore, the records of hospitals and clinics where infants might have been
taken to die were examined. More than one-half of infants were 1 year
old (cohorts recruited from September 19, 1979, through September 18,
1980), and the remaining were older than 6 months at the time of the
present analysis. No additional deaths were likely to occur. An infant
mortality rate of 4 per 1000 live births for Puriscal is 82% less than the
national figure and 50% less than the Puriscal rate before the Puriscal
study began. Before the rooming-in, colostrum, and early stimulation
interventions, the difference between the national infant mortality and
that of Puriscal had remained rather constant.

Table IX.   Main Attributed Causes of Neonatal Deaths, San Juan de Dios Hospital

		Deaths per 1000 live births				
Year	Intervention[a]	Acute infections	Immaturity	Congenital defects	Asphyxia	Hyaline membrane disease
1976	A	16(2.1)[b]	30(3.9)	9(1.2)	14(1.8)	46(6.0)
1977	B	18(2.1)	51(2.9)	13(1.5)	25(2.9)	37(4.3)
1978	B + C	9(1.0)	29(3.2)	10(1.1)	33(3.7)	32(3.6)
1979	B + C + D	7(0.8)	31(3.6)	12(1.4)	39(4.5)	31(3.6)
1980	B + C + D	8(0.9)	22(2.4)	15(1.7)	26(2.9)	16(1.8)
% reduction in rates 1976–1980		57.1	38			71[c]

[a]See Table III and text.
[b]Deaths (rate per 1000 live births), number of live-borns as in Table VI.
[c]Percent reduction in rates 1976–1979, because severe cases of HMD after 1979 were quickly referred to the National Children's Hospital.

Table X. Infant Mortality Per 1000 Live Births

Year	Rate per 1000 live births		Percent difference C.R.-Puriscal	Intervention[b]
	Costa Rica	Puriscal		
1970	61	49	20	
1973	45	30	33	Rural health (RH)
1975	37	28	24	RH + supplementary feeding (SF)
1977	27	15	44	RH + SF + rooming-in (B)
1980	22[a]	4	82	RH + SF + B + colostrum + early stimulation[c]

[a]Estimated.
[b]For description of interventions see Table III and text.
[c]Affects about 95% of Puriscal infants, or about 13% of infants nationwide.

It is worth noting here that several social, economic, and health measures have been under way in Costa Rica for several years, and they have influenced, and are still influencing, the decline in infant deaths in the country. Among the health interventions, the Rural Health Program and the Nutrition Program (feeding centers) cover more than 80% of the dispersed rural population. The Rural Health Program emphasizes primary health care[31] and should not have strongly affected survival in the neonatal period. The Feeding Program emphasizes food distribution for preschool children,[32] but evidently infants have not been a target. Thus, the rooming-in, colostrum and breast-feeding, and early stimulation interventions are most probably responsible for a considerable part of the remarkable increase in survival, as infant mortality in Puriscal is now considerably below the national figure, and even below that of developed urban areas of Costa Rica (unpublished data).

Child Abandonment. Since there appears to be a relationship between bonding and breast-feeding and an increased capacity of the mother to protect the infant, the rate of abandonment was investigated. A significant reduction in abandonment of normal term infants was demonstrated,[33] correlated with rooming-in, skin-to-skin proximity, and breast-feeding interventions (Table XI). The decline in abandonment of hospitalized infants with some form of pathology was less, but nevertheless significant, and in accord with the theory of bonding.[2,9,26,34] A reduction in abandoned children prevents malnutrition and premature death, as well as the complications stemming from the social pathology that often surrounds abandoned children.

Resistance to Infection. The significant increase in prevalence of breast-feeding in Puriscal, especially in subcohort 1.1, should have been

Table XI.   Nosocomial Interventions and Child Abandonment,[a] San Juan de
Dios Hospital

Period (October–September)	Intervention	Condition of infant		
		Term	Ill[a]	Total
1976–1977 $N = 8988^b$	A	9(10.0)[c]	10(11.1)	19(21.1)
1977–1978 $N = 9143$	B	3 (3.3)	7 (7.7)	10(10.9)
1978–1979 $N = 8737$	B + C	1 (1.1)	5 (5.7)	6 (6.9)
1979–1980 $N = 8972$	B + C + D	1 (1.1)	5 (5.6)	6 (6.7)
% reduction in rates 1976-1980		89	50	68

[a]Seven infants were abandoned because of maternal death, mental illness, or mental retardation; they were excluded from table.
[b]Number of infants varied from those in preceding tables because they were computed for the period October–September.
[c]Infants abandoned (rate per 10,000 live births).
[d]Hospitalized, preterm, or with various pathologies.

accompanied by an increased protection against enteric infection, an improved capacity to recover from diarrhea and dehydration, better nutrition, and a better state of health derived from the direct benefits of breast milk,[1,5,6] as well as indirect effects, such as increased sharing of time with the infant and a greater degree of parental affection and care.[7] In fact, weight gain in Puriscal infants with rotavirus diarrhea varied according to feeding regimens.[18] Among infants with similar birth weights, the weaned tended to exhibit a larger negative response to rotavirus diarrhea than the supplemented, and in turn had a greater negative response than the exclusively breast-fed, taking age into account. Furthermore, the incidence of diarrhea for subcohort 1.1, which received the benefit of support from our health personnel, was significantly smaller than that of subcohort 1.2, which did not.[18]

Physical Growth. The relationship of feeding pattern and weight gain was explored for all infants of subcohorts 1.1 and 1.3 who were at least 1 year old and who had rather complete anthropometric data at birth and at 3, 6, 9, and 12 months. Low-birth-weight infants (less than 2.5 kg) were not included in the analysis. Mean weights were contrasted for breast-fed (including those receiving supplements) and weaned infants with the 25th and 50th percentiles of the NCHS-CDC (Fels Research Institute) curves[35] (Tables XII and XIII). Supplementation in this society often begins at 3 months; by 6 months most infants already receive supplements to breast milk. The weight of breast-fed infants was slightly better, as a group, than that of non-breast-fed infants at 3 and 6 months. At 12

Table XII. Weight of Infants from Birth to 12 Months, by Type of Feeding, Puriscal (Subcohort 1.1), 1979–1981

Age (months)	At the breast[a] (N) $\bar{x}$ weight, kg	Weaned (N) $\bar{x}$ weight, kg	Breast–weaned difference, kg	Fels Research Institute 25th P	50th P
Boys					
Birth	(21)3.19			3.06	3.40
3	(18)6.43	(3)5.75	+0.68	5.35	6.01
6	(15)7.94	(6)7.52	+0.42	7.17	8.50
9	(12)8.71	(9)9.04	−0.33	8.59	9.28
12	(11)9.35	(6)10.15	−0.80	9.51	10.10
Girls					
Birth	(14)3.15			2.89	3.25
3	(14)5.86			4.86	5.41
6	(13)7.47	(1)7.80	−0.33	6.61	7.20
9	(11)8.40	(2)8.70	−0.30	7.89	8.54
12	(6)9.32	(4)9.30	+0.02	8.81	9.57

[a]Supplementation generally was started at 3 months.

Table XIII. Weight of Infants from Birth to 12 Months, by Type of Feeding, Puriscal (Subcohort 1.3), 1979–1981

Age (months)	At the breast (N) $\bar{x}$ weight, kg	Weaned (N) $\bar{x}$ weight, kg	Breast-weaned difference, kg	Fels Research Institute 25th P	50th P
Boys					
Birth	(18)3.15			3.06	3.40
3	(10)6.55	(9)6.02	+0.53	5.35	6.01
6	(4)8.01	(14)7.80	+0.21	7.17	8.50
9	(4)8.81	(13)9.13	−0.32	8.59	9.28
12	(3)9.93	(14)9.83	+0.10	9.51	10.10
Girls					
Birth	(34)3.24			2.89	3.25
3	(26)5.83	(6)5.53	+0.30	4.86	5.41
6	(21)7.61	(13)7.31	+0.30	6.61	7.20
9	(11)8.63	(23)8.55	+0.08	7.89	8.54
12	(8)9.39	(21)9.55	−0.16	8.81	9.57

[a]Supplementation generally was started a 3 months.

months, the weight for the weaned was, as a group, similar to that of the breast-fed group, except weaned boys of subcohort 1.1, who, at 12 months, were slightly heavier than breast-fed boys. These differences were not significant. It should be kept in mind that breast-fed infants shifted to the weaned group as they got older. The important consideration is that, during the critical first 6 months of life, breast-fed infants fared better compared with the reference standard than did weaned children.

COMMENT

Rural infants in Puriscal and many other localities of Costa Rica live under much better socioeconomic conditions than those in other developing areas of the world. Central and local governments have promoted construction of water supplies and latrines and have developed health education programs and an adequate infrastructure of health services.[27,36,37]

Puriscal, like most of rural Costa Rica, had experienced a decline in breast-feeding, revealed by recent surveys.[10,16] With this background, interventions were started to promote breast-feeding in an attempt to diminish morbidity and mortality caused by diarrhea. The reason to intervene in the maternity ward stems from the known effect of early mother–infant interaction on breast-feeding and bonding that influences child growth, performance, and survival.[2,4,7,9] Most Puriscal infants are delivered at the San Juan de Dios Hospital. The interventions effected in hospital cannot be considered optimal, since complete skin-to-skin contact and complete rooming-in were not attained; however, they seemed capable of inducing an increased incidence of breast-feeding, and an apparently related reduction in perinatal morbidity and mortality and child abandonment. A significant reduction in the rate of diarrhea had already been demonstrated by Larguía and co-workers[28,29] after administration of colostrum to neonates.

A decrease in incidence of HMD suggests that colostrum and human milk may have an effect on maturation that prevents or ameliorates this disease. This hypothesis could explain the relatively high rate of lethal HMD in nations where neonates do not receive colostrum.

The influence of early mother–infant stimulation apparently was effective for several months postpartum. While a control was not established beforehand, mainly because such striking changes were not anticipated, prevalence surveys conducted in other localities showed similar results if mothers delivered infants in the hospital where the interventions were effected. Furthermore, prevalence surveys in similar rural localities served by another hospital, where separation of mothers and infants is the norm, revealed a high incidence of early weaning, a much deteriorated situation as compared with Puriscal, and as bad as or worse than that of rural Costa Rica 1 year prior to the interventions and the beginning of the Puriscal study. Stimulation by field workers also seems important, since differences were noted in the incidence of breast-feeding within the cohort population of Puriscal, in that breast-feeding was more prevalent in subcohort 1.1, where mothers were in closer contact with our field staff. It should be stressed that information on feeding practices was obtained on a monthly basis, employing the same procedure for interview and data-recording for all populations studied.

In addition to improved breast-feeding, there was a lower rate of diarrheal disease in breast-fed than in weaned infants. Furthermore, diarrhea had a greater negative effect on growth in weaned than in breast-fed infants,[18] and the incidence of diarrhea was in general low in the population of breast-fed infants.

The two deaths observed were neonatal, accounting for the very low infant mortality. Puriscal has enjoyed a marked improvement in health, as have other rural areas of Costa Rica[31,36,37] and may be deriving further gains from its distinct ruralism.[38] Nevertheless, the virtual absence of postneonatal infant deaths among 1000 consecutive newborns in about 18 months of prospective observation strongly suggests an effect of interventions in the hospital and in the Puriscal study. Survival has been carefully monitored, including all infants in emigrating families. Additional infant deaths might occur, but even if they double, the infant mortality would still be below the expected rate.

The hospital interventions are not expensive, except for the breast pumps, but two pumps can serve an obstetrics service attending 8000 deliveries per year. The field intervention is expensive because it is part of an ongoing, long-term, prospective field study. The intervention could become incorporated into the duties of existing health personnel.

The significant improvement in breast-feeding in this transitional society, the lower attack rate of diarrheal diseases, diminished rate of abandonment, and increased survival are findings that should prompt implementation of measures to promote bonding, breast-feeding, and nutrition, especially in developing nations undergoing transition and experiencing an increase in institutionalized childbirth, consumption of formula milk, and other ills disruptive of mother–infant health and well-being.

ACKNOWLEDGMENTS

Aid has been obtained from the Vice-Rectorship of Research Affairs of the University of Costa Rica, the Ministry of Health, the Social Security System, and the president's office. Also, support was obtained from the U.S.A.I.D. (Loan 515-T-026), the British O.D.A., and the National Council for Scientific Research and Technology (CONICIT). The cooperation of Drs. Hernán Collado, Max Terán, and José Rafael Araya (San Juan de Dios Hospital, Costa Rica) and of Drs. Guillermo Contreras and Carlos Díaz (Ministry of Health, Costa Rica) is fully appreciated. The technical assistance of the personnel of INISA, the San Juan de Dios Hospital, and the Ministry of Health is recognized, especially that of R.N. Nancy Sabean, Lic. Francisco Sánchez, Dr. Marcela Vives, Louis Blanco, Eliceth León, Teresa Arce, Enilda Campos, Ana C. Vargas, María M. Jiménez, Carlos Rodríguez, and Giovanna Carrillo.

REFERENCES

1. Jelliffe, D. B., and Jelliffe, E. F. P. The uniqueness of human milk. Symposium. *Am. J. Clin. Nutr.* **24**:968, 1971.
2. Porter, R., and O'Connor, M. Parent-infant interaction, Ciba Foundation Symposium No. 33 (new series). Elsevier/Excerpta Medica, Amsterdam, 1975.
3. Elliot, K., and Knight, J. Acute diarrhoea in childhood, Ciba Foundation Symposium No. 42 (new series). Elsevier/Excerpta, Amsterdam, 1976.
4. Elliott, K., and Fitzsimons, D. W. Breast-feeding and the mother, Ciba Foundation Symposium No. 46 (new series). Elsevier/Excerpta, Amsterdam, 1976.
5. Hambraeus, L., and Hanson, L. A. Food and immunology, Swedish Nutrition Foundation Symposium No. 12. Stockholm, 1977.
6. Waletzky, L. R. Symposium on human lactation. DHEW Pub. No. (HSA) 79-5107, Washington, D.C., 1979.
7. Jelliffe, D. B., and Jelliffe, E. F. P. Human milk in the modern world. Psychological, nutritional and economic significance. Oxford University Press, New York, 1978.
8. Puffer, R. R., and Serrano, C. V. *Patterns of Mortality in Childhood*, PAHO Sci. Pub. No. 262, Washington, D.C., 1973.
9. Klaus, M. H., and Kennell, J. H. Maternal-infant bonding. C. V. Mosby, St. Louis, 1976.
10. Díaz, C., Brenes, H., Córdoba, M., García, P., and Quirós, J. Encuesta nacional antropométrica y de hábitos alimentarios en Costa Rica. Ministry of Health, Costa Rica, 1975.
11. Comité Técnico de Alimentación y Nutrición (CTAN). Encuesta basal sobre la situación nutricional. Managua, Nicaragua, 1979.
12. Comité Hondureño sobre Lactancia Natural. Lactancia natural y alimentación materno-infantil en Honduras. Tegucigalpa, Honduras, 1980.
13. Rohlf, K. L. *An exploratory study of breast-feeding in Costa Rica.* Thesis, Iowa State University, Ames, 1978.

14. Popkin, B. M., Bilbsborrow, R. E., Yamamoto, M. E., and Akim, J. Breast-feeding practice in low income countries: Patterns and determinants, Carolina Population Center Papers, No. 11. University of North Carolina, October 1979.
15. Mata, L., Murillo, S., Jiménez, P., Vargas, W., Allen, M. A., and García, B. Child feeding in less developed countries. Induced breast-feeding in a transitional society. In: *Clinical Disorders in Pediatric Nutrition*. Marcel Dekker, New York, 1981, p. 35.
16. Ministerio de Salud. Encuesta nacional de nutrición 1978. Departamento de Nutrición, Ministerio de Salud, Costa Rica, 1980.
17. Mata, L. Epidemiologic perspective of diarrheal disease in Costa Rica and current efforts in control, prevention, and research. *Rev. Latinoam. Microbiol.* **23**:109, 1981.
18. Mata, L., Jiménez, P., Allen, M. A., Vargas, W., García, M. E., Urrutia, J. J., and Wyatt, R. G. Diarrhea and malnutrition: Breast-feeding intervention in a transitional population. In: *Acute Enteric Infections in Children: New Prospects for Treatment and Prevention*. Saltsjobaden, Stockholm, in T. Holme, J. Holmgren, and M. H. Merson, (Eds.), Amsterdam. Elsevier/North Holland, 1981, p. 233.
19. Mata, L., Villegas, H., Albertazzi, C., and Mohs, E. Crecimiento fetal humano en Costa Rica, 1970–75. *Rev. Biol. Trop.* **26**:431, 1978.
20. Chavez, A., and Martínez, C. *Nutrición y Desarrollo Infantil. Un Estudio Eco-etológico sobre la Problemática del Niño Campesino en una Comunidad Rural Pobre*. Interamericana, México, 1979.
21. Cravioto, J., and Delicardie, E. R. Mother-infant relationship prior to the development of clinically severe malnutrition in the child. *Proceedings of the Western Hemisphere Nutritional Congress IV.*, P. L. White and N. Selvey (Eds.) p. 127. Pub. Sc. Group, Acton, Massachusetts, 1975.
22. Mata, L. J. *The Children of Santa María Cauqué. A Prospective Field Study of Health and Growth*. M.I.T. Press, Cambridge, 1978.
23. Wyon, J. B., and Gordon, J. E. *The Khanna Study. Population Problems in the Rural Punjab*. Harvard University Press, Cambridge, 1971.
24. Kielmann, A. A., Taylor, C. E., and Parker, P. L. The Narangwal nutrition study: A summary review. *Am. J. Clin. Nutr.* **31**:2040, 1978.
25. Chen, L. C., Rahman, M., and Sarker, A. M. Epidemiology and causes of death among children in a rural area of Bangladesh. *Int. J. Epidemiol.* **9**:25–33, 1980.
26. Winikoff, B., and E. C. Baer. The obstetrician's opportunity: Translating "breast is best" from theory to practice. *Am. J. Obstet. Gynecol.* **138**:105, 1980.
27. Allen, M. A., Araya, J. R., Terán, M., Collado, H., and Mata, L. Evolución de la mortalidad neonatal en función de intervenciones nosocomiales, Hospital San Juan de Dios, 1976–1980. *Rev. Méd. Hosp. Nac. Niños* (Costa Rica) 1982.
28. Larguía, A. M., Urman, J., Ceriani, J. M., O'Donnell, A., Stoliar, O., Martínez, J. C., Buscaglia, J. C., Weils, S., Quiroga, A., and Irazu, M. Inmunidad local en el recién nacido. Primera experiencia con la administración de calostro humano a recién nacidos pretérmino. *Arch. Argent. Pediatr.* **72**:109, 1974.
29. Larguía, A. M., Urman, J., Stolinar, O. A., Ceriani, J. M., O'Donnell, A., Buscaglia, J. C., and Martínez, J. C. Fresh human colostrum for the prevention of E. coli diarrhea— A clinical experience. *J. Trop. Pediatr.* **23**:289, 1977.
30. Ogra, P. L., and Dayton, D. H. Immunology of breast milk, NICHD, NIH. Raven Press, New York, 1979.
31. Mata, L., and Mohs, E. Cambios culturales y nutricionales en Costa Rica. *Bol. Méd. Hosp. Inf.* (Méx.) **33**:579, 1976.
32. Díaz, C., and Novigrod, R. Programa nacional de nutrición. Ministerio de Salud, Costa Rica. 1980.

33. Matamoros, L., Ortiz, J., Rodríguez, M. E., and Mata, L. Estudio de 48 casos de abandono de recién nacidos, Hospital San Juan de Dios, 1976–1980. *Rev. Méd. Hosp. Nal. Niños* (Costa Rica) (in press) 1982.
34. Bowlby, J. *Attachment and Loss,* Vol. 1. Basic Books, New York, 1969.
35. National Center for Health Statistics–Center for Disease Control. NCHS growth curves for children, Birth–18 years, United States. DHEW Pub. No. (PHS) 78-1650, Washington, D.C., 1974.
36. Mohs, E. Evolution of nutrition in a transitional society: Costa Rica. In: *Nutrition in Transition.* (Proceedings of the Western Hemisphere Nutritional Congress, (P. L. White and N. Selvey, *eds.*). American Medical Association, Monroe, Wisconsin, 1978.
37. Villegas, H. Extensión y cobertura de salud en Costa Rica. *Bol. Of. Sanit. Panam.* 83:537, 1977.
38. Mata, L. Sociocultural factors in the control and prevention of parasitic diseases. *Res. Infect. Dis.* 4:871, 1982.

13

Oral Rehydration in the Treatment of Diarrhea:

Issues in the Implementation of Diarrhea Treatment Programs

RICHARD A. CASH

The purpose of this chapter is twofold: (1) to examine the modes of treatment of diarrheal disease, with particular emphasis on oral therapy, and (2) to explore the issues involved in the implementation of treatment programs, with the focus on community-based programs.

THE CLINICAL EFFECTS OF DIARRHEAL DISEASE

Acute watery diarrhea leads to deficits in water and electrolytes. Acidosis and potassium and sodium deficiency result from a loss of bicarbonate, potassium, and sodium in the stool and urine. Extracellular fluid diminishes with increasing stool loss, and the clinical signs of dehydration begin to appear. When the deficit is over 5% of the body weight, the following symptoms may begin to occur in rather rapid succession: tachycardia, decreased skin turgor, postural hypotension, oliguria, anuria, severe thirst, stupor, and finally, coma. When the deficit exceeds 10% of body weight, shock occurs. Vomiting may be present at any time in the course of the diarrhea, though it tends to be most common in the early phases of the disease. Children, especially those who are malnourished, may develop severe hypoglycemia that can lead to convulsions, coma, and death. A summary of these findings may be found in Table I.

RICHARD A. CASH • Harvard Institute for International Development, Cambridge, Massachusetts.

Table I. Assessment of Dehydration and Fluid Deficit[a]

Signs and symptoms	Mild dehydration	Moderate dehydration	Severe dehydration
General appearance			
Infants and young children	Thirsty; alert; restless	Thirsty; restless, or lethargic but irritable when touched	Drowsy; limp, cold, sweaty cyanotic extremities; may be comatose
Older children and adults	Thirsty; alert; restless	Thirsty; alert; giddiness with postural changes	Usually conscious; apprehensive; cold, sweaty, cyanotic extremities; wrinkled skin of fingers and toes; muscle cramps
Radial pulse[b]	Normal rate and volume	Rapid and weak	Rapid, feeble, sometimes impalpable
Systolic blood pressure	Normal	Normal-low	May be unrecordable
Respiration	Normal	Deep, may be rapid	Deep and rapid
Anterior fontanelle	Normal	Sunken	Very sunken
Skin elasticity[c]	Retracts immediately	Retracts slowly	Retracts very slowly
Eyes	Normal	Sunken	Deeply sunken
Mucous membranes	Moist	Dry	Very dry
Urine flow	Normal	Reduced amount and dark	None passed for several hours; empty bladder
Percent body weight loss	4–5%	6–9%	10% or more
Estimated fluid deficit	40–51 ml/kg	60–90 ml/kg	100–110 ml/kg

[a]Source: adapted from reference 2.
[b]If radial pulse cannot be felt, listen to heart with stethoscope.
[c]Not useful in marasmic malnutrition or obesity.

It is important to emphasize that the dehydration is primarily isotonic, and very few infants, especially in less developed countries, ever develop serious hypertonic dehydration (serum sodium over 160 meq/liter). The fact that hypernatremia is so uncommon in developing countries may be because most children are breast-fed; breast milk has a much lower solute load than cow's milk, and feeding volumes tend to be smaller.[1] In addition to the loss of water and electrolytes, diarrhea affects the nutritional status of the child. The nutritional effects of diarrhea are noted elsewhere, but to summarize, they may be as follows: a loss of appetite, the withholding of food and the inappropriate use of certain foods in treating the patient, the catabolic effect, direct loss of nutrients in the stool, and intestinal malabsorption.

TREATMENT

Guidelines for treatment of diarrhea have been well established and there are a number of good reviews on the subject[2-4] (Table II). Replacement of initial fluid and electrolyte deficits, continued maintenance of a normal state of hydration by replacing continuing fluid and electrolyte losses, and proper feeding of the child during the acute and convalescent phases of diarrhea are the principles of diarrhea therapy (see Table III). The effective use of intravenous (IV) therapy for the treatment of diarrhea goes back to the turn of the century. During ensuing years, treatment was refined to the point where, in the 1960s, the use of intravenous fluids was able to reduce the mortality from cholera to less than 1%.

An ideal IV polyelectrolyte solution for treating cholera and gastroenteritis in patients of all ages is DTS (Diarrhea Treatment Solution), which is recommended by WHO. This solution (not commercially available) contains, per liter of distilled water, 8 g glucose, 4 g sodium chloride, 6.5 g sodium acetate (or 5.4 g sodium lactate), and 1 g of potassium chloride. Other acceptable solutions are Ringer's lactate (to which potassium must be added), or 5:4:1 (Dacca solution—not commercially available).

Initial fluid deficits are rapidly corrected with I.V. fluid, and, by carefully monitoring the output of stool and urine, a normal state of hydration can be maintained with additional fluid. Intravenous fluid is particularly effective in treating those with very severe dehydration and excessive purging. There are real limitations, however, to the use of I.V. fluid. The fluid itself and the equipment needed to administer it (I.V. tubing and needles) are often not available, particularly in the peripheral

Table II. Guidelines for Rehydration Therapy[a]

Degree of dehydration	Age group	Type of fluid	Volume of fluid (per kg body weight)	Time of administration
Mild	All	ORT solution	50 ml/kg	Within 4 hours
Moderate	All	ORT solution	100 ml/kg[b]	Within 4 hours
Severe		I.V. such as Ringer's lactate	30 ml/kg	Within 1 hour
Infants		Followed by I.V. such as Ringer's lactate	40 ml/kg	Within next 2 hours
		Followed by ORT solution	40 ml/kg	Within next 3 hours
Older children and adults		I.V. such as Ringer's lactate	110 ml/kg	Within 4 hours; initially as fast as possible until radial pulse is palpable

Source: adapted from reference 2.
[b]During the initial stages of therapy, adults can usually consume up to 750 ml per hour and children up to 300 ml per hour.

Table III.   Guidelines for Maintenance Therapy[a]

Amount of diarrhea	Kind of therapy	Administration	Amount of fluid
Mild diarrhea (not more than one stool every 2 hours or less than 5 ml stool per kg per hour)	ORT	By mouth; at home	100 ml/kg body weight per day until diarrhea stops[b]
Severe diarrhea (more than one stool every 2 hours, or more than 5 ml of stool per kg per hour)	ORT	By mouth; at treatment facility	Replace stool losses volume for volume; if not measurable, give 10-15 ml/kg body weight per hour
Severe diarrhea with recurrence of signs of dehydration	Treat as for severe dehydration in Table II		

[a]Source: adapted from reference 2.
[b]In infants, as an alternative, mothers can be advised to give 10 ml/kg body weight for each diarrheal stool. In older children and adults, thirst is an adequate guide for fluid needs; they can be told to drink as much as they want to satisfy their thirst.

clinics and at the community level in developing countries. If the fluid is available, it may not be of the right composition and its relative cost may be prohibitive. In Bangladesh, for example, the intravenous fluid required to treat an adult with a severe case of cholera may cost the equivalent of 4 months of a laborer's wages. In addition to its relative expense, intravenous fluid must be administered by a well-trained health provider; being able to insert a pediatric scalp vein (if it is available) takes extra skill and patience. Lastly, children treated with I.V. replacement are totally dependent on the skill of health workers; over- or underhydration is all too common when I.V. fluid is used.

Because of the limitations of I.V. fluid, there was a continuing search for an effective means of oral hydration. Oral therapy found a small role in a few hospital centers in the treatment of dehydration in the late 1940s and early 1950s in children with milder cases. The routine use of an oral solution, particularly in moderately and sometimes seriously dehydrated patients with severe diarrhea, was not begun until the late 1960s, when the physiological basis for oral therapy was demonstrated and was shown to be clinically effective in treating cholera.[5] It was then recognized that the substrate glucose was necessary to aid the transport of sodium across the intestinal lumen.[6] Earlier studies involving membrane transport, and finally intestinal lavage, had demonstrated that the transport of glucose was not impaired by cholera toxin. The clinical application of oral therapy for cholera was clearly suggested in well-controlled balance studies.[5,7,8] Even in the most severely ill cholera patient, up to 80% of intravenous fluid can be saved if oral therapy is used effectively.

A series of observations followed, including field trials for oral therapy,[9] the use of oral therapy in children,[10,11] and the use of other substrates such as glycine.[12,13] The applicability of using oral therapy in diarrhea of varying etiologies has been clearly shown.[14,15] Furthermore, it was demonstrated that oral therapy alone could treat patients who were moderately dehydrated.[16] It proved very effective even when used under the extremely adverse conditions of a crowded refugee camp.[17]

It is important at this point to summarize the advantages of oral therapy solution. Oral therapy is an effective means of treating most cases of diarrheal disease. Because it requires no special equipment and is made from inexpensive ingredients and available drinking water, its low cost is ensured; it has the potential of greater availability in areas that are far from treatment centers; technical skills required for administering oral therapy are minimal; and it is safer to use than intravenous fluid.

There are certain limitations, however. Those patients in shock or with altered states of consciousness cannot be rehydrated with oral therapy alone but require intravenous fluids; there are some patients (especially those with severe cholera) who may not be able to maintain normal hydration with oral therapy alone; a few patients may have a transient glucose malabsorption that will limit absorption of the oral therapy solution; intractable emesis, though uncommon, may necessitate giving fluid I.V.; and lastly, there may be problems associated with the actual preparation and delivery of the solution in peripheral, hard-to-reach rural areas.

An integral part of any diarrhea treatment program, particularly an oral therapy program, is proper instruction on the feeding of children. Infants and children who are breast-feeding should continue nursing uninterrupted. Children taking milk formula should not interrupt feeding for more than 6 hours, and thereafter may receive full-strength milk.[18] Preferably, the milk should be mixed with food and given in smaller doses. If the child has a negative reaction to full-strength formula, milk can be withdrawn. This is not a common finding, however. Recent studies have shown that when normal levels of lactose were given to lactase-deficient children, absorption was normal and no significant diarrhea resulted.[19] Feeding of other foods such as cereals should continue, and feeding should be increased during convalescence to make up for reduced nutrient intake during the course of the illness.[20] Whereas the appetite of the child may be poor during diarrhea,[21] the intestinal absorption of nutrients is only partially affected (see chapter 9, this volume). These ideas may contradict long-standing folk beliefs, or beliefs of Western-oriented health practitioners.

Antibiotics are generally not recommended for the treatment of diarrhea except when the patient has clinical symptoms of an illness known to be responsive, such as shigellosis or cholera. The fundamental principles of treatment are still the replacement of lost fluids, the continuing maintenance of a state of hydration, and appropriate feeding of the afflicted individual. There is no role for absorbing agents such as kaolin and pectin, agents that reduce motility such as paregoric, or any drug that increases blood pressure.

FORMULA OF THE ORAL THERAPY MIX

The formula that has been recommended by the World Health Organization has the following composition: sodium chloride (table salt), 3.5 grams; sodium bicarbonate, 2.5 grams; potassium chloride, 1.5 grams; glucose, 20 grams; and water, 1 liter. This gives the following electrolyte composition: sodium 90 meq/liter; potassium 20 meq/liter; chloride 80 meq/liter; bicarbonate 30 meq/liter, and glucose 110 millimoles/liter.

QUESTIONS REGARDING ADDITIONS, SUBSTITUTIONS, OR ELIMINATION OF VARIOUS COMPONENTS OF THE ORAL THERAPY MIX

Early use of oral therapy, especially in the home, may arrest and/or reverse progress to the severe dehydration that leads to hospitalization or death. To extend oral therapy beyond the hospital or clinic into the community may require the alteration of the oral therapy formula. The following section examines the effects of the two variables to be considered: the amount of salt and sugar, and the volume in which they are dissolved.

Glucose, Sucrose, and/or Other Substrates. For treating most cases of diarrhea, glucose and sucrose are almost equivalent,[22] but for more severe cases of dehydration and diarrhea, glucose is preferred. Sucrose is usually easier to obtain than glucose, especially in the community that is far away from a central production unit. It would be incorrect to assume, however, that sucrose is always available. Recently there have been several sugar shortages in some countries, and it is almost certain that these will occur again. Twice as much sucrose as glucose must be used. If oral therapy packets are to be produced centrally, glucose is preferred. Glucose, however, is more hydroscopic than sucrose, so glucose must be packaged in foil—a more expensive material. As water absorption by sucrose as well as by glucose is substantial in warm climates and at relative humidity greater than 85%, the comparative economic advantage of the packaging disappears under these conditions.[23]

Rice water is another substrate that has been used. Rice has been made into a powder and then dissolved in water; when the other electrolytes were added, the resulting solution proved to be very effective (see chapter 17, this volume). Early reports indicate that it may be even better absorbed than glucose alone. Amino acids, such as glycine, have also been used and found to be effective.[13] Glycine seems to act synergistically with glucose to decrease the duration of diarrhea. The addition of amino acids, however, will add to the cost and may enhance bacterial growth in contaminated solutions.

Sodium. With the exception of severe cholera in adults, the WHO-recommended level of sodium is suitable for all age groups. Some have expressed concern, however, that this is too much sodium, especially for infants with immature kidneys.[24] They argue that the stool electrolyte composition in much of pediatric diarrhea is less than 50 meq/liter. Furthermore, it is felt that the 90 meq/liter that are recommended do not provide enough margin of safety if the formula is not properly prepared. Concern over possible hypernatremia may be the result of a number of reports of its occurrence in the 1950s when children in the United States were given concentrated cow's milk during diarrhea, leading to loss of water but not salt in the large bowel.[1] As noted earlier, this is rarely the case in developing countries where breast milk, in frequent feedings, is the general practice (breast milk has a sodium concentration of 2 to 3 meq/liter). If water or breast milk is given *ad lib* (not added to oral therapy) with oral rehydration therapy (ORT) to children and infants, the concentration of sodium will approximate 50 meq/liter. Others have advocated a two-for-one regimen; that is, two parts of oral therapy for one part of plain water. Such a formulation, however, makes treatment more complicated, and the recommendations of breast milk for the nursing child or *ad lib* water for the non-breast-fed seem to be much more consistent with the simplified treatment regimen.

Recently, a study was conducted comparing ORT solutions of 50 and 90 meq/liter of sodium. A number of children in the low-sodium group developed hyponatremia.[25] In an earlier study in India, however, a solution containing 50 meq/liter of sodium proved to be effective.[26] In a large oral therapy field trial in Bangladesh involving over 5000 patients, no clinical cases of hypernatremia were seen that could be attributed to the oral therapy (J. Snyder, personal communication, 1981).

From a programmatic point of view, it is much easier to recommend one formula rather than multiple formulas. It is difficult enough for a local concern to produce one well-recognized packet, much less packets designed for particular age groups. It is this desire to simplify that has led to the single formula.

Potassium. There are significant losses of potassium with diarrhea. As diarrhea increases in volume, the concentration of potassium diminishes, but the deficit will rise. When potassium is not included in the ORT mix, hypokalemia may occur. In a recent study in Honduras, a simple sugar-salt solution corrected dehydration, but hypokalemia was a persistent problem.[27] This is particularly true in the more severe cases of diarrhea.[28] There are dietary sources for potassium such as bananas, coconut water, and citrus fruit juice. Bananas are the best source, but a large number would have to be consumed if the potassium deficits were to be made up.[27] Breast milk contains 13 meq/liter of potassium. The loss of potassium in large amounts will lead to the recognized signs of flaccidity, decreased bowel tone, and possible cardiac arrhythmias. The effects of low body potassium on appetite have not been well defined.

Bicarbonate. Bicarbonate replacement may not be necessary in the mild to moderate cases. In recent studies in Bangladesh, however, it was shown that when fluid loss exceeded 50 ml per kg, acidosis was only slowly corrected by renal or respiratory mechanisms. The consequences of prolonged acidosis are not well defined. When the patient is acidotic, hypokalemia may be masked, though it will become evident the minute acidosis is corrected. True potassium deficiency may not be noted in patients treated with ORT that is deficient in bicarbonate.

Water. Some have advocated that water used in the preparation of oral therapy must be pathogen-free. If this policy were to be followed, the water would have to be boiled, disinfected, or taken from a clean source. In many areas of the developing world, the fuel needed to heat water is not available. In addition, heating water may give it a different character in those areas where there is a hot and cold categorization of food.[29] Potable water, such as that which is chemically treated or from a tube well, is often not available, or it may have a taste or quality that is unacceptable. Just how does contaminated water affect the bacterial growth of an oral therapy solution? The presence of glucose or sucrose supports the multiplication of organisms in contaminated water. In laboratory studies it has been shown that significant growth of fecal coliform organisms from one to five logs occurs in oral therapy solution prepared from naturally contaminated water.[30] These studies, however, do not duplicate field conditions. In Gambia, patients treated with oral therapy solution made with contaminated water had diarrhea that was equal in duration to that in patients treated with ORT made with sterile water.[31] It was estimated that excess *E. coli* ingested in the oral therapy was no more than 5% of the *E. coli* commonly ingested in food. There do not

seem to be any studies that indicate what happens when enteric pathogens are ingested by an individual already experiencing diarrhea caused
by another pathogen.

The overall recommendation by WHO is that ORT be made with
ordinary drinking water, and that prepared oral therapy should not be
kept more than 24 hours. There is no apparent reason to alter this
recommendation.

CONTAINERS AND VOLUMES FOR THE ORAL THERAPY MIX

The volume size may determine use patterns and product safety. The
smaller the volume prepared, the more likely the oral therapy solution
will be used within a short period of time. The less standing, the less
chance for bacterial growth. However, making up smaller packets will
increase the price, as packaging constitutes a significant cost of production. Smaller packets may also create the impression that only a small
volume is required to treat diarrhea.

An equally important issue is the volume in which the oral therapy
mix is to be dissolved. Salts are one-half of the equation; the volume is
the other half. A standardized packet requires a standardized volume in
which it will be dissolved. In much of the world a standardized measure
is not available. If there is a standard measure, such as a beer bottle, the
packet will have to be adapted to this. A standardized container could be
produced and sold commercially, though this would greatly increase the
initial (but one-time) cost of the oral therapy. The solution could be put
into plastic containers that would expand to the appropriate volume
when liquid is added, or premixed and sold in fluid form. The lack of
standardized measures will present a problem in any country that wishes
to extend oral therapy beyond health centers into the community.

FORMS IN WHICH SALTS ARE DELIVERED

Table IV summarizes the advantages and disadvantages of different
methods of delivering ORT.

Packets. Production of packets at some central facility has the major
advantage of providing a complete, standardized formula. The use of
glucose as substrate is more feasible in this situation than in programs
that stress home preparation from market ingredients. A packet can be
designed so that it is easily distinguished by populations, and as such,
advertising campaigns can use this to sensitize the population to the use
of oral therapy. When the commercial sector is part of a countrywide
program, packet recognition is essential. The disadvantages are equally

Table IV. Advantages and Disadvantages of the Different Methods of Delivering ORT
Ingredients to the Community[a]

Plan	Advantages	Disadvantages[b]	Situation
Prepackaged WHO formula	Standardized; highly visible and identifiable, effective for severe and mild diarrhea	More expensive; ingredients may not be locally available	Effective for a health delivery system that can reach the bulk of the population
Prepackaged WHO formula with sucrose	Sucrose may be more readily available	Less effective for severe diarrhea; may be more vomiting; ineffective if sucrose deficiency develops	Effective for a health system that can reach the bulk of the population
Local mixing using WHO formula (spoon set)	No dependence on central facilities; no packaging costs	Increased risk of error; storage of ingredients may be a problem	Effective for a system of urban and rural clinics with outreach to patients
Home mixing using salt/sugar formula (double spoon)	Reduced costs; direct participation of community and family; less dependence on health system; may permit earlier institution of treatment at home	Not as effective as WHO formula; measurement of ingredients variable; requires individual instruction of users	Effective where majority has no access to an organized health service but where there is strong community involvement in health
Local mixing using salt/sugar (no spoons)	Requires no packets, spoons, or devices; minimum investment; encourages self-reliance	Not as effective as WHO formula; needs individual instruction of users; measurement of ingredients is more variable	Effective where provision of measuring spoons is not practical
Any distribution scheme using formula with lower sodium content (e.g., 60 meq/liter)	Decreased risk of hypernatremia	Risk of hyponatremia; less effective in severe diarrhea caused by *V. cholerae* or *E. coli*	Effective where supervision and surveillance is impossible

[a]Source: adapted from reference 23.
[b]For home use, all methods require a standard container or standardization of a home container; individual instruction and frequent follow-up are required for any home-based program.

clear. The packaging greatly increases the cost of an oral therapy mix, and once packaged, it must be distributed. The primary care system of most countries often falls short in properly distributing commodities. If packets are prepared at the periphery, i.e., in the clinic, some of the logistical problems may be decreased.

Spoons. Spoons have been developed that measure each of the ingredients. If multiple spoons are used, all the ingredients must be available and spoons should be color-coded to correspond to the color of the particular salt container. The cost of packaging may be eliminated, but the population will still be dependent upon distribution of preweighed salts through the health centers.

An even simpler modification has been a spoon that measures only sucrose and salt (NaCl). Spoons have been produced for containers of 200 to 1,000 cc. The advantages of the spoon are that it is identified with the use of oral therapy and it is a one-time distribution. The limitations are that the spoons may be lost, they produce an incomplete formula, the correct volume of water must also be determined, and the volumes of salt and sugar will vary depending on how filled the spoon is. These spoons have been used extensively in Indonesia.

Pinch and Scoop. An individual can be taught to prepare the oral therapy mix by using the hand to measure the correct amount of salt and sugar (sucrose); this is the pinch and scoop method. The advantages are that no implements are required, and once taught the method, the individual is far less dependent on the health delivery system. The disadvantages are similar to those of the spoon in that there may be greater variation in the amounts of ingredients supplied, only salt and sugar are used, and a standardized volume must be available or known to the population. Some reports on the use of this method or other village-based programs have indicated extreme variability in the electrolyte composition, and in a number of solutions sodium levels were high.[32,33]

More recent studies from Bangladesh demonstrate that the variability of sodium levels in the pinch and scoop method[34,35] or other home-based preparations[36] can be kept at a minimum with well-designed, personal instruction. In addition, by lowering the desired sodium level to approximately 60 meq/liter, solutions with sodium above 120 meq/liter were prevented in this pinch and scoop program.[35]

FACTORS TO CONSIDER IN DEVELOPING A NATIONAL DIARRHEA TREATMENT PROGRAM

The key to reduction of mortality and morbidity from diarrhea is accessibility to an effective ORT mixture that is appropriately used. Studies in Bangladesh,[37] India,[38] and Egypt[39] have indicated that a reduction in diarrhea-related mortality of up to 50% may be achievable when the public has complete access to, and uses, ORT. Early use of ORT may also lead to a reduction in malnutrition[40] (Imran Ozalp, personal communication, 1981).

Making ORT more accessible will require making some of the trade-offs discussed earlier. For example, a packet of ORT salts will give a more uniform and complete mix than the double spoon method of preparation, but the packet may be less accessible. The program a country introduces will depend on health sector and non–health sector variables.

Health sector factors might include the following: the number of health personnel; the location and accessibility of clinics; the availability, training, and attitudes of health personnel; the degree of integration of health services; the importance given to primary care; and the sensitivity of the population to its health problems. Health personnel would include private physicians, pharmacists, and traditional healers in addition to government health workers. If, as noted earlier, the population has limited access to the official health providers, a community-based program may be developed.

Such a program could emphasize a variety of approaches, such as designating a volunteer worker to be distributor of packets, or teaching all mothers the pinch and scoop method. Factors outside the health system that might influence access to health services would include the role of women in the society; the education level of different groups in the population; the physical infrastructure of a country, including roads and waterways; the population density; the methods of communication, and the degree to which mass media reach the population; and the distribution of income and purchasing power of the urban and rural poor. Each society, then, will have a different mix of health sector and non–health sector resources that will determine its diarrhea treatment program. Lessons learned elsewhere can be adapted. The experiences of a number of diarrheal programs emphasizing ORT have recently been reviewed.[41]

Limitations of the health sector are frequently discussed; thus, it might be worthwhile to examine in greater detail those factors outside the health system that might shape an ORT program.

WOMEN'S ROLE

As diarrhea programs are generally aimed at providing care for children, the role of women is crucial. It includes responsibility for childcare, e.g., providing treatment, determining feeding practices, and being a major decision-maker in seeking health care. If women are confined to their homes or compound, there may be problems in educating them about diarrhea treatment or encouraging early treatment at a health facility.

In Bangladesh, a program has been developed by the Bangladesh Rural Advancement Committee (BRAC), which tries to deal with a female population that is largely illiterate and not very mobile.[35] Oral replacement workers (ORWs), women 20 to 50 years of age who can read and write Bengali, go house-to-house in their program area, teaching one woman in each household how to prepare and use oral therapy (see Figure 1). After engaging the village woman in friendly conversation, the

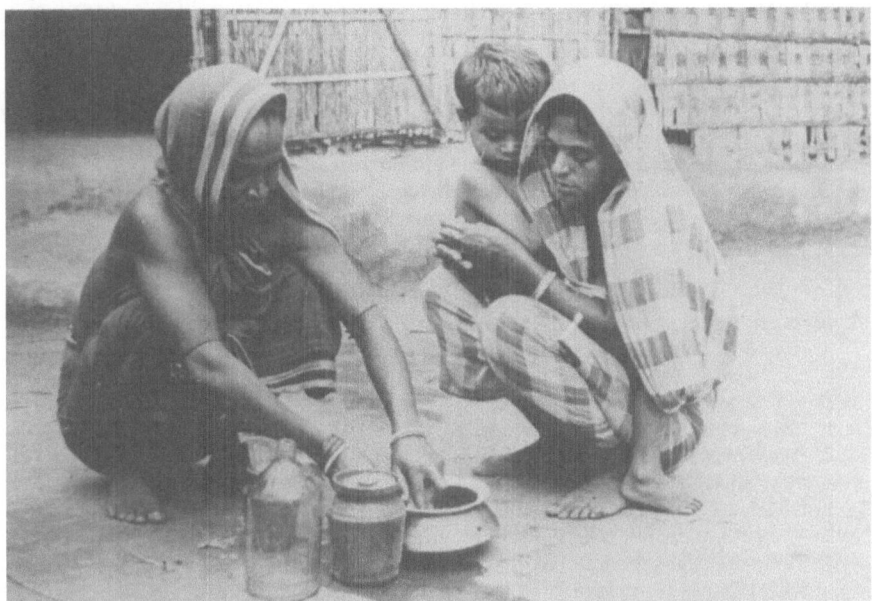

Figure 1. A village health worker in Bangladesh shows a mother how to prepare oral therapy.

ORW shifts the topic to the treatment of diarrheal disease and gives the woman 10 points to remember (Table V). The ORW shows the woman how to measure sugar and salt (the pinch and scoop method) and accurately marks one of the home containers for the correct volume to use. The visit lasts 20 to 30 minutes. Follow-up visits 3 to 4 weeks later indicate that 98% of village women remember seven or more points. Samples of 996 oral therapy mixes from 1079 randomly selected households showed a mean sodium of 47 meq/liter, with only 0.4% above 120 meq/liter (expected Na was 66 meq/liter).

If women participate in the marketplace, as they do in Indonesia,[42] they are more accessible. As many Indonesian women are involved in the commercial sector, they have greater awareness of weights and measures—important skills in preparing ORT at home. A woman's worth in society may determine the level of illness necessary for the family to seek outside assistance. There is evidence that in those societies where male children are more highly valued, males are brought to health facilities more frequently than females.[43] This is further reflected in higher female mortality rates. A home-based program, by decreasing the need for clinic visits, may help reduce the mortality differentials.

Table V. Message Given to Mothers by Oral Therapy Workers of BRAC[a]

Ten points to remember

1. *Diarrhea*—more than one watery stool in a day.
2. *Transmission*—occurs when the feces of an infected person or carrier enters someone else's mouth.
3. *Treatment*—of diarrhea is oral replacement mixture, fluid, and food.
4. *Oral replacement mixture*—is a mixture of sugar and salt in water. *Lobon-gur*[b] is one kind of oral replacement mixture.
5. *Lobon-gur mixture*—is made by mixing a three-finger pinch of salt (up to first crease of index finger) with two four-finger scoops of gur in one-half seer[c] of tube well or boiled water and stirring.
6. *Begin* giving *lobon-gur* mixture after the first watery stool.
7. *Amount* of lobon-gur mixture for children should equal the amount of water in the stools. If the mother does not know, let the child have as much as desired.
8. *Danger* of lobon-gur mixture when:
   1. *Too much salt* is added to mixture.
   2. *Small, frequent feedings* are not given to infants and small children.
9. *A doctor* should be consulted when:
   1. Diarrhea lasts more than 2 days.
   2. The patient cannot take fluid by mouth.
   3. The patient has severe diarrhea and cannot replace the water lost in the stools with lobon-gur mixture.
10. *Nutritional advice* for patients with diarrhea includes the following:
    1. *During* diarrhea continue to take food and fluid.
    2. *After* diarrhea take more than normal amount of food and fluid for 7 days.

[a]Source: adapted from Bangladesh Rural Advancement Committee (BRAC) Oral Therapy Program, Dacca, Bangladesh, September 1979.
[b]*Lobon* is salt and *gur* is unrefined sugar.
[c]One-half *seer* is equivalent to 500 cc.

EDUCATION

The education level of the population will determine the type of training and the sophistication of health messages. Literacy levels generally reflect the degree of development of any society. Health education programs also will have to take into account the fact that women generally have a much lower literacy level than men. Schoolchildren may serve as a good entry point for the introduction of health ideas to the family. Introducing ideas of ORT into primary school curriculums has been used effectively in Indonesia.[44]

PHYSICAL INFRASTRUCTURE AND POPULATION DENSITY

Distribution of the population and the physical infrastructure of roads and waterways will determine the accessibility to the population.

Because of density and roads, urban populations are easier to serve than those in rural areas. In some parts of the world, especially those countries in Saharan and sub-Saharan Africa, populations are widely dispersed and roads are few and often impassable for part of the year. Providing health services to these populations and distributing supplies, such as ORT packets, are difficult and costly. Over 50% of the cost of providing primary health care in these rural settings may go to transport, and keeping health personnel in these environments is difficult.

Contrast this with the situation that exists in a country such as Egypt, where 99% of the population lives on 3.5% of the land, and where over 90% of the population is within 4 kilometers of some type of government health facility. Providing supplies and personnel should be easier in this environment.

High population density does not necessarily ensure easy access. In Bangladesh, for example, the country is so laced with rivers and farm-land is so valuable, it is costly to build roads and bridges. Much travel is by foot or by hand- and wind-powered boats. Considerable time is spent going short distances, and as women are restricted in land travel, distances are effectively longer. Services and supplies are not always easy to provide in such an environment.

MASS COMMUNICATION

Availability of mass media will enhance a society's ability to disseminate information on proper therapy. Statistics on the number of radios and televisions, and the circulation rates of newspapers, may mislead those wanting to increase appropriate use of ORT. Whereas the population may be stimulated to seek oral therapy, unless there is direct instruction of the mother in either a clinic or pharmacy, or at home, there will be inappropriate use of ORT, especially in its preparation and administration. To the extent that programs such as those in Bangladesh[35-37] or Egypt[39] are successful, credit must be given to the quality of individual instruction, not to any mass media campaign.

INCOME LEVELS

There are few countries in the developing world where health care is completely free. Although government services may be free, they are accessible (open) for only limited times of the day, with health care personnel, especially physicians, available for even less time. This is particularly true in rural areas. Patients may be seen free of charge, but drugs are frequently unavailable except at private pharmacies and small shops.

Even when drugs are available, extra costs such as injection fees are often solicited. It should be noted that in many societies, a large percentage of government physicians spend an equal or greater amount of time in the private sector, where payment is required. The ability to pay for services, especially in the poorer areas where enteric disease is more of a problem, is critical to having access to care.

CONCLUSION

Oral therapy is a very effective means of treating diarrhea. It is inexpensive, easy to prepare and use, accessible, and relatively safe if combined with better dietary practices such as continued feeding during illness (especially breast-feeding) and a compensatory increase in intake following recovery. The ORT formula recommended by WHO is the best one now available for all age groups. Various components can be changed (sucrose for glucose) or eliminated (bicarbonate or potassium), but the effectiveness of the ORT will be altered.

There are a number of ways that ORT can be packaged or delivered to the health sector or community. The method of delivery will be determined by two major factors: (1) the state of the health sector, including the number, availability, and knowledge of health personnel; the cost of treatment; and the degree of integration of the health services; and (2) the non–health sector where crucial factors include the role of women; the education levels of the society; the physical infrastructure and population distribution; and levels of income and purchasing power. There will always be a trade-off involving safety, effectiveness of treatment, and accessibility of ORT. Each society has a different combination of the above and will have to adapt an ORT program to its own resources. By the same token, a number of observations of ORT programs in a variety of settings have been made and each has some degree of transferability. It is crucial that lessons gained from these many hospital, clinic, and field-based experiences be examined for those elements that are usable in other programs.

REFERENCES

1. Hirschhorn, N. The treatment of acute diarrhea in children: An historical and physiological perspective. *Am. J. Clin. Nutr.* 33:637–663, 1980.
2. World Health Organization. *Diarrheal Disease Control Program: A Manual for the Treatment of Acute Diarrhea.* WHO, Geneva, Switzerland, 1980.

3. Cash, R. A. Oral therapy for diarrhoea. *Trop. Doctor* **9**:25-30, 1979.

4. Pierce, N. F., and Hirschhorn, N. Oral fluid—A simple weapon against dehydration in diarrhea: How it works and how to use it. *WHO Chronicle* **31**:87-93, 1977.

5. Nalin, D. R., Cash, R. A., Islam, R., Molla, M., and Phillips, R. A. Oral maintenance therapy for cholera in adults. *Lancet* **ii**:370-373, 1968.

6. Curran, P. F. Ion transport in the intestine and its coupling to other transport processes. *Fed. Proc.* **24**(4), Part I:993-999, 1965.

7. Hirschhorn, N., Kinzie, J. L., Sachan, D. B., Northrup, R. S., Taylor, J. O., Ahmad, S. Z., and Phillips, R. A. Decrease in net stool output in cholera during intestinal perfusion with glucose-containing solutions. *N. Engl. J. Med.* **279**:176-180, 1968.

8. Pierce, N. F., Banwell, J. G., Mitra, R. C., Caranasos, G. J., Keirnowitz, R. I., Mondal, A., and Maryi, P. M. Effect of intragastric glucose-electrolyte perfusion upon water and electrolyte balance in Asiatic cholera. *Gastroenterology* **55**:333-343, 1968.

9. Cash, R. A., Nalin, D. R., Rochat, R., Reller, L. B., Hague, Z. A., and Rahman, A. S. M. M. A clinical trial of oral therapy in a rural cholera-treatment center. *Am. J. Trop. Med. Hyg.* **19**:653-656, 1970.

10. Nalin, D. R., and Cash, R. A. Oral or nasogastric maintenance therapy in pediatric cholera patients. *J. Pediat.* **78**:355-358, 1971.

11. Mahalanabis, D., Sack, R. B., Jacobs, B., Moudal, A., and Thomas, J. Use of an oral glucose-electrolyte solution in the treatment of pediatric cholera: A controlled study. *J. Trop. Pediat. Environ. Child Health* **20**:82-87, 1974.

12. Rohde, J. E., and Cash, R. A. Transport of glucose and amino acids in human jejunum during Asiatic cholera. *J. Infect. Dis.* **127**:190-192, 1973.

13. Nalin, D. R., Cash, R. A., Rahaman, M., and Yunus, M. Effect of glycine and glucose on sodium and water absorption in patients with cholera. *Gut* **11**:768-772, 1970.

14. Nalin, D. R., Levine, M. M., Mata, L., De Cespedes, C., Vargas, W., Lizano, C., Loria, A. R., Simhon, A., and Mohs, E. Oral rehydration and maintenance of children with rotavirus and bacterial diarrhoeas. *Bull. WHO* **57**:453-459, 1979.

15. Sack, D. A., Chowdhury, A. M. A. K., Eusof, A., Ali, M. A., Merson, M. H., Islam, S., Black, R. E., and Brown, K. H. Oral hydration in rotavirus diarrhoea: A double blind comparison of sucrose with glucose electrolyte solution. *Lancet* **ii**:280-283, 1978.

16. Cash, R. A., Nalin, D. R., Forrest, J. N., and Abrutyn, E. Rapid correction of acidosis and dehydration of cholera with oral glucose and electrolyte solution. *Lancet* **ii**:549-550, 1970.

17. Mahalanabis, D., Choudhuri, A. B., Bagchi, N. G., Bhattacharya, A. K., and Simpson, T. W. Oral fluid therapy of cholera among Bangladesh refugees. *Johns Hopkins Med. J.* **132**:197-205, 1973.

18. Rees, L., and Brook, C. G. D. Gradual reintroduction of full-strength milk after acute gastroenteritis in children. *Lancet* **i**:770-771, 1979.

19. Brown, K. H., Parry, L., Khatun, M. D., and Ahmed, M. G. Lactose malabsorption in Bangladeshi village children: Relation with age, history of recent diarrhea, nutritional status and breast-feeding. *Am. J. Clin. Nutr.* **32**:1962-1969, 1979.

20. Rohde, J. E. Preparing for the next round: Convalescent care after acute infection. *Am. J. Clin. Nutr.* **31**:2258-2268, 1978.

21. Hoyle, B., Yunus, M., and Chen, L. C. Breast-feeding and food intake among children with acute diarrheal disease. *Am. J. Clin. Nutr.* **33**:2365-2371, 1980.

22. Sack, D. A., Islam, S., Brown, K. J., Islam, A., Kabir, A. K. M. I., Chowdhury, A. M. A. K., and Ali, M. A. Oral therapy in children with cholera: A comparison of sucrose and glucose electrolyte solutions. *J. Pediatr.* **96**:20-25, 1980.

23. National Academy of Sciences, Committee on International Nutrition Programs. *Man-*

agement of the Diarrheal Diseases at the Community Level. NAS/NRC, Washington, D. C., 1981.

24. Bart, K. J., Finberg, L., Single solution for oral therapy of diarrhea (Letter). Lancet ii:633-634, 1976.

25. Nalin, D. R., Harland, E., Ramlal, A., Swaby, D., McDonald, J., Gangarosa, R., Levine, M., Akierman, A., Antoine, M., MacKenzie, K., and Johnson, B. Comparison of low and high sodium and potassium content in oral rehydration solutions. J. Pediatr. 97:848-853, 1980.

26. Chatterjee, A., Mahalanabis, D., Jalan, K. N., Matra, T. K., Agarwal, S. K., Dutta, B., Khatua, S. P., and Bagclu, D. K. Oral rehydration in infantile diarrhea: Controlled trial of a low sodium glucose electrolyte solution. Arch. Dis. Child. 53:284-289, 1978.

27. Clements, M. L., Levine, M. M., Black, R. E., Hughes, T. P., Rust, J., and Tome, F. C. Potassium supplements for oral diarrhoea regimens (Letter). Lancet ii:854, 1980.

28. Islam, M. R., Greenough, W. B., III, Rahaman, M. M., Choudhury, A. K. A., and Sack, D. A. Lobon-gur (common salt and brown sugar) oral rehydration solution in the diarrhoea of adults, Scientific Report No. 36, p. 17. International Centre for Diarrhoeal Disease Research, Bangladesh (ICDDR,B), Dacca, Bangladesh, 1980.

29. Wellin, E. Water-boiling in a Peruvian town. In: Health, Culture and Community, B. Paul (Ed.). Russell Sage Foundation, New York, 1955.

30. Shields, D. S., Shields, M. N., Guerrant, R. L., Araiyo, J. G., Brown, S. E., de Sousa, M. A., and Hook, E. W. Electrolyte/glucose concentration and bacterial contamination in home-prepared oral rehydration: A field experience in Northeastern Brazil. J. Pediatr. (in press) 1981.

31. Watkinson, M., Lloyd-Evans, N., and Watkinson, A. The use of oral glucose electrolyte solution prepared with untreated well water in acute non-specific childhood diarrhea. Trans. Roy. Soc. Trop. Med. Hyg. 74:657-662, 1980.

32. Harland, P. S. E. G., Cox, D. L., Lyew, M., and Luido, F. Composition of oral solutions prepared by Jamaican mothers for treatment of diarrhea. Lancet i:601, 1981.

33. Levine, M. M., Hughes, T. P., Black, R. E., Clements, M. L., Matheny, S., Siegel, A., Cleaves, F., Gutierrez, C., Foote, D. P., and Smith, W. A. Variability of sodium and sucrose levels of simple sugar/salt oral rehydration solutions prepared under optimal and field conditions. J. Pediatr. 97:324-327, 1980.

34. Cutting, W. A. M., and Ellerbrook, T. V. Homemade oral solutions for diarrhea (Letter). Lancet i:998, 1981.

35. Bangladesh Rural Advancement Committee (BRAC). Oral Therapy Program. Mohakhali C/A, Dacca, Bangladesh, September 1979.

36. Chen, L. C., Black, R. E., Sarder, A. M., Merson, M. H., Bhatia, S., Yunus, M., and Chakraborty, J. Village-based distribution of oral rehydration therapy in Bangladesh. Am. J. Trop. Med. Hyg. 29:285-290, 1980.

37. Rahaman, M. M. Aziz, K. M. S., Patwari, Y., and Munshi, M. H. Diarrhoeal mortality in two Bangladeshi villages with and without community-based oral rehydration therapy. Lancet ii:809-812, 1979.

38. Kielmann, A. A., and McCord, C. Home treatment of childhood diarrhea in Punjab villages. Environ. Child Health 23:197-201, 1977.

39. Diarrheal Disease Control Study—Final Report on Phase 1, SRHD Project, Rural Health Department, Ministry of Health, Arab Republic of Egypt, to USAID and WHO (EMRO), April 1981.

40. Republic of the Philippines, World Health Organization, John Snow Public Health Group, and International Study Group. A positive effect on the nutrition of Philip-

pine children of an oral glucose-electrolyte solution given at home for the treatment of diarrhoea: Report on a field trial. *Bull. WHO* **55**:87–94, 1977.

41. Oral rehydration therapy (ORT) for childhood diarhhea. *Popul. Rep.* Series L(2), November-December, 1980.

42. Rohde, J. E., Ismail, D., Sadjimin, T., Suyadi, A., and Tugerin, Training course for village nutrition programs. *Trop. Pediatr. Environ. Child Health* **25**:83–96, 1979.

43. Chen, L. C., Huq, E., and D'Souza, S. Sex bias in the family allocation of food and health care in rural Bangladesh. *Pop. Dev. Rev.* **7**:55–70, 1981.

44. Rohde, J. E., and Sadjimin, T. Elementary school pupils as health educators: Role of school health programmes in primary health care. *Lancet* i:1350–1352, 1980.

14

Feeding Practices in Relation to Childhood Diarrhea and Malnutrition

DILIP MAHALANABIS

INTRODUCTION—CHILDHOOD DIARRHEA: MAGNITUDE AND NUTRITIONAL IMPACT

A recent analysis of the findings from 27 active surveillance studies conducted for a year or more suggests that about 750 million children below 5 years of age in Asia, Africa, and Latin America suffer from acute diarrhea each year.[1] It has also been estimated that between 3 and 6 million in this age group die from acute diarrhea each year; 80% of these deaths occur in the first 2 years of life. Repeated attacks of diarrhea are thought to produce malnutrition and growth retardation, presumably because of (a) associated food restriction by mothers, (b) anorexia, (c) malabsorption and direct nutrient losses in the feces, and (d) catabolic effects of the infection causing diarrhea. For example, a careful longitudinal study by Martorell and co-workers in Guatemalan children 7 years old and under showed that repeated attacks of diarrhea lead to significantly more growth retardation in both height and weight compared to that associated with other illnesses.[2] Rowland et al.[3] reported that diarrhea is the most significant infection retarding growth of Gambian children. Using the multiple regression technique, they have also shown that had there been no diarrhea, the growth velocity of the Gambian children would have been similar to that of affluent societies.

DILIP MAHALANABIS • Kothari Centre of Research in Gastroenterology, Calcutta Medical Research Institute, Calcutta, India.

A significant development in recent years has been the discovery that dehydration from acute diarrhea of all etiologies and in all age groups can be safely and effectively treated by the simple method of oral rehydration using a single formula. The global diarrheal disease control program initiated by the World Health Organization has identified oral rehydration therapy (ORT) as a primary public health tool, and major efforts are under way to use ORT as an immediate strategy for reducing deaths from acute diarrheas and diarrhea-associated malnutrition. ORT may also serve as an effective entry point for the promotion of appropriate child care and environmental health practices for reducing morbidity, the latter being a long-term goal. These initiatives raise the critical issue: What constitutes appropriate child-care practices in terms of nutrition during episodes of diarrhea?

Breast-Feeding and Diarrhea

The importance of breast-feeding in preventing morbidity and mortality from diarrhea has been dramatically demonstrated in Europe and North America since the Industrial Revolution until recent decades. "Bottle feeding in resource-poor countries increases the risks of certain infections greatly, especially diarrheal disease."[4] The subject has been extensively reviewed by Jelliffe and Jelliffe.[4] As an example, Kanaaneh[5] has recently demonstrated a striking difference in the number of infants from three Arab villages in Israel hospitalized for diarrheal disease in relation to breast-feeding. The effect of breast-feeding in reducing hospital admission for diarrhea was most apparent in those solely breast-fed for 6 months.

Given the existing evidence, we are not in a position to separate the direct effect of the well-known protective properties of breast milk from the indirect effect of preventing large doses of environmental infective agents entering through the introduction of foods other than breast milk. Data on deaths from diarrheal diseases in relation to breast-feeding practices are available from eight Latin American countries (13 projects).[6] Our analysis of these data (Table I) shows that the difference in the percentage of deaths due to diarrhea in infants 28 days to 5 months old is lower in the group breast-fed and never weaned, the difference being highly significant. However, the group breast-fed for at least 1 month did not enjoy this advantage when compared with the group never breast-fed. Strikingly similar results were obtained when deaths caused by nutritional deficiency were compared according to breast-feeding practices (Table II). Those who were breast-fed and never weaned had a signifi-

Table I. Deaths (Expressed as Percentage of Deaths from All Causes) from Diarrheal Diseases as Underlying Cause, According to Breast-Feeding Patterns in Infants Dying at 28 Days to 5 Months of Age in Eight Latin American Countries (13 Projects)[a]

Breast-fed	Breast-fed		
Never weaned	≥ 1 month	< 1 month	Not breast-fed
(a)	(b)	(c)	(d)
31.7%	51.4%	54.2%	51.7%

X^2: Between (a) and (b) = 136.9
Between (a) and (c) = 179.9
Between (a) and (d) = 132.2
Between (b) and (c) = 3.66
Between (b) and (d) = 0.043
(Degree of freedom = 1)

[a]Source: reference 6.

cantly lower infant death rate (percent of total) when compared to those never breast-fed or breast-fed for a brief period. This effect is apparent in 28-day to 5-month age groups as well as in those 6 to 11 months old (Table II). It would only be fair to assume that both nutritional consequences and diarrhea-related mortality, depending on breast-feeding practices, are closely related to each other.[7]

Table II. Infant Deaths (Expressed as Percent of Total Infant Deaths) from Nutritional Deficiency as Underlying or Associated Cause According to Breast-Feeding Patterns in Eight Latin American Countries (13 Projects)[a]

	Breast-fed	Breast-fed		
	Never weaned	≥ 1 month	< 1 month	Not breast-fed
	(a)	(b)	(c)	(d)
28 days–5 months (1)	34.1%	49.2%	50.0%	51.5%
6–11 months (2)	45.3%	58.6%	59.2%	64.6%

X^2 1. Between (a) and (b) = 80.51
Between (a) and (c) + (d) = 116.37
Between (a) and (d) = 132.54
2. Between (a) and (c) + (d) = 37.85
Between (a) and (b) = 29.98
(Degree of freedom = 1)

[a]Source: our analysis of data of Puffer and Serrano, reference 6.

FEEDING PRACTICES AND ORAL REHYDRATION

Almost all recent trials with oral rehydration therapy for acute diarrhea in infants and children followed a policy of early feeding (i.e., as soon as signs of dehydration are corrected and before diarrhea ends) and unrestricted breast-feeding. All studies showed a highly successful general outcome in terms of cessation of diarrhea, weight gain in the acute phase, and early end to fluid therapy. Quantitative information on the intake of food and its absorption and metabolism are, however, not available. Steady weight gain in a group of 40 infants and small children with moderate to severe dehydration receiving oral therapy along with food and unrestricted breast-feeding in those breast-fed (43%) is shown in Table III as an example of such an approach. Hirschhorn and Denny[8] compared the discharge weight of a group of Apache Indian infants treated with oral rehydration and liberal food intake during the acute phase of recovery with a comparable group treated earlier in the same hospital with intravenous fluids and a slow return to normal diet. Better weight gain was observed in the former group. This favorable impact is a likely outcome of a liberal feeding program during the early phase of treatment of acute diarrhea, since a large part of the food consumed during the acute phase of diarrhea is absorbed, as discussed later. Our unpublished data on pediatric cholera patients suggest that excellent weight gain without any adverse effect on the course of diarrhea is obtainable by allowing a more liberal intake of food as soon as the patient is able to eat, without waiting for the diarrhea to cease.

In the Philippines, an international study group compared the effect

Table III. Mean Weight Gain (Percent Increase after Admission) in 40 Children 3 Months to 6 Years Old during Acute Phase of Treatment for Moderate to Severe Dehydration with Oral Rehydration and Continued Feeding after Initial Hydration[a]

6 hours	24 hours	48 hours	72 hours
5.1%	8.2%	9.4	10.4%

Etiologies: *V. cholerae* el Tor, 9; enterotoxigenic *E. coli*, 19; rotavirus, 7

Food: All breast-fed babies (43%) continued breast-feeding beginning within 8 hours; all babies on formula milk at home received cow's milk formula with added rice-based cereal. Older children were put on adult hospital diet (boiled rice, fish, lentils, potatoes, etc.). No significant diarrhea was noted after 48 hours except in 5 patients: (cholera, 2; rotavirus, 1; rotavirus + ETEC: LT & ST, 1; ETEC: LT, 1).

[a]Source: Patra, Jalan, and Mahalanabis, unpublished data, 1980.

Table IV. Effect of Continued Feeding with or without Oral Rehydration during Episodes of Diarrhea in a Community Study over a 7 Month Period[a]

Group	Relative weight gain (%) over controls	Significance Y
With 2 attacks of diarrhea	5.9	$p < 0.01$
With 1 attack of diarrhea	3.9	$p < 0.025$
The whole group		
1–5 years old	3.6	$p < 0.001$
< 1 year old	6.5	n.s.

[a]Source: reference 9.

of promoting continued feeding with or without oral rehydration therapy during episodes of diarrhea in children.[9] The group treated with oral rehydration therapy showed a better weight gain compared to the controls (Table IV). This favorable impact could have resulted for several reasons: (a) the oral rehydration therapy, other variables being common, (b) greater confidence in continued feeding with oral rehydration support, and (c) the possibility of dietary intervention being more forceful in the group treated with oral rehydration. Even if we reject the proposition that oral rehydration therapy alone was responsible for the improved weight gain, it would still be reasonable to conclude that optimum use of oral rehydration therapy probably imparts greater confidence to the health worker and the mother in enforcing the policy of continued feeding during and after diarrhea.

EVOLUTION OF THE MEDICAL MANAGEMENT OF DIET DURING ACUTE DIARRHEA

I cannot help quoting from a paper by Arthur W. Chung, published in 1948[10]:

> The policy of sharply reducing the oral intake or eliminating oral food entirely at the onset of the attack [of diarrhea] with a very cautious and gradual increase after a period of days has been the generally accepted procedure both in this country and abroad. When an increasing oral intake was followed by an exacerbation of the diarrhea it was generally assumed that the food was increased too rapidly, and a second period of therapeutic starvation was tried and sometimes even a third. This regimen is based on theoretical concepts that have never been critically tested. Our predecessors placed their reliance on the appearance and number of stools as the criterion of success of treatment, and since withholding food reduced the volume and

frequency of the stools it was assumed that this was beneficial. This point of
view was sharply challenged in 1924 by Park, who maintained that the child
rather than the stools should be taken as criterion for evaluating therapy. . . .
The fact remains that changes in the stools are more readily assessed than
changes in the clinical state of the patient; the possible benefit from
increased feeding is not sufficiently apparent to outweigh the emotions
engendered in the spectators by an increased number of stools and the stools
still tend to dominate therapy.

For the past 50 years this attitude formed the basis of dietary practice
by the medical profession during and after episodes of acute diarrhea in
infants. Such a practice may have been responsible for the bulk of iatrogenic malnutrition. Available data as early as the late 1940s suggest that
full advantage has not been taken of the substantial absorption of
nutrients (in absolute terms) on a relatively high food intake even during
the acute phase of diarrhea.[10] In 1948 Chung and Viščorová[11] compared a
group of infants with acute diarrhea treated with full feeding with cow's
milk-based formula along with hydration procedures with a group
treated similarly except that food was introduced gradually (Table V).
The former group recovered with a better weight gain and a significantly
reduced duration of diarrhea.

We have come across one other interesting early study in which the
effect of ripe, dehydrated banana fed during the acute phase of infantile
diarrhea was compared with a control group treated conventionally with
gradual introduction of food.[12] The study, in retrospect, is a good example
of the beneficial effect of early feeding during acute episodes of diarrhea
in infants (in this instance food consisted solely of bananas). The treated
group received from banana as much as 50 calories per kg over the first
24 hours of hydration therapy. Mean duration of diarrhea was significantly lower and mean weight gain was significantly higher in the
treated group compared to controls (Table VI).

Table V.   Effect of Early Feeding on the Course of Acute Diarrhea in Infants[a]

	Group fed early	Group fed late (conventional therapy)
Mean age (range) in months	7.3 (1–24)	7.9 (2–23)
Number	53	50
Mean duration of diarrhea (days)	6.9[b]	7.74
± S.E.M.	±0.57	±0.48

[a]Source: reference 11.
[b]$p < 0.05$ (Student's t test)—our analysis of the data.

Table VI.   Early Feeding with Ripe (Dehydrated) Banana (50 calories/kg) Over
First 24 Hours[a]

Age	Treated 1 to 12 months	Control 1 to 7 months
Mean duration of diarrhea (days)	2.90[b] (≤ 4 days = 20)[c] (> 4 days = 0)	4.84[b] ± 0.61 (≤ 4 days = 10)[c] (> 4 days = 9)
Mean weight gain on recovery (g) ± S.E.	94 g[d] ± 65 g	72 g[d] ± 58 g

[a]Source: our analysis of data of Fries *et al.*, reference 12.
[b]$p < 0.01$ (*t* test).
[c]Fisher's exact probability = 0.004.
[d]$p < 0.05$ (*t* test).

NUTRIENT ABSORPTION AND METABOLISM DURING DIARRHEA

As early as 1915, Emmet Holt and his colleagues[13] demonstrated that the percentage absorption of nitrogen ingested during acute diarrhea in infants was as high as 75%, while fat absorption was about 60% of the intake. Chung[10] reported results of careful metabolic balance studies in infants with acute diarrhea and compared the effect of low, moderate, and high intake in the early acute phase. He showed that introduction of a cow's milk-based formula with added corn syrup at 80 to 100 calories per kg body weight promptly led to positive nitrogen balance, nearly 60% absorption of ingested fat, positive calcium and potassium balance, and an improvement in the sodium and chloride balance. Feeding at this level, however, led to an impressive increase in the frequency and bulk of stools.

Even lower intakes of similar feeds at 30 to 60 calories per kg per day produced a marked improvement in the nutrient and mineral balance compared with periods of starvation. Early metabolic balance studies of Darrow *et al.*[14] in infants with moderate to severe dehydration during the acute recovery phase showed that even a modest intake of nutrients at 30 to 40 calories per kg per day, using a cow's-milk-based formula, promptly induced positive nitrogen balance. In spite of these observations, however, Darrow was discouraged from recommending a more liberal dietary intake in the scheme of management of acute diarrhea in view of the associated increase in the volume and frequency of stool. If frequency and volume of stool are used as the sole criteria of successful therapy, then feeding during acute diarrhea could be regarded as harmful.

With the data so far reviewed, it may be stated that, in most acute diarrheas in infants, effective intestinal absorption of all important nutrients occurs even in the most severe cases, and that absorption is roughly proportional to intake. This statement refers to the amount absorbed and does not focus attention on the amount not absorbed, and it ignores the economic issues of food requirements.

Thus far we have referred to early studies on acute diarrheas of undetermined etiology in infants. A recent expansion in our knowledge on the etiology and mechanism of acute diarrheas has stimulated renewed interest in studying nutrient absorption and metabolism in acute diarrheas of specific etiology. Our studies conducted in 1967 in six children aged 12 to 24 months with severe dehydration associated with cholera showed that, when cow's-milk-based formula was introduced within about 24 hours after initiation of fluid replacement therapy, positive nitrogen balance was promptly achieved and there was no recrudescence of diarrhea (Table VII). In the first three patients a more cautious introduction of food (milk) was compared with *ad libitum* milk intake (except for the first 24 hours of nothing by mouth) in the last three patients. In the latter group, intake from 48 hours on was supernormal in both protein and calories. Recently generated data on etiology-specific diarrheas (particularly rotavirus and enterotoxigenic *Escherichia coli*) at the International Centre for Diarrhoeal Disease Research-B in Dacca will be of utmost relevance (Molla and Molla, personal communication, 1981.)

FEEDING PRACTICES AND INTESTINAL DISACCHARIDASE DEFICIENCY

Low intestinal disaccharidase levels, particularly lactase, have been demonstrated during the acute phase of diarrhea[15] and during immediate convalescence.[16] However, even in the ethnic groups known to have primary low lactase activity, significant lactase deficiency does not develop in infants and small children under 2 years of age—the age group most vulnerable to episodes of acute diarrhea.[16] Also, there is no hard evidence of milk intolerance in breast-fed infants during acute diarrhea. Transient depression of lactase, if it occurs at all during acute diarrhea, has not been documented to be of any practical significance if such infants are allowed a moderate intake of milk soon after initial dehydration has been corrected. Further studies to define the optimum dietary pattern during and after acute episodes of diarrhea are of paramount importance.

Table VII.   Nitrogen Intake and Output (mg/kg per 48 hr) during Recovery from Severe, Dehydrating Diarrhea from Cholera in Six Children 11 to 24 Months Old Fed Cow's Milk Formula

Patient[a]		0–48 hr	48–96 hr	96–144 hr	144–192 hr
P-9	Intake	22	678	608	
	Output: urine	367	540	681	
	stool	105	168	58	
	Percent absorption	(−45)	(75)	(90)	
	Retention	−450	−30	−131	
P-10	Intake	0	438	537	
	Output: urine	262	246	186	
	stool	49	38	45	
	Percent absorption	(−)	(91)	(92)	
	Retention	−301	+154	+306	
P-11[b]	Intake	0	206	2981	986
	Output: urine	485	305	357	1075
	stool	45	5	5	71
	Percent absorption	(−)	(97)	(98)	(93)
	Retention	−530	−104	−71	−288
P-12	Intake	458	1154		
	Output: urine	590	1048		
	stool	5	0		
	Percent absorption	(88)	(100)		
	Retention	−219	+106		
P-13	Intake	231	1742	3094	
	Output: urine	468	807	1368	
	stool	25	20	29	
	Percent absorption	(89)	(98)	(99)	
	Retention	−262	+915	+697	
P-14	Intake	229	1387	1478	
	Output: urine	447	647	961	
	stool	295	382	312	
	Percent absorption	(−28)	(+72)	(+79)	
	Retention	−513	+357	+205	

[a]In the first three patients (P-9, P-10, P-11), a cautious introduction of food (milk) is contrasted with *ad libitum* milk intake (except for the first 24 hours of nothing p.o.) in the last three patients (P-12, P-13, P-14). In the latter group, intake from 48 hours on was supernormal in terms of both protein and calories.

[b]All children treated with tetracycline for 48 hours except P-11, whose case was complicated by parotitis with fever (probably explaining the catabolic effect).

CATABOLIC EFFECT OF INFECTIOUS DIARRHEA

No gross catabolic phase caused by infection itself was discernible in the studies discussed in the preceding section. Beisel and his colleagues[17] have shown that the catabolic response to infection is relatively independent of the nature of the infection and that fever is the major stimulus for initiating catabolic losses during an acute infectious fever, and the magnitude of the catabolic losses is related to the degree and duration of fever. In pure secretory diarrhea such as cholera or enterotoxigenic E. coli, fever is not a prominent feature, and when present it is short-lived. Studies on catabolic losses are lacking in acute diarrheas caused by invasive pathogens.

FOOD INTAKE AND ANOREXIA DURING ACUTE DIARRHEA

To the clinician, "conventional wisdom" suggests that acute infectious diarrheas often cause anorexia. This is, however, difficult to quantify. Although hard data are lacking, it is also the general consensus that during convalescence from acute diarrhea, appetite often returns to supernormal levels. Recently, Chen and his colleagues in Bangladesh have studied the quantity of breast milk ingested during acute attacks of diarrhea and after recovery. Quantity of breast milk ingestion was remarkably good. Active promotion of other foods, on the other hand, did not lead to any improved intake compared to the control group. The latter finding may, however, reflect the inevitable delay in accepting unaccustomed food to which the infant has not been exposed before the diarrhea episode rather than anorexia *per se*.

A recent prospective study by MacLean et al.[18] showed the presence of steatorrhea during convalescence in eight infants who had a single episode of acute diarrhea (mean age of onset, 28 days) compared to prediarrhea fecal fat excretion. In spite of steatorrhea, the percentage of fat absorption was as high as 72. Intake of energy in these infants was higher during the postdiarrhea collection periods, and they were gaining in weight steadily.

Quantitative data on the effect of different infections on the food intake of children are sparse. Martorell and colleagues[19] calculated the impact of ordinary illnesses on the dietary intake of children 15 to 60 months old in rural Guatemala and showed a 19% reduction in food intake, which was more pronounced during diarrheal illnesses than during episodes of respiratory illness. However, data are lacking in the most vulnerable age group, i.e., 6 to 18 months.

Using the data on Gambian children,[3] Briscoe (20) compared the actual weight losses with the expected losses from metabolic effects alone. The comparison suggests that, while there is no implied food reduction during malaria, about 75% of the weight loss during diarrhea can only be explained by changes in food intake. His calculations suggest that children suffering from diarrhea appear to consume about 22% less food than their healthy counterparts. In these instances of indirect estimates, the impact of anorexia cannot be separated from effects of imposed restriction of food intake.

REFERENCES

1. World Health Organization. *A Manual for the Treatment of Acute Diarrhoea*. WHO/CDD/SER/80.2, Geneva, Switzerland, 1980.
2. Martorell, R., Habicht, J. P., Yarbrough, C., Lechtig, A., Klein, R. E., and Western, K. A. Acute morbidity and physical growth in rural Guatemalan children. *Am. J. Dis. Child.* 129:1296, 1975.
3. Rowland, M. G. M., Cole, T. J., and Whitehead, R. G. A quantitative study into the role of infection in determining nutritional status in Gambian village children. *Br. J. Nutr.* 37:437, 1977.
4. Jelliffe, D. B., and Jelliffe, E. F. P. *Human Milk in the Modern World. Psychological, Nutritional, and Economic Significance*, pp. 284–291. Oxford University Press, Oxford, England, 1978.
5. Kanaaneh, H. The relationship of bottle-feeding to malnutrition and gastroenteritis in a preindustrialised setting. *J. Trop. Pediatr. Environ. Child Health* 18:302, 1972.
6. Puffer, R. R., and Serrano, C. V. *Patterns of Mortality in Childhood*, Pan American Health Organization Scientific Publication No. 262, pp. 265–271. PAHO, Washington, D.C., 1975.
7. Scrimshaw, N. S., Taylor, C. E., and Gordon, J. E. *Interactions of Nutrition and Infection*, World Health Organization Monograph Series No. 57. WHO, Geneva, Switzerland, 1968.
8. Hirschhorn, N., and Denny, K. M., Oral glucose electrolyte therapy for diarrhea. A means to maintain or improve nutrition? *Am. J. Clin. Nutr.* 28:189, 1975.
9. The International Study Group. A positive effect on the nutrition of Philippine children of an oral glucose-electrolyte solution given at home for the treatment of diarrhea. *Bull. WHO* 55:87–94, 1977.
10. Chung, A. W. The effect of oral feeding at different levels on the absorption of foodstuffs in infantile diarrhea. *J. Pediatr.* 33:1–13, 1948.
11. Chung, A. W., and Viščorová, B. The effect of early oral feeding versus early oral starvation on the course of infantile diarrhea. *J. Pediatr.* 33:14–22, 1948.
12. Fries, J., II., Chiara, N. J., and Waldron, R. J. Dehydrated banana in the dietetic management of diarrheas of infancy. *J. Pediatr.* 35:367–372, 1950.
13. Holt, L. E., Courtney, A. M., and Fales, H. L. The chemical composition of diarrheal as compared with normal stools in infants. *Am. J. Dis. Child.* 9:213, 1915.
14. Darrow, D. C., Pratt, E. L., Flett, J., Gamble, A. H., and Weise, H. F. Disturbances of water and electrolytes in infantile diarrhea. *Pediatrics* 3:129, 1949.
15. Chatterjee. A., Mahalanabis, D., Jalan, K. N., Maitra, T. K., and Bagchi, D. Evaluation of a sucrose/electrolyte solution for oral rehydration in acute infantile diarrhea. *Lancet* i:1333–1335, 1977.
16. Brown, K. H., Parry, L., Khatun, M., and Ahmed, G. Lactose malabsorption in Bangladesh village children. Relation with age, history of recent diarrhea, nutritional status, and breast-feeding. *Am. J. Clin. Nutr.* 32:1962, 1979.

17. Beisel, W. R., Sawyer, W. D., Ryll, E. D., and Crozier, D. Metabolic effects of intracellular infections in man. *Ann. Intern. Med.* **67**:744, 1967.
18. MacLean, W., Klein, G. L., Lopez de Romana, G., Massa, E., and Graham, G. G. Transient steatorrhea following episodes of mild diarrhea in early infancy. *J. Pediatr.* **93**:562–565, 1978.
19. Martorell, R., Yarbrough, C., Yarbrough, S., and Klein, R. E. The impact of ordinary illnesses on the dietary intakes of malnourished children. *Am. J. Clin. Nutr.* **33**:345–350, 1980.
20. Briscoe, J. The quantitative effect of infection on the use of food by young children in poor countries. *Am. J. Clin. Nutr.* **32**:648–676, 1979.

15

Environmental and Educational Interventions against Diarrhea in Guatemala

Benjamin Torún

Introduction

Diarrheal diseases play an important role in the incidence of malnutrition. Diarrhea and malabsorption in association with malnutrition are best documented and most devastating in young children.[1,2] Data presented and discussed in a workshop sponsored 10 years ago by the U.S. National Academy of Sciences[3] supported the concept that improved nutrition would result from the prevention of enteric infection and enteric diseases because (a) infections decrease food intake and increase metabolic losses, (b) diarrhea produces malabsorption of nutrients, and (c) chronic, subclinical enteric disease is associated with impaired tests of intestinal function, such as the absorption of D-xylose and vitamin B_{12}, and with morphologic abnormalities of the intestinal mucosa. It is believed that these abnormalities are related to alterations in microbial colonization of the gut or to chronic or recurrent intestinal infections. Lindenbaum and co-workers[4,5] showed that the structural and functional gastrointestinal changes observed in an indigenous population and visitors living in developing countries where sanitation is poor and there is a high incidence of diarrheal diseases can revert to normal after the individuals live for several months or years in a more sanitary environment.

Benjamin Torún • Institute of Nutrition of Central America and Panama (INCAP), Division of Human Nutrition and Biology, Guatemala City, Guatemala.

It is also conceivable that the incidence and severity of malabsorption and diarrhea can be decreased in developing countries by improving environmental conditions. Diarrheal diseases are frequently associated with the environmental, dietary, and educational conditions that accompany poverty. Although the ideal solution would be a substantial improvement in income and educational levels, there is some evidence that the transmission of diarrheal disease in poor communities can be reduced over a relatively short period by improving water supply and environmental hygiene, coupled with behavioral changes through education, before any reduction in poverty and deprivation over the longer term.[6]

METHOD

The improvements in water supply and environmental hygiene must be accompanied by appropriate educational measures in order to achieve a reduction in diarrheal morbidity and an improvement in nutrient absorption, as shown in Figure 1. Such achievements will, in turn, result in improved nutritional status and better health and growth of children. This should be particularly apparent in populations that have a marginal nutritional intake, because mild to moderate malabsorption may not have a serious impact on the health and other functional aspects of well-fed individuals.

The importance of education to close the gap shown in Figure 1 is stressed by reports that improvements in water supply and physical facilities for excreta disposal without adequate behavioral changes in the tar-

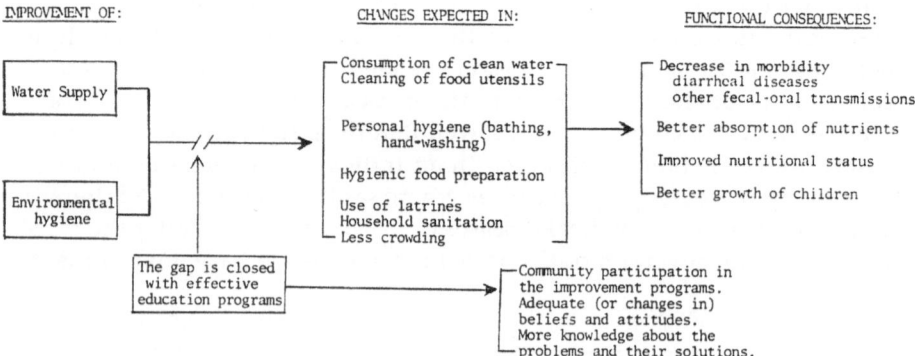

Figure 1. Conceptual linkage between environmental and health improvements.

get population did not result in important reductions of diarrheal incidence.[7-9] What follows is a summation of the results of investigations recently carried out by the Institute of Nutrition of Central America and Panama (INCAP) in Guatemala, supporting the need for *both* sanitation and education. These investigations were on the effects that water supply improvement had on gut absorptive functions and on the effects that a community education program had on the incidence of diarrhea in children.

IMPROVEMENT OF WATER SUPPLY AND EFFECT ON INTESTINAL ABSORPTION*

The objectives of the project were to test the following hypotheses: (a) A population living under unsanitary conditions would have an increased prevalence of diarrheal morbidity and improvements in sanitation, with emphasis on water supply, would diminish diarrheal morbidity. (b) A population with a high prevalence of diarrheal morbidity may waste more food than a population with a lower prevalence of diarrheal morbidity would, and such waste would be a consequence not only of the acute diarrheal episodes but also of chronic, subclinical malabsorption.

Setting and Population. The studies were conducted between 1973 and 1976 in two villages located in the Pacific lowlands of Guatemala (Guanagazapa, or GU, as it will be referred to here, and Florida Aceituno, FA). The villages were 30 kilometers apart and they were comparable with respect to population size (1006 and 1097 inhabitants), age, and sex distribution; family structure; mobility because of seasonal occupational requirements; and climate (warm temperatures with annual means of 27 to 29°C, altitudes of 200 to 250 meters above sea level, and high annual rainfall of about 2000 mm, mainly between April and November). Both villages had a high morbidity rate; respiratory and diarrheal morbidity accounted for 70% of all reported illnesses.

Because one of the objectives was to determine the intestinal absorptive capacity of these populations compared to a population with a lower prevalence of diarrheal morbidity, absorption tests were also carried out in a group of soldiers who were from areas similar to GU and FA, with similar ethnic, sociocultural, and environmental backgrounds, who had been inducted into the army and stationed for at least 6 months in a garrison in Guatemala City (Mariscal Zavala, MZ). Their diets provided bet-

*These studies were carried out by INCAP and the University of North Carolina (Chapel Hill) under the direction of Drs. Roberto Schneider and Morris A. Shiffman, sponsored by the U.S. Agency for International Development.[10]

ter nutrition, mainly in terms of total energy and animal protein, and diarrheal morbidity was significantly lower.

Living Conditions and Sanitation. The two villages had poor sanitary and housing conditions. The streets were of earth, becoming very muddy in the rainy season. Most houses had only one or two rooms. Eating, sleeping, and leisure activities usually took place in the same room. The cooking hearth (usually an open fire) was located outside many of these homes. Most houses had cane or bamboo walls, tin roofs, and earth floors.

Most latrines were poorly kept, and many houses had none. Garbage and trash were carelessly handled, domestic animals were frequently present in the kitchen, eating utensils were not stored to prevent contamination, and housekeeping was also poor.

Water Supply. In 1973 the principal water sources in both villages were shallow wells, generally hand-dug with no casing, without covers or curbstones (the parapet was usually an old automobile tire). A small proportion of the people used water from nearby rivers and creeks. The rivers were also used for clothes-washing and bathing. These conditions did not change in FA throughout the study. There were a few communal faucets in GU in 1973, part of a water supply system built by the Ministry of Public Works. Its construction started in mid-1972 and was completed at the end of 1973. Water was piped into the yards of 164 houses (65% of all houses in GU) in 1974–1975. The water treatment and distribution system consisted of a protected source (spring), chlorination facilities, adequate storage, and water mains with faucets in the yards of 164 homes. This system provided unlimited quantities of high-quality water (chemically and bacteriologically) at a small cost, and did not adversely affect the environment (breeding of vectors). However, it required outside assistance for future maintenance. It was therefore designed for health and environmental appropriateness rather than for functional appropriateness as defined by Pacey.[11]

Health Education. A health education component was introduced in GU in mid-1975. Its overall purpose was to change sanitation behavior in order to optimize the benefits from the potable water system. Its specific objectives were to (a) reduce the fecal wastes of animal and human origin in the home and surrounding yard, (b) install gates to keep domestic animals out of the kitchen and home, (c) promote the construction and use of latrines, (d) improve food and water storage practices, and (e) increase water use for hygienic purposes (personal and home cleanliness and food preparation).

The program was directed mainly to housewives, who met each week for 2 hours with project personnel, and toward adult men, who formed a Betterment Committee that also met each week for 2 to 3 hours. The program was designed and organized by a Health Education Consultant. The field team responsible for health education was formed by two women with a high school education, with support from the Health Post physician, a sanitary inspector, and two Health Post auxiliary nurses who participated on a part-time basis. The program was designed to maximize villager involvement and to have a group-multiplier effect to increase community participation.

The results were evaluated through periodic home visits during which information was solicited from the housewives, and the interviewers looked for specific items. Sixteen objective criteria of sanitary behavior at home (Table I) were used to assess the situation initially (1975). The eight variables pointed out in Table I, plus observation on the cleanliness of the informant's shoes and the protection (covering) of water containers, were analyzed to evaluate changes after 1 year of health education.

Morbidity. The incidence of morbidity was explored through monthly surveys, eliciting information about disease episodes and symptoms of any illness during the 2 weeks that preceded the survey. Questions were asked regarding the health of all family members.

Table I. Home Sanitation in the Two Study Villages before Health Education Program In GU—Mean Frequency of Satisfactory Observations (%)

Environmental variables	GU	FA
Cleanliness of informant's clothes[a,b]	76	85
Animals in the kitchen	46	42
Kitchen barrier present	8	1
Glasses and cups properly stored	19	10
Cooked food protected[a]	94	94
Fecal material on kitchen floor[a]	67	52
Flies seen on food	66	61
Garbage on kitchen floor[a]	62	42
Plates for food protected from animals	96	95
Garbage and trash burned	1	3
Garbage in the yard[a]	47	41
Latrine clean[a]	61	50
Yard recently swept[a]	50	40
Cleanliness of family's clothes[a,b]	72	83
Cleanliness of the house[b]	50	45
Soap observed in house	61	36

[a]One of the 10 criteria used to evaluate the results of the health education program.
[b]Met the norm for the village.

Water Quality. Several hundred samples were collected at 15 different times in 3.5 years in each village during the study period. They were subjected to chemical and bacteriological analyses. The latter was done in the field using the Colitester® (Millipore Corp., U.S.A.) method and standard laboratory procedures for the examination of water.

Absorption studies. More details of these studies have been reported elsewhere.[12]

SOLDIERS. Thirteen soldiers 18 to 22 years old, who had been born in and had lived all their lives in the lowlands of Guatemala, and who had been at an army station (MZ) near Guatemala City for 2 years, were interviewed and evaluated clinically. Besides being exposed during this period to improved environmental sanitation, these men had been eating a better diet than the one commonly eaten in rural areas. All fulfilled the following criteria: (a) no history of acute or chronic gastrointestinal diseases, (b) normal physical checkup, (c) normal urinary excretion of D-xylose 5 hours after an oral dose of 25 g, and (d) two direct examinations of fresh stools negative for ova and parasites.

During the experimental period they lived in a metabolic unit set up at the military post infirmary (altitude: 1500 m; temperature 19 to 22°C; low humidity). After 2 days of adaptation to the rural-type metabolic diet (Table II), sequential 3-day metabolic studies were done. The results of balance II (i.e., days 6 to 8) were used to compare with the studies done in men from GU and FA.

VILLAGERS. In 1973, 60 male volunteers aged 14 to 45 years were randomly chosen in each community among those men who had lived there for at least 10 years. By 1974 some had emigrated and were replaced by others of the same ages, also chosen at random, in order to study 120 men each year. The same procedure was followed in 1975 and 1976. Therefore, at the end of the 4 years there was a "longitudinal" group that had been examined each year and a "nonlongitudinal" group formed by men who participated one, two, or three times in the study. All were healthy at the time of the studies. All men had mild or moderate infestations with one or more of the following intestinal parasites: *Ascaris lumbricoides*, *Trichuris trichiura*, and/or hookworm.

Absorption studies were carried out between May and November of 4 consecutive years beginning in 1973. The men were housed in groups of 8 or 10 in a rural Metabolic Unit adjoining the hospital of a nearby city (Escuintla) with the same climate as that in the study villages. The groups alternated between men of each village, and they lived in the Metabolic Unit for 5 days in 1973 and 8 days in each of the succeeding years. Metabolic balance studies began on the day after admission; in

Table II. Amount of Foods Prepared and Ready to Eat
Offered Daily at the Metabolic Unit to Men from Mariscal
Zavala (MZ), Guanagazapa (GU), and Florida Aceituno (FA)

	Amount of food g/day
Cooked beans[a]	307
Fried beans[a]	40
Corn tortilla	570
Rice	200
Bread	45
Sweet rolls	66
Meat	107
Cheese	109
Chayote[a]	100
Squash	68
Carrots	66
Sugar	37

Total energy 2800 kcal
Total protein 95 g = 380 kcal (13.6% energy); 34% animal protein
Total fat   35 g = 315 kcal (11.2% energy); 22% animal fat

[a]Black beans = *Phaseolus vulgaris;* chayote = *Sechium edule.*

1973 only one 3-day metabolic balance study was performed, and in each of the following years, two consecutive 3-day balance studies were done. Results of the second balance study were used for comparison purposes. During the last 2 days fecal collections were completed and D-xylose absorption tests were carried out.

Metabolic balance tests. The diet shown in Table II, divided into three daily meals, was used for all men. It was prepared with the foods and recipes used in GU and FA, except that it included certain amounts of commercial, canned black beans and more animal protein, because meat is not eaten every day at home. The men were encouraged but not forced to eat all the food served in the Metabolic Unit.

The amounts of each food eaten by each man were weighed at every meal and nutrient intake was calculated from the analyses of representative food aliquots. Complete urine and fecal collections were also obtained, using carmine red as a fecal marker. Aliquots of the foods and of the 3-day stool collections from each balance period were analyzed, and their contents of total energy (bomb calorimetry), nitrogen (macro-Kjeldahl), and fat (Van de Kamer) were used to calculate apparent absorptions. Urinary nitrogen was also determined (micro-Kjeldahl) to calculate apparent nitrogen balance.

RESULTS

Morbidity. There were no differences between GU and FA in terms of total morbidity or in morbidity divided into four groups: diarrheal diseases, respiratory diseases, skin infections, and other infectious diseases. The analyses failed to show an effect of the interventions in GU in absolute terms or adjusted for age, sex, family size, and season. Diarrheal disease was significantly higher in both villages during the rainy season, mainly from April to September.

Water Quality. Potable water in both villages met all chemical quality criteria. Drinking water was "soft," with few total solids and a neutral pH. Bacteriological tests showed that only 3% of 698 samples collected from the GU water distribution system had coliform bacteria, compared with 52% of 505 well-water samples from FA. The frequency of contamination increased in GU when water was sampled from the home yard faucets: 35% of 753 samples had coliform bacteria. The situation was worse in water kept in containers in the house for drinking and cooking purposes: 34 to 52% of the samples collected throughout the 3.5 years were contaminated. No improvements were detected in association with the implementation of the water delivery system or the health education program.

In FA the proportion of contaminated water samples increased from 52% in the wells to 59% ($N = 875$) in home containers.

Health Education. There were improvements in GU related to a decrease in feces on the kitchen floor, better storage of cooked food and drinking water, cleaner yards and latrines, and more health knowledge. There were no changes in FA. This indicated that a health education program can induce behavioral changes leading to improved sanitation.

Metabolic Balance Studies. Within each village there were no differences between the "longitudinal" and "nonlongitudinal" groups of men. The results in 1973 did not differ from balance I in 1974 and there were no consistent differences between 1974, 1975, and 1976 in FA nor between 1974 and 1975 in GU. Absorption of nutrients was higher in GU in 1976 than in other years (Tables III and IV).

The men from FA had larger stool volumes throughout the 4 years of the study than those from GU and MZ, although the differences were not always statistically significant. The apparent absorption of nutrients (i.e., without accounting for obligatory fecal losses) were lower in 1974

Table III. Results of Metabolic Balance Studies in Rural Guatemalan Men after 3 Days in the Metabolic Unit (Balance Period II, Longitudinal Group) and Comparison with Soldiers[a]

Measurement	FA-1974 N = 28[b]	GU-1974 N = 34	FA-1976 N = 28	GU-1976 N = 34	MZ - II N = 13
Body weight, kg	50.35 ± 5.67[c]	58.86 ± 10.39	51.02 ± 5.51	60.69 ± 10.53	62.77 ± 3.02
Stool weight, g/3 days	1056 ± 422	776 ± 238	928 ± 442	759 ± 229	627 ± 291
Nitrogen, mg/kg per day					
Intake	324 ± 46	300 ± 62	329 ± 42	303 ± 49	285 ± 14
Fecal	83 ± 32	70 ± 29	71 ± 24	44 ± 20	40 ± 20
Urinary	194 ± 40	171 ± 51	220 ± 37	225 ± 46	193 ± 21
Apparent balance	59 ± 62	79 ± 25	34 ± 39	31 ± 26	52 ± 22
Apparent absorption, %	75 ± 8	77 ± 8	78 ± 9	84 ± 6	86 ± 6
Energy, kcal/kg per day					
Intake	57 ± 8	53 ± 10	56 ± 6	49 ± 8	50 ± 2
Fecal	7 ± 3	5 ± 2	6 ± 3	3 ± 1	4 ± 2
Apparent absorption, %	88 ± 5	90 ± 3	89 ± 6	95 ± 2	93 ± 4
Fat, mg/kg per day					
Intake	702 ± 78	589 ± 106	574 ± 60	573 ± 89	583 ± 28
Fecal	150 ± 51	115 ± 45	96 ± 46	54 ± 26	87 ± 34
Apparent absorption, %	79 ± 6	81 ± 6	84 ± 7	91 ± 4	85 ± 3

[a]Men from villages FA and GU in 1974 and 1976, and soldiers from MZ (balance period II).
[b]Number of men.
[c]Mean ± SD Results of comparisons between groups shown in Table VII.

Table IV.   Comparisons between Metabolic Balance Period II in Rural Men (FA and GU, in both 1974 and 1976) and Soldiers (MZ)[a]

	FA, 1974, compared with				GU, 1974, compared with			GU, 1976, compared with	
Measurement	GU 1974	MZ	FA 1976	GU 1976	MZ	GU 1976	FA 1976	MZ	FA 1976
Stool weight, g/3 days	↑[b,d]	↑[d]	—	↑[d]	—	—	—	—	—
Apparent absorption									
Nitrogen	—	↓[d]	—	↓[d]	↓[d]	↓[d]	—	—	↑[d]
Total energy	—	↓[d]	—	↓[d]	↓[d]	↓[d]	—	↑[c]	↑[d]
Fat	—	↓[d]	↓[d]	↓[d]	↓[d]	↓[d]	—	↑[d]	↑[d]
Nitrogen balance, mg/kg per day									
Intake	—	↑[d]	—	—	—	—	↓[c]	—	↓[c]
Fecal	—	↑[d]	—	↑[d]	↑[d]	↑[d]	—	—	↓[d]
Urinary	—	—	↓[d]	↓[d]	—	↓[d]	↓[d]	↑[c]	—
Balance	—	—	—	↑[c]	↑[d]	↑[d]	↓[d]	↓[c]	—

[a]From data shown in Table III.
[b]Mean values were higher (↑) or lower (↓) based on Student's grouped *t* test.
[c]$P < 0.05$.
[d]$P < 0.01$.

and 1975 in both villages than in MZ. In 1976, however, the men from GU absorbed dietary protein and energy as well as those from MZ.

All men from GU and FA had between one and seven intestinal parasite species at the time of the metabolic balance studies (*Ascaris lumbricoides, Trichuris trichiura,* hookworm, *Enterobius vermicularis, Giardia lamblia, Escherichia coli, Entamoeba histolytica*). All were asymptomatic, and ova counts suggested mild to moderate infections. There was no correlation between apparent absorption of nitrogen or total energy and the number of parasitic species in the host's intestine.

The results indicate that adult men from rural areas of a developing country who live under conditions of poor sanitation, without appropriate use of potable water, and who eat diets largely based on corn and black beans with some animal protein and low fat (about 11% of total energy intake) have apparent absorptions of the order of 90% of total energy, 75 to 80% of protein, and 75 to 85% of fat. If we assume fecal obligatory losses of 12 to 14 mg N/kg per day, the "true" nitrogen digestibilities would be around 5% higher than apparent digestibilities. Environmental changes and health education seem to improve the absorption of nutrients.

The diets used in this study were typical of the region, although their protein content (P% around 13.6) and the contribution made by protein of animal origin (about 34% of total protein) were higher than those in the diets of most men of similar ethnic, cultural, and socioeconomic conditions in other parts of the country. It is conceivable that protein absorption may be somewhat lower in the latter, whose diets have a P% closer to 10 than 13, and animal proteins contribute to the total by only 20 to 25%.

D-Xylose Absorption. The absorption of D-xylose in FA ranged between 17.8 and 20.0% of the oral dose, with coefficients of variation of 30 to 38%. There were no tendencies toward change throughout the study. In GU, absorption ranged from 19.7 to 23.7%, with coefficients of variation of 25 to 36%. Although there was a trend toward better absorption in 1976, the large year-to-year variability in both villages casts doubt about the significance and consistency of that trend if other tests were done in 1977. It should be noted, however, that a large proportion of men in both villages (29 to 31%) had low absorptions (i.e., < 16% of the oral dose) throughout the study.

CONCLUSIONS FROM THIS STUDY

The introduction of a good water supply system did not seem to be associated with a decrease in the incidence of waterborne diseases. However, it is possible that the assessment of morbidity changes through 2-week recall surveys performed on a monthly basis is not sensitive enough to detect small or moderate changes in communities where there is a high endemic prevalence of diarrheal disease.

The bacteriological monitoring of water sources and at intermediate points in water supply systems in communities with poor sanitation can be misleading. Contamination is, at least in part, a function of home and individual cleanliness and it occurs frequently in the home environment. It is necessary to monitor the quality of water from home faucets and in containers used to keep water for drinking and food preparation.

Health education programs can induce favorable changes in the hygienic behavior and environmental sanitation of rural communities in developing countries.

Absorption of dietary protein and energy is higher in men who have lived for 2 years in environments with better sanitation and who have modified their hygiene habits through education. Improvements of the water supply systems in these men's home environments seems to have a similar effect, especially if it is accompanied by an education component that modifies hygiene behavior.

SANITARY EDUCATION, ENVIRONMENTAL CONTAMINATION, AND INCIDENCE OF
DIARRHEA*

This project was carried out in 1979 and 1980, prompted by the
results of the preceding investigations.

Most programs that intend to reduce diarrheal disease in developing
countries are based on the development of potable water systems, environmental sanitation, and/or construction of latrines. These programs
are expensive and their implementation is beyond the current technical
or financial means of many countries with large numbers of people living in small villages or in widely scattered rural areas. It is, therefore,
necessary to find practical alternatives to reduce fecal-oral contamination.

Extradomiciliary contamination is usually compounded by a highly
contaminated environment within the homes, mainly because of poor
hygiene. Just as education programs must accompany water and sanitation improvements to assure adequate use of clean water and the new
sanitary facilities, it seemed possible that a health education program oriented to change the behavior of mothers and other family members to
reduce domiciliary contamination might reduce diarrheal disease in rural
families and their communities. This might have an effect even without
the introduction of other public health measures. Based on these considerations, a study was designed to test the hypothesis that a health education program, as the sole intervention, would reduce fecal contamination in the home and thus the incidence and prevalence of diarrhea.

Setting and Population. The study was carried out in Florida Aceituno,
a village with 1194 inhabitants, located in the Pacific lowlands of Guatemala. Its altitude is 235 m above sea level, it has a warm climate (mean
annual temperature 27°C), and its annual rainfall between April and
November is 2000 mm. This was the "control" village evaluated in the
project described earlier.

The original settlers of Florida Aceituno, about 70% of its 263 families, own and live on small plots of land (about 1500 m²) located in the
flat central section of the village (Plain). The remaining 30% are newcomers who live on the slopes of a small hill that surrounds part of the central area (Slope). They are poorer than most Plain dwellers. They all have
some fruit trees and they raise a few hens, ducks, geese, and hogs. About
80% of the adult men are migrant agricultural laborers who work some

*These studies were done under the direction of Drs. Fernando Viteri, Leonel Gallardo,
Luis Octavio Angel, and Juan Jose Urrutia, sponsored by the International Development
Research Centre, Ottawa, Canada.

seasons in various parts of the country and are unemployed 3 to 4 months of the year. About 40% of the families lease plots from surrounding landowners to grow corn and black beans, mainly for home consumption. Ninety-six percent of women 15 years old or older engage in home chores without pay. Mean per capita annual income, aside from the family's agricultural production, is about Q 150 (1 Q = $1 U.S.).

Among the adult population (defined as 15 years of age and older), 53% of the men and 75% of the women are illiterate. Almost all who read and write have had only 1 to 3 years of schooling. There is now a primary school (grades 1 to 6) in the village with three teachers who cater to a population of 268 children 6 to 14 years old, although not all of them attend school.

Forty-two percent of the 95 deaths between 1973 and 1977 were caused by, or associated with, gastrointestinal diseases. Of those dying, 82% were children under 5 years of age and 42% were less than 1 year old. Childhood mortality (i.e., between 0 and 5 years of age) during that 5-year period was 235 per 1000 live births. Fifty-one percent of the deceased children died before they were 1 year old.

Living Conditions and Sanitation. The village does not have electric power, although a dozen of the "wealthiest" families have electricity in their homes through wiring that connects them to posts about 300 meters away. Streets are unpaved and become muddy or flooded when it rains. The baseline information obtained on sanitation and water supply is shown in Table V.

It should be stressed that the construction of latrines requires technical considerations because water wells are shallow (at a depth of less than 2 m in the rainy season) and the yards surrounding the houses are usually small and do not allow for an adequate distance between the latrine and the well. Most (75%) existing latrines were found without lids, dirty, and without protection from domestic animals.

Assessment of the Environment. Surveys were carried out to obtain the initial (baseline) demographic, sanitary, and sociocultural information described above. Special care was paid to beliefs and behavioral aspects that might influence fecal contamination and diarrheal morbidity. Based on this information, a visual survey was designed to obtain objective data. For example, the surveyor looked for the presence of garbage in the kitchen while conducting a morbidity survey, rather than relying on the housewife's statements concerning garbage disposal.

Educational Program. The educational program was directed primarily to families with at least one child under 6 years of age. There were 153 such families with 274 children in that age group at the beginning of the study. The program was based on the women's knowledge, the village's

Table V. Sanitary Conditions and Habits fo 263 Families in Florida
Aceituno—1979

Characteristics	% of families
Housing	
Poor general conditions	51
Tin roofs	97
Earth floor	34
Walls made of canes and sticks	44
Wooden walls	37
Water supply (50% of all wells are poorly kept)	
Well in home yard	50
Well away from home	41
Springs and creeks	9
Use of water	
Do not boil drinking water	88
Hand-washing (housewives)	
Only once a day	48
Before preparing foods	22
After defecating	11
After cleansing soiled infants	4
Excreta and garbage disposal	
Latrines (75% in unsanitary conditions)	30
Children under 7 defecate in or around house	89
Feces observed inside the house	20
Feces observed in the yard	70
Soiled diapers mixed with other clothes	87
Garbage observed in the house or yard	95
Kitchen and food-handling	
Animals roam freely in the kitchen	56
Dirty dishes in kitchen	96
Clean dishes prone to contamination (poor storage)	85
Proportion of cooked food left uncovered	54
Infant feeding	
Feed colostrum to newborns	None
Newborns suck a cloth with chickory solution	53
Bottle-feeding to supplement breast-feeding	
Supplemented breast-fed infants	73
In first month of life	59
Solutions of cornstarch, barley, or sugar	64

sociocultural reality, and the baseline information obtained by INCAP. The educational contents and objectives were based on the behavioral aspects listed in Table VI. Figure 2 summarizes the educational methodology that was followed.

The teaching methods were based on a process of *reflection* and *action*, eliminating traditional classroom methods. People were led to reflect about the problems and their solutions. Among the techniques used for reflection, real-life histories related to diarrheal disease were used in radio-theater dramatizations so that people, mainly housewives, would discuss and analyze the situations. Another technique was showing large pictures (e.g., Figures 3 and 4) to housewives and asking them to think about the details related to health. Nine figures with negative and 45 with positive messages were used.

Table VI. Knowledge and Behavior Contents in Educational Program Related to Fecal Contamination and Diarrheal Disease

1. Recognizing when a child has diarrhea
2. Recognizing when a child is dehydrated
3. Immediate handling of a child with diarrhea
4. Oral rehydration
5. Importance of taking the child to the Health Post
6. Preventive measures related to feces
   Use of diapers and underwear and changing as soon as child soils or wets
   Keeping soiled diapers and underwear in closed containers, separated from other clothes; soaking in lime water[a]
   Washing soiled diapers every day
   Teaching toddlers to use a chamber pot; emptying feces into the latrine or burying them and washing the chamber pot immediately
   Playpens for toddlers to avoid deposition of feces in the house
   Looking after latrines: cleaning, covering with a lid; a door that can be securely shut; covered wastebasket for papers; burning soiled paper
   Washing hands with soap under a faucet after defecating or handling soiled diapers
7. Hand-washing to prevent fecal contamination: how, when, why
8. Cleansing of breasts before nursing
9. Food hygiene
   Covering corn meal *(masa)* and cooked foods until eaten
   Washing and protecting (covering) grinding stones, dishes, and cooking utensils
   Washing, boiling, and protecting babies' bottles
10. Caring for drinking water
    Maintenance of wells: curbstones, lids, cleanliness
    Keeping well ropes, buckets, and water containers clean
    Keeping drinking water in closed containers and boiling, especially before giving to babies
11. Food and nutrition[b]
    Nutritive value of foods
    Taking advantage of the most nutritious foods in the household
    Increasing food availability: raising chicks, family orchards, wild plants, etc.
    Nutrition of pregnant women
    Breast-feeding
    Bean pastes to supplement breast milk after 3 months of age

[a]This concept was introduced based on findings of Viteri andTorún (Unpublished observations, 1980).
[b]This section was included because of the relationship between diarrheal disease and malnutrition.

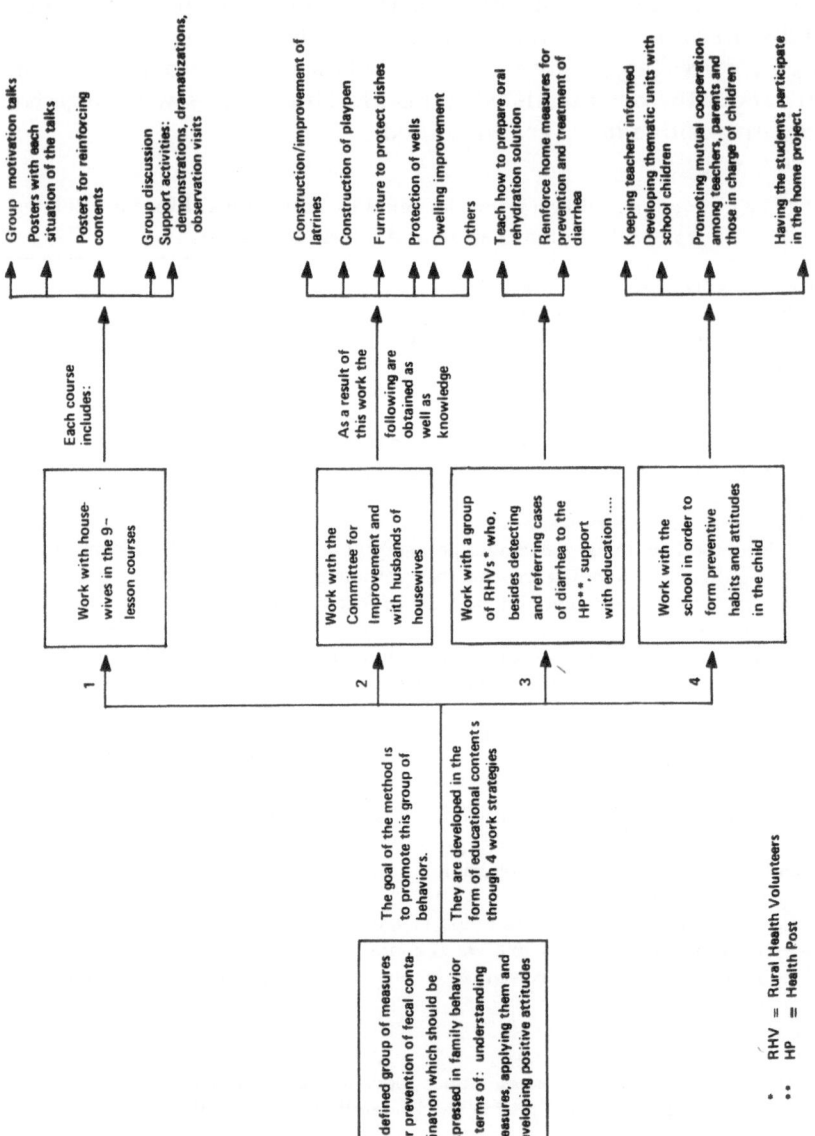

Figure 2. A reflection–action educational methodology to influence behavior of groups and aid in the decrease of fecal contamination of the environment.

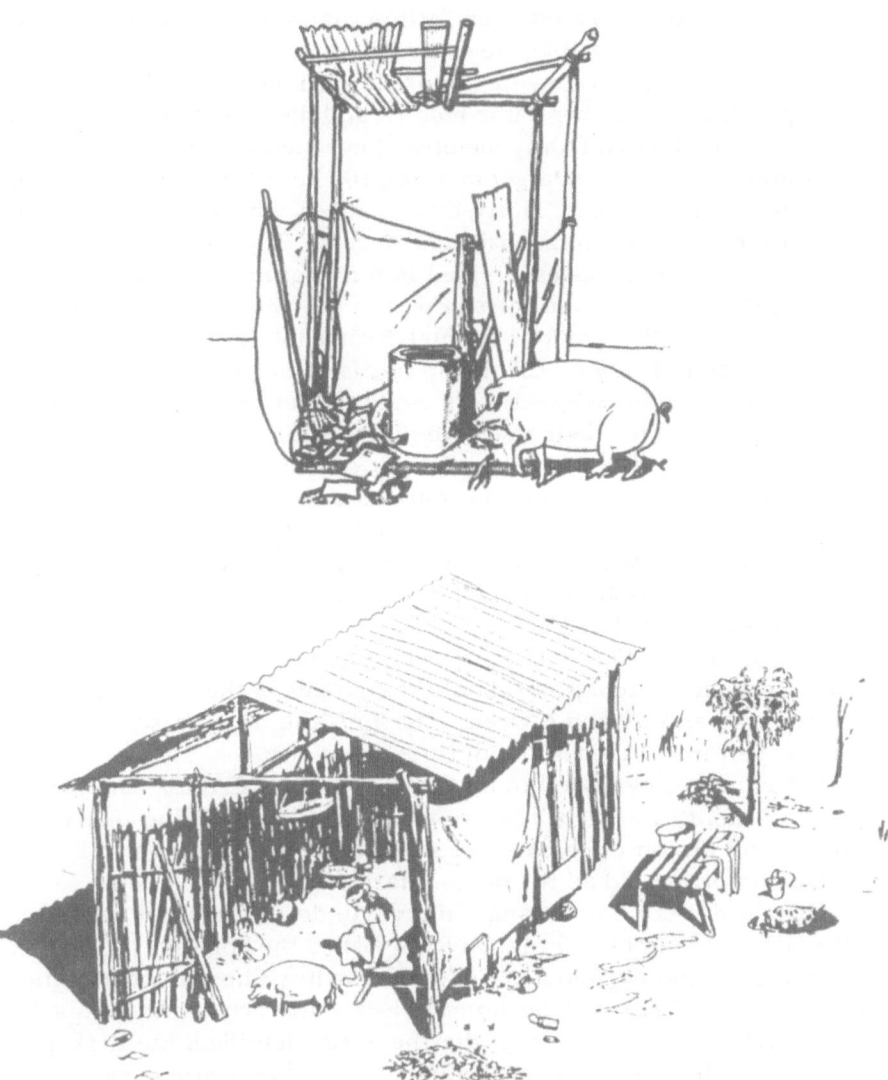

Figures 3 and 4. These pictures were shown to housewives who were then asked to think about the details related to health. The actual pictures were ten times larger.

The *action* centered around an "action commitment" by family members. They pledged to participate every day in the tasks shown in a graph form provided to the housewife (Figure 5). Each person was represented on the graph with a rubber stamp picture, and the housewife was responsible for seeing that all family members kept their pledges.

Among the 153 main target families, 106 housewives participated in the educational program. Thirty-two of those who refused education agreed to the periodic home visits and surveys. The 106 women participated in nine 1-hour classes, divided into five groups of 9 to 27 women each, identified throughout the study with the abbreviations CAMSA 1 to CAMSA 6. CAMSA groups 1 through 5 came into the study at intervals of approximately 1 month. CAMSA 6 consisted of 14 women who could read and write, who accepted work as Rural Health Volunteers (RHV); they were trained for their roles 3 months before beginning the study with CAMSA 1, and they took the 9-hour course 4 months later. The 32 women who acted as the control group were identified by the abbreviation NOCAMSA. Twelve of these women were better off than the average; they were the wives of storeowners, evangelist preachers, or community leaders and lived in better houses in the Plain. They were identified as NOCAMSA ELITE.

Evaluation of Results. Retention of knowledge was evaluated by testing the women in each group about the contents of the CAMSA courses before, at the end of, and 6 weeks after finishing the course. The same observer performed the test on all three occasions.

Behavior was evaluated in all CAMSA and NOCAMSA families six times at 2-month intervals, based on observed items during interviews at home and not on the women's subjective statements. Two well-standardized observers did all the home interviews.

Diarrheal morbidity among children under 6 years was evaluated twice each week for 14 months. An RHV visited the homes of all families under study to inquire about episodes of diarrhea. She was accompanied by a member of the project personnel at least once each month for quality control. Whenever a child with diarrhea was identified, the RHV provided the mother with powdered mineral mix, gave instructions on how to prepare and administer the oral hydration solution, and reported the case to the project personnel, who confirmed the diagnosis and, whenever necessary, referred the child to the Health Post. A stool specimen was obtained for microbiological analysis. Information was recorded about the number of diarrheal episodes and the number of days that each lasted.

Domiciliary bacterial contamination was investigated in 32 CAMSA families. Specimens for bacteriological cultures were obtained initially

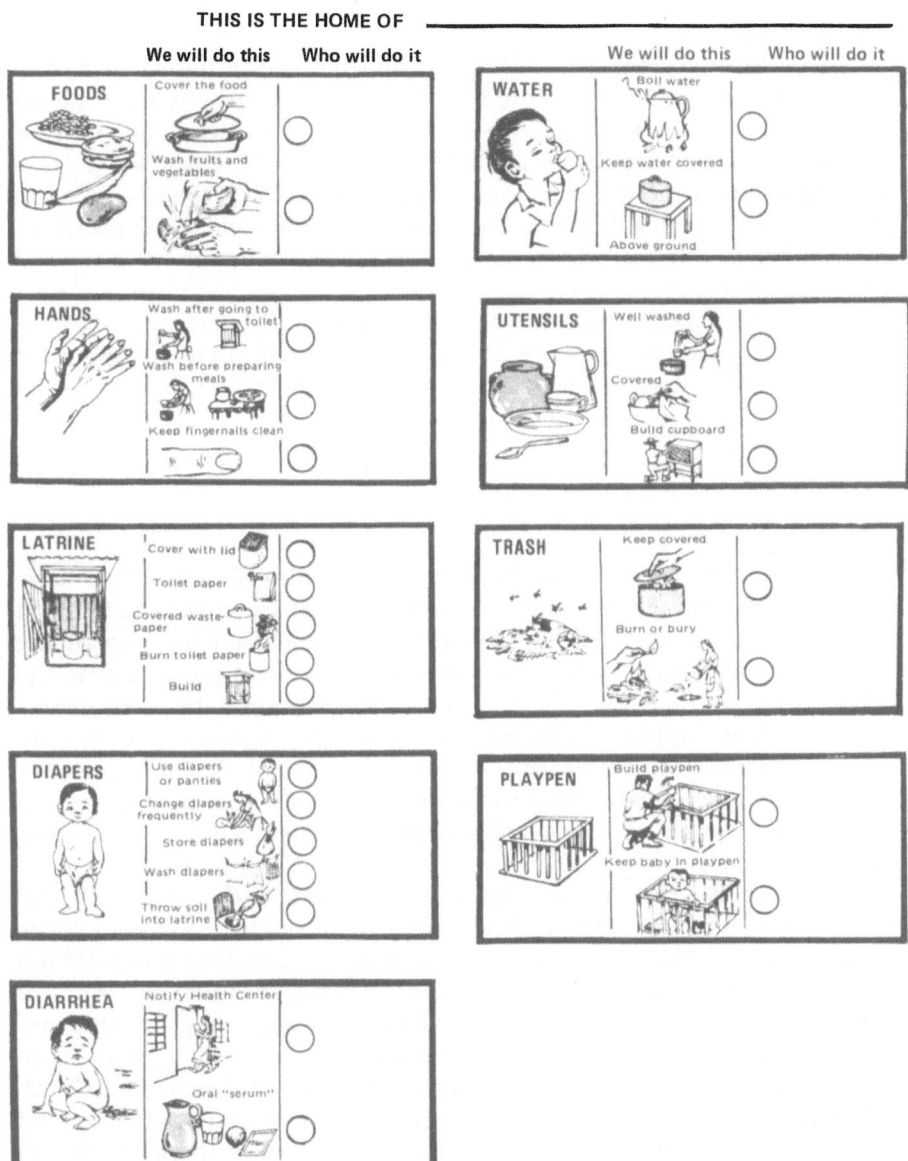

Figure 5. Guide for looking after the family's health; poster of commitments.

and five more times at 2-month intervals from the housewives' hands, drinking water in the home containers, dishware, corn tortillas, and cooked black beans.

The urinary excretion of D-xylose and the concentration of hydrogen in the breath were explored as field tests for carbohydrate malabsorption that might be related to changes in fecal-oral contamination or to alterations in gastrointestinal-tract bacterial ecology. Urinary excretion of D-xylose was measured 5 hours after feeding 25 g D-xylose to adult men randomly selected among the CAMSA (39 men) and NOCAMSA (23 men) families. The test was performed at the beginning, the middle, and the end of the experimental year.

Hydrogen concentration was determined in exhaled air of 37 children 3 to 5 years old from the 32 families subjected to measurements of bacterial contamination in the home. Exhaled air was collected after an overnight fast for 6 consecutive days at the beginning, middle, and end of the experimental year.

RESULTS

Learning and Retention of New Knowledge. Table VII shows that there was an increase in the acquisition and retention of knowledge before and after the course ($p < 0.001$). The differences between the end of the course and 6 weeks later were not significant. CAMSA group 6 were the RHVs who had received a short training course 3 months earlier; this explains their higher results before the course. Groups 1 to 5 were trained in chronological order at 1-month intervals, between September 1979 and January 1980. The tendency toward better results in the initial test as time went by can be attributed to "reflex education" in the community.

Hygiene Behavior at Home. Figure 6 shows the changes observed at the end of the study in each of 27 objective items evaluated. It should be noted that the 19 items that improved among the CAMSA groups did not involve additional expenditures, whereas among the items that did not improve, several would have implied buying such things as chamber pots or materials to make a curbstone and lid for the well, a shack to enclose the latrine, or pens to keep animals out of the kitchen and yard. The lack of change related to the use of diapers and underpants was not surprising, since more than 90% of the children used them before the course. It is thus conceivable that the results might have been better if there had been no economic constraints.

Table VIII shows the proportions of adequate (i.e., positive) observations recorded, pooling all 28 items, in the first and last objective obser-

Table VII. Proportion (%) of Correct Answers Obtained before and after the Courses Given to Housewives about Diagnosis and Causes of Diarrhea, Measures to Prevent Diarrhea, and Child-Feeding

Groups	Test before course			Test at end of course			Test 6 weeks later		
	Diagnosis	Prevention	Feeding	Diagnosis	Prevention	Feeding	Diagnosis	Prevention	Feeding
CAMSA 1 22[a]	36.5 ± 9.6[b]	48.7 ± 9.5	51.5 ± 13.2	79.4 ± 11.9	85.4 ± 6.5	82.7 ± 16.0	78.9 ± 9.7	84.6 ± 6.8	82.7 ± 15.9
CAMSA 2 11	31.5 ± 7.9	54.2 ± 7.3	50.5 ± 11.7	84.9 ± 14.7	86.9 ± 6.2	95.2 ± 5.2	84.9 ± 8.4	86.2 ± 3.9	87.4 ± 8.3
CAMSA 3 22	42.0 ± 10.0	53.5 ± 5.7	52.4 ± 14.1	87.3 ± 7.5	91.1 ± 3.8	92.7 ± 7.5	84.5 ± 8.6	88.4 ± 4.6	92.9 ± 8.3
CAMSA 4 24	41.4 ± 8.8	58.7 ± 5.8	58.7 ± 13.4	87.7 ± 8.4	91.3 ± 3.6	92.8 ± 6.9	81.7 ± 8.1	86.8 ± 4.6	89.0 ± 11.6
CAMSA 5 7	41.0 ± 9.8	58.6 ± 8.4	61.1 ± 21.1	85.7 ± 7.1	93.1 ± 6.1	100.0 ± 0.0	87.8 ± 8.1	88.3 ± 3.3	97.4 ± 6.0
CAMSA 6 14	58.1 ± 12.1	65.6 ± 4.7	71.6 ± 11.8	96.1 ± 4.3	94.6 ± 2.7	95.9 ± 11.3	92.2 ± 7.3	92.6 ± 4.0	97.6 ± 7.7
TOTAL 100	41.7 ± 12.1	55.8 ± 8.7	56.8 ± 15.1	86.5 ± 10.5	90.0 ± 5.7	91.7 ± 11.1	83.9 ± 9.3	87.5 ± 5.4	90.1 ± 12.0

[a]Number of women in each group.
[b]Mean ± SD.

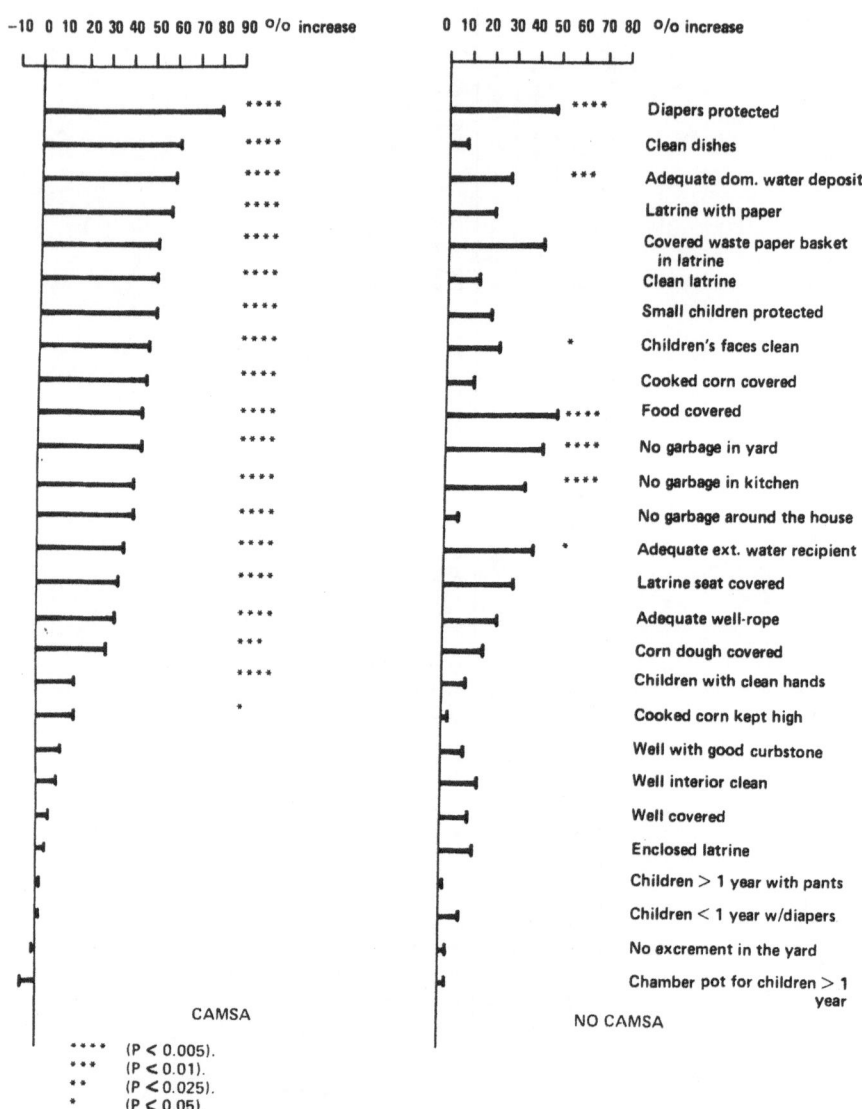

Figure 6. Change in specific behaviors in relation to baseline survey (1979) and final survey (1980) of CAMSA and NOCAMSA groups.

Table VIII. Distribution of CAMSA and NOCAMSA Families according to the Proportion of Adequate Behavior in the First and Last Objective Observation Surveys

Proportion of adequate results %	All CAMSA families				All NOCAMSA families				All families studied			
	First		Last		First		Last		First		Last	
	N	%	N	%	N	%	N	%	N	%	N	%
80–90	0	0	5	4.8	0	0	0	0	0	—	5	3.0
71–80	0	0	13	12.5	0	0	6	9.4	0	0	19	11.3
61–70	3	3.1	34	32.7	1	2.6	6	9.4	4	2.9	40	23.8
51–60	9	9.3	30	28.8	6	15.4	13	20.3	15	11.0	43	25.6
50 and less	85	87.6	22	21.1	32	82.0	39	60.9	117	86.0	61	36.3
Total	97	100.0	104	100.0	39	100.0	64	100.0	136	100.0	168	100.0

vation surveys. It must be noted that the NOCAMSA group included the 12 elite families whose initial behavior was at a higher level than that of the nonelite families and similar to that of the RHVs who formed one of the CAMSA groups. Initially, only 3% of the CAMSA or NOCAMSA families had a score of 60% or better. At the end, one-half of the CAMSA families and one-fifth of the NOCAMSA had such scores. The small, but significant, improvement among the latter may be because (a) although only the CAMSA groups received systematic education, all families under study may have been influenced by the project activities, mainly the home visits and interviews; and (b) the interaction and communication among all inhabitants of the village (CAMSA and NOCAMSA) may have resulted in some degree of "reflex education."

Incidence of Diarrhea. Data from the NOCAMSA, elite and CAMSA 6 (RHV) groups were excluded from the analysis. The incidence of diarrheal disease was high in the village, with 10 to 36% of all children under 6 affected every month over a 12-month period. Initially, it was higher among the CAMSA groups, which may be an artifact because of the small number of children in this group during the first 2 months of the study (Table IX). There was an increase in the incidence of diarrheal disease with the onset of the rains, and this "epidemic" superimposed on the endemic picture peaked in June 1980. Similar epidemics had been recorded in the village from 1973 to 1976.[10] Although there were small differences in the overall endemic situation between the CAMSA and NOCAMSA groups, the epidemic increase was significantly lower among the CAMSA children (Table IX and Figure 7). This was true whether expressed as the proportion of children with diarrhea or as the ratio of child-days with diarrhea/child-days studied. The differences were mainly due to the incidence of diarrheal disease among children 0 to 24 months old (Table X). There were only slight variations in the diarrheal incidence observed in CAMSA and NOCAMSA children 2 to 6 years old.

Similar results were obtained when data from the Plain dwellers and the poorer Slope dwellers were analyzed separately. However, although in both geographical locations the CAMSA children fared better than the NOCAMSA, the epidemic increase was higher in the Slope than in the Plain area. This suggests that the educational measures had a greater impact among those families who lived under relatively better conditions.

Stool Cultures. Bacteriological investigations were done on 451 specimens collected during 49% of the 929 diarrheal episodes recorded. *Escherichia coli* (stable toxin), *Shigella*, and *Salmonella* were identified in 18.7, 4.0, and 0.7% of the specimens, respectively. Because of technical difficulties it was not possible to investigate the presence of labile-toxin *E. coli*. Rotavirus was found in 3.8% of the specimens.

Stable-toxin *E. coli* was identified in 28% of the cultures obtained between September 1979 and March 1980, with transient decreases in October and January. It decreased gradually to less than 10% from March to August 1980, which coincided with the diarrhea epidemic period. In July and August 1979 it was also found in less than 10% of the feces from children with diarrhea. The incidence of diarrhea was relatively high in those 2 months (Tables IX and X). Rotavirus was found in 10 to 23% of the specimens in September, October, January, February, and April. They were absent in all other months, including those with peak diarrheal incidence. This suggests that, although rotavirus and the three bacteria mentioned above were responsible for one-third of the diarrheal episodes during the nonepidemic months, other agents were probably responsible for the epidemic peak. These may have been labile-toxin *E. coli*, enteroviruses other than rotavirus, or other bacteria.

Bacterial Contamination of Hands, Foods, and Dishware. Drinking water was contaminated with enteric bacteria, mainly *E. coli* and *Klebsiella*, in 84 to 100% of the specimens sampled six times throughout the study in the homes of CAMSA group 1. However, *E. coli* was found in 44% of the specimens in September and November 1979, and only in 3 to 12% in February, March, May, and August 1980.

There were no consistent changes in the frequency with which *E. coli* was identified in corn tortillas or cooked beans, ranging from 6 to 70% of the time, or in dishware (22 to 94%), or on the housewife's hands (19 to 88%). *Clostridium*, however, was found most frequently in tortillas, beans and dishes, and on hands in the months of August and October 1979, and with the least frequency at the end of the study (May and July 1980). The latter corresponded to the epidemic period.

In general terms, tortillas were contaminated more often than cooked beans. Bacterial counts were $10^{4.5}$ to $10^{7.8}$/g in tortillas and $10^{3.6}$ to $10^{7.6}$/g in cooked beans. *Klebsiella* and *E. coli* were the predominant bacteria. They were also predominant in dishware, with total bacterial counts of $10^{4.3}$ to $10^{7.8}$/cm^2 of surface area. The same was true on the hands of housewives washed with sterile water. Except for the evaluation done in August, enterobacteriae ($10^{4.3}$ to $10^{7.8}$/ml of wash water) were found more than 56% of the time. It must be noted that housewives normally washed their hands with household water that, as mentioned above, was contaminated 84 to 100% of the times tested.

Malabsorption Tests. The absorption of D-xylose was relatively low: urinary excretion (mean ± *SD*) was 18 ± 9% of the ingested dose in 155 tests performed. There were no differences between men from CAMSA

Table IX. Incidence of Diarrheal Disease in Children Under 6 Years of Age (1979–1980)

Per thousand Child Month	Children studied	Children with diarrhea		Child-days studied	Child-days with diarrhea		Diarrheal episodes		
Month		N	%		N	per thousand days	N	Per child with diarrhea, mean	Days duration, mean
CAMSA									
1979									
September	53	17	32	1533	78	51	19	1.1	4.1
October	72	18	25	2117	56	26	22	1.2	2.5
November	112	25	22	3297	116	35	33	1.3	3.5
December	153	24	16	4499	100	22	28	1.2	3.6
1980									
January	157	44	28	4688	233	50	52	1.2	4.5
February	158	30	19	4424	73	16	33	1.1	2.2
March	185	35	19	5180	112	22	39	1.1	2.9
April	186	39	21	5445	108	20	42	1.1	2.6
May	183	36	20	5480	146	27	47	1.3	3.1
June	186	45	24	5408	210	39	57	1.3	3.7
July	188	32	17	5689	181	32	39	1.2	4.6
August	188	19	10	5725	81	14	18	0.9	4.5

NOCAMSA

1979								
July	201	84	42	5694	242	42	119	1.4	2.0
August	223	61	27	6277	260	41	71	1.2	3.7
September	182	41	23	5018	157	31	48	1.2	3.3
October	149	29	19	4332	152	35	41	1.4	3.7
November	98	24	24	2683	107	40	33	1.4	3.2
December	69	8	12	1923	22	11	10	1.2	2.2
1980								
January	48	12	25	1385	38	27	15	1.2	2.5
February	49	8	16	1347	23	17	9	1.1	2.6
March	82	17	21	1870	72	38	20	1.2	3.6
April	83	24	29	2332	115	49	31	1.3	3.7
May	80	22	28	2374	111	47	27	1.2	4.1
June	84	30	36	2437	177	73	44	1.5	4.0
July	87	22	25	2563	66	26	22	1.0	3.0
August	90	9	10	2660	29	11	10	1.1	2.9

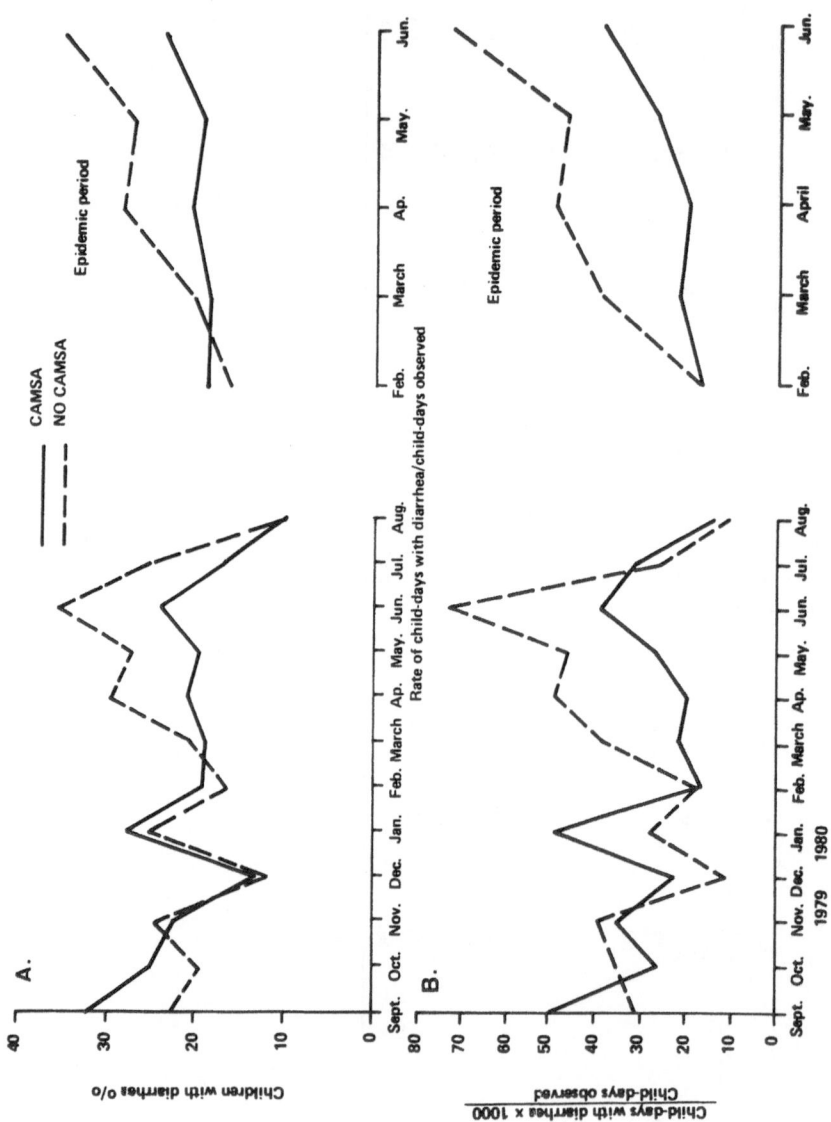

Figure 7. Diarrhea incidence in children under 6 years of age. A: percentage (%) of children with diarrhea. B: rate of child-days with diarrhea/child-days observed.

and NOCAMSA families or at the beginning, middle, or end of the study year.

H_2 concentration in exhaled air ranged from 8 to 32 ppm throughout the year, and there were no changes related to the education program.

Therefore, the educational program with its concomitant sanitary behavior changes did not affect the absorption of D-xylose or the concentration of exhaled hydrogen while fasting, at least under the prevailing experimental conditions.

CONCLUSIONS

The educational program induced behavioral changes that resulted in improved domiciliary hygiene conditions. There were indications that the improvements might have been greater had there been no economic constraints. Some degree of improvement was observed among the families that were not subjected to the systematic educational program. This may have been because of reflex education as a consequence of the interaction and communication among all village inhabitants.

The endemic level of diarrheal disease showed a slight tendency to decrease with the educational program. The program prevented or diminished the diarrhea epidemic superimposed on the endemic diarrhea background. This preventive role of education was seen mainly in children 0 to 24 months old, and it was greater among families who lived under relatively better conditions.

The educational program did not reduce the contamination of hands, dishware, food, and drinking water with E. coli and Klebsiella. However, neither stable-toxin E. coli, Salmonella, Shigella, nor rotavirus was responsible for the epidemic rise in diarrheal disease. It is possible that the methods used to investigate contamination with microorganisms and to identify the etiological agents of diarrhea were not the most suitable to relate the two types of information. It may be that the diarrheal epidemic was caused by a virus or an unidentified agent.

Nevertheless, education as the sole intervention did protect children from an increase in the incidence of diarrheal disease. Its effect would probably be greater if it were combined with measures such as improvements in water supply and environmental sanitation.

CONCLUSIONS FROM BOTH STUDIES

The studies summarized in this chapter demonstrate that changes in behavior associated with improvements in water supply or environmen-

Table X. Incidence of Diarrheal Disease in Children Under 24 Months of Age (1979–1980)

Month	Children studied	Children with diarrhea		Child-days studied	Child-days with diarrhea		Diarrheal episodes		
		N	%		N	per thousand Child-days	N	Per child with diarrhea, means	Days duration, mean
CAMSA									
September	13	5	38	377	28	74	5	1.0	5.6
October	16	5	31	460	12	26	6	1.2	2.0
November	32	12	38	940	67	71	18	1.5	3.7
December	48	13	27	1437	52	36	15	1.2	3.5
January	54	19	35	1562	134	86	24	1.3	5.6
February	54	11	20	1492	34	23	14	1.3	2.4
March	59	19	32	1729	56	32	22	1.2	2.5
April	60	19	32	1743	66	38	20	1.1	3.3
May	58	14	24	1770	72	41	20	1.4	3.6
June	61	23	38	1764	92	52	28	1.2	3.3
July	63	17	27	1939	91	47	21	1.2	4.3
August	65	7	11	1986	30	15	7	1.0	4.3

NOCAMSA

July	52	22	42	1438	103	72	34	1.5	3.0
August	57	23	40	1593	101	64	25	1.1	4.0
September	52	12	23	1438	73	51	15	1.2	4.9
October	46	11	24	1332	64	48	15	1.4	4.3
November	28	10	36	757	59	78	14	1.4	4.2
December	24	3	12	645	12	19	4	1.3	3.0
January	20	7	35	569	28	49	10	1.4	2.8
February	20	5	25	552	15	27	6	1.2	2.5
March	30	9	30	734	50	68	11	1.2	4.5
April	33	15	45	919	87	95	20	1.3	4.4
May	30	13	43	880	67	77	17	1.3	3.9
June	33	17	52	956	123	129	27	1.6	4.6
July	35	14	40	1036	45	43	14	1.0	3.2
August	36	4	11	1053	19	18	5	1.2	3.8

tal sanitation will have a favorable impact on the incidence of diarrheal disease and the absorption of nutrients in populations of developing countries. This, in turn, will aid and enhance other measures tending to ameliorate the population's nutritional status, as hypothesized in Figure 1. The implementation of sanitary or educational measures as isolated interventions will usually have a small impact or none at all. Conversely, the association of these interventions may have a synergistic effect. As Gordon et al.[7] pointed out years ago, "control [of acute diarrheal disease] depends to a great extent on individuals. . . . The argument is for equal attention to people and to things, to babies as well as to water. . . . The provision of physical facilities without the sympathy and understanding of the people who are to use them has repeatedly proved ineffective. The cultivation of a hygienic way of living creates demand for the physical facilities with which to achieve it."

REFERENCES

1. Scrimshaw, N. S., Taylor, C. E., and Gordon, J. E. *Interactions of Nutrition and Infection*, World Health Organization Monograph Series No. 57. WHO, Geneva, Switzerland, 1968.
2. Viteri, F. E., and Schneider, R. E. Gastrointestinal alterations in protein-calorie malnutrition. *Med. Clin. North Am.* **58**:1487–1505, 1974.
3. Rosenberg, I. H., and Scrimshaw, N. S. (Eds.). Malabsorption and nutrition. *Am. J. Clin. Nutr.* **25**:1045–1289, (Oct., Nov.), 1972.
4. Lindenbaum, J., Gerson, C. D., and Kent, T. H. Recovery of small-intestinal structure and function after residence in the tropics. I. Studies in Peace Corps volunteers. *Ann. Intern. Med.* **74**:218, 1971.
5. Gerson, C. D., Kent, T. H., Saha, J. R., Siddiqui, N., and Lindenbaum, J. Recovery of small-intestinal structure and function after residence in the tropics. II. Studies in Indians and Pakistanis living in New York City. *Ann. Intern. Med.* **75**:41, 1971.
6. Feachem, R. Priorities for diarrhoeal disease control: Water, excreta, behaviour and diarrhoea. *Diarrhoea Dialogue* **4**:4–5, 1981.
7. Gordon, J. E., Béhar, M., and Scrimshaw, N. S. Acute diarrheal disease in less developed countries. 3. Methods for prevention and control. *Bull. WHO* **31**:21–28, 1964.
8. Levine, R. J., Khan, M. R., D'Souza, S., and Nalin, D. R. Failure of sanitary wells to protect against cholera and other diarrhoeas in Bangladesh. *Lancet* **ii**:86–89, 1976.
9. Feachem, R. *Water, Health and Development*. Tri-Med Books, London, England, 1978.
10. Shiffman, M. A., Schneider, R., Faigenblum, J. M., Helms, R., and Turner, A. Field studies on water sanitation and health education in relation to health status in Central America. *Prog. Water Technol.* **11**:143–150, 1978.
11. Pacey, A. (Ed.). Technology is not enough: The provision and maintenance of appropriate water supplies. *Aqua* **1**:1–58, 1977.
12. Schneider, R. E., Torún, B., Shiffman, M., Anderson, C., and Helms, R. Absorptive capacity of adult Guatemalan rural males living under different conditions of sanitation. In: *Protein-Energy Requirements of Developing Countries: Evaluation of New Data*, B. Torún, V. R. Young, and W. M. Rand (Eds.), pp. 139–149. United Nations University World Hunger Programme, Food and Nutrition Bulletin Supplement No. 5, 1981.

V

Policy, Planning, and Implementation

16

Diarrhea and Nutrient Requirements

NEVIN S. SCRIMSHAW, OSCAR BRUNSER, GERALD KEUSCH, AYESHA MOLLA, IMRAN OZALP, AND BENJAMIN TORÚN

INTRODUCTION

The high prevalence rates, particularly among young children in most developing countries, make the influence of diarrhea on nutritional requirements of major concern. The multiple mechanisms whereby diarrhea of infectious origin can affect dietary requirements for calories and protein are listed in Table I. Estimation of the consequences for nutritional requirements is complicated by large quantitative and qualitative variations in the disease burden among different population and age groups. The effects depend on the type of diarrhea as well as on its frequency, severity, and duration. Moreover, available quantitative data are extremely limited. Those available under each of the categories indicated are examined separately in the text that follows.

NEVIN S. SCRIMSHAW • The United Nations University World Hunger Programme, Massachusetts Institute of Technology, Cambridge, Massachusetts. OSCAR BRUNSER • Laboratorio de Investigaciones Pediatricas, Santiago, Chile. GERALD KEUSCH • Division of Geographic Medicine, Tufts University School of Medicine, Boston, Massachusetts. AYESHA MOLLA • International Centre for Diarrhoeal Disease Research, Dacca, Bangladesh. IMRAN OZALP • Hacettepe University, Faculty of Medicine, Department of Biochemistry, Hacettepe, Ankara, Turkey. BENJAMIN TORÚN • Institute of Nutrition of Central America and Panama, Division of Physiology and Clinical Nutrition, Guatemala City, Guatemala.

Table I. Potential Nutritional Effects of Diarrhea[a]

Effect	Mechanism	Nitrogen	Calories	Vitamins and minerals
1. Anorexia	Unknown	+ +	+ +	+ +
2. Altered diet	Cultural practices	+ +	+	+ +
3. Malabsorption	Morphological, functional			Variable
Acute	changes—G. I. Hurry	+	+	Unknown
Chronic	"Tropical jejunitis"	+	+	
4. Losses				
Urine—metabolic	Stress response	+	—	Variable
pathological	Not relevant to diarrhea	—	—	—
Feces—pathological	Protein-losing enteropathy, blood	+	±	—
Skin	Not relevant to diarrhea	—	—	—
Other	Vomiting	±	±	
5. Internal sequestering	Variable	—	—	Variable
6. Internal synthesis	C-reactive protein, immunoglobulins, etc.	*	±	—
7. Fever	Increased BMR	—	+#	—

[a]These vary with the etiology, duration, and severity of diarrhea and with the age and physiological and nutritional state of the individual and the diet during the acute episode.
+ = Mild effect.
* = Moderate effect.
# = Proportional to fever.
± = Minimal effect.
— = Negative effect

CLASSIFICATION AND DEFINITIONS

Investigators of diarrheal disease have repeatedly lamented the difficulty, if not the impossibility, of having a universally applicable definition of diarrhea. This is in part because dietary factors (e.g., fiber) will affect the bulk and water content of the stool without necessarily altering intestinal physiology, and also in part because morphology and consistency of stool is only grossly reflective of its water content. In addition, individual sensitivity or stoicism ("observational threshold") conditions the awareness of daily changes in defecation patterns, although the bloody, mucoid stool of dysentery or diarrhea is readily recognized.

For these reasons, either definitions have been arbitrarily set (e.g., four or more liquid or semiliquid stools per day) or the individual is asked to take note of a change in his habitual pattern in the number or nature of the stools. While the former may well underestimate the incidence of diarrheal disease, the latter approach may be too subjective for the purpose of quantitative scientific study. Methods appropriate for the metabolic ward will often not be feasible in the field. The dilemma is heightened by the fact that infections with known enteric pathogens result in a clinical spectrum of illness from the asymptomatic to severe.

All of these factors affect the perception of illness and the decision of patients to seek help from the available health facilities. Since the duration of symptoms enters into this decision making, the time dimension becomes an important variable as well. Recognizing all of this, it is clear that diarrhea is a clinical concept that encompasses a range from a rapidly fatal disease to a subtle distinction from the normal, or accepted, state.

For the purpose of a standard, minimal definition, we propose that diarrhea be defined as an increase in the frequency by two or more times of the usual daily number of stools that are, in addition, loose, extending over a period of 24 hours or more. The presence of nausea, vomiting, fever, abdominal cramps, dehydration, or bloody-mucoid stools is consistent with, but not necessary for, the diagnosis. In practice, however, the perception of the patient, or the mother (or surrogate) of the infant or child, of changes in the quantity or quality of the stool is the most reliable guide.

The dysenteric diseases are usually separated from the diarrheas. The latter are fluid-losing enteric processes, whether clear or bloody, whereas dysentery is a syndrome recognized by the presence of multiple, small-volume stools consisting largely of blood and mucus, accompanied by cramps and tenesmus. Diarrhea may precede dysentery, or the clinical distinction may be blurred, as in some cases of shigellosis. The two entities are also generally attributable to lesions of the proximal small bowel and colon, respectively.

In consideration of nutrient requirements during and after an episode of diarrhea or dysentery as defined, it is desirable to separate one etiology from another, for the pathogenesis of illness varies considerably, and with it the nutritional impact in both the short and long term. Determination of etiology, however, requires technology that may not be readily available and, under the best of circumstances, is at present possible in only a portion of the patients, whether in hospital or field studies (see Black *et al.*, chapter 4, this volume). The remainder will be composed of a mixed group of other etiologies as well as unrecognized cases of the identifiable diseases.

From the standpoint of nutritional requirements, however, the specific etiology is less important than is the nature of the resulting pathophysiological lesion. In addition, some cases of diarrhea, particularly in

Table II.   Physiological Classification of Diarrheas

Category	Pathophysiology	Site	Example
Electrolyte-losing	Net accumulation of isotonic fluid in gut lumen	Proximal small bowel	*V. cholerae*
Nutrient malabsorption	Villus cell damage or loss	Proximal small bowel	Rotavirus
Inflammatory	Mucosal inflammation and necrosis	Ileum and/or colon	*Shigella* sp.

children, are nonenteric in origin. Diarrhea may be associated with measles, otitis media, malaria, and other common systemic or localized infections, and may contribute to their adverse impact on nutritional status.

A physiological classification will, in fact, reflect the specific etiology and the predominant mechanism(s) involved in pathogenesis. The potential nutritional consequences of illness, and the implications for nutrient requirements, can be considered under three headings: electrolyte-losing, nutrient malabsorption, and inflammatory (exudative) diarrheas (Table II). Chapters 2 and 3 in this volume review the major enteric bacterial and viral pathogens and provide the background data on pathogenesis and pathophysiology for this classification. It is important to remember that any one pathogen can affect more than one pathway.

The hallmark of the electrolyte-losing diarrheas is the excretion of large volumes of isotonic fluids with a resulting problem in body fluid homeostasis. There is no histologically demonstrable damage to the mucosa and no inflammatory exudate in the stool, which contains little or no protein.

In addition to electrolyte losses, agents that damage the proximal small bowel mucosa and reduce the absorptive surface and/or the absorptive function of individual villous epithelial cells may cause a defect in absorption of various nutrients, including nitrogen, carbohydrate, and fat. The data reported in chapter 9 indicate a markedly depressed coefficient of absorption for nitrogen, carbohydrate, and fat in rotavirus infection, presumably by the suggested mechanism, although this is not directly demonstrated.

In addition to causing electrolyte and nutrient losses, agents that damage the distal small bowel and colon, and that induce ulcerative lesions of the epithelial cell lining, promote the exudation and loss from the body of leukocytes, erythrocytes, glycoprotein-rich intestinal mucus, and plasma proteins (see chapter 10). Exudative losses of nutrients will exacerbate the nutritional consequences of absorptive losses and must be accounted for in calculation of nutrient requirements.

We operationally define chronic diarrhea as the persistence of symptoms for 3 weeks or longer, with or without positive cultures for the original (or another) recognized pathogen. Similarly, the beginning of the recovery or convalescent period corresponds to the earliest return of stools to a normal or near normal pattern, usually with a diminution in subjective (anorexia, apathy, etc.) or objective (fever, cramps, etc.) signs or symptoms.

DIARRHEAL DISEASE MORBIDITY

Diarrhea is rarely a significant health problem during the early months of life for the breast-fed infant because weight loss, if it occurs, is rapidly made up. Once breast milk is no longer an adequate source of food, complementary feeding is inadequate and often contaminated, and growth falters, diarrhea becomes so frequent and nutritionally significant that it has received the name "weanling diarrhea." Some typical morbidity rates are shown in Table III. These amount to about eight attacks of diarrheal disease per child per year.[1]

Since all available evidence suggests a convalescent period several times longer than the acute episode, the effects of diarrhea alone on the growth of children under 2 years of age can be considerable. Field studies demonstrated a strong longitudinal correlation between days ill with diarrhea and depressed weight gain (see chapter 8, this volume).

Table III. Days of Diarrhea Experienced by 45 Cohort Children, Santa María Cauqué[a]

Age (months)	Person-days of observation	Total days with diarrhea	Percent of life experience ill with diarrhea
0–5	8,213	466	5.7
6–11	8,213	788	9.6
12–17	8,213	1,236	15.0
18–23	8,213	1,487	18.1
24–29	7,757[b]	1,184	15.3
30–35	7,605[b]	972	12.8
Total	48,214	6,133	12.7

[a]Source: reference 1.
[b]Attrition due to deaths.

For older children, diarrheal episodes become less frequent, but for individuals at the higher end of the frequency distribution, diarrhea may still have serious adverse effects on nutritional and health status. Much the same statement can be made for diarrheal disease morbidity in adults. For the individual in borderline nutritional status, and with an inadequate diet, the additional burden of acute diarrhea can be significant.

EXTERNAL LOSSES

REDUCED FOOD INTAKE

Anorexia. The effects of diarrhea on nutrient intakes operate through several mechanisms. Anorexia during episodes of acute diarrhea is a leading cause for decreased food intake. Dehydration, electrolyte losses, abdominal distention, acidosis, and vomiting may contribute to anorexia. Anorexia often results in a drastic reduction in food intake or even cessation of breast-feeding for the young infant.

Many authors have shown that, in the lower socioeconomic groups of most developing countries, infectious diseases are responsible for anorexia and marked reduction in food intake during the second year of life when children are commonly being weaned. A strong inverse correlation has also been reported between infectious disease and calorie intake during this period of a child's life (Table IV).[2] Martorell and Yarbrough (chapter 8) found, in a Guatemalan village, an average daily reduction of calorie and protein intake of 20%, equivalent to 175 kcal and 4.8 g protein per day. The effect of diarrhea on food intake was significantly greater than that from other infections.

Hoyle *et al.*[3] studied three groups of matched children in rural Bangladesh (control, acute diarrhea, and acute diarrhea with feeding encouragement). Calorie and protein intake in the control children was 129.9 kcal/kg and 1.9 g protein/kg, respectively. In a group of children with acute diarrhea whose mothers did not receive dietary education, intake of calories and protein was 75.0 kcal/kg and 0.96 g/kg, respectively. In another group with diarrhea whose mothers received dietary education, average intakes were 60.9 kcal/kg and 0.70 g protein/kg per day, respectively. These results suggest that, even with intensive encouragement, increased food intake was not possible, mainly because of child anorexia.

Recently, A. M. Molla *et al.* (chapter 7) studied the intake of protein and metabolizable calories during and after acute diarrhea of various etiologies (Table II). These results confirm that anorexia plays an impor-

Table IV. Calorie Intake by Village Children *during Illness* and Periods *Free* of Symptoms[a]

Child no.	Mean % recommended calories			Mean % recommended calories associated with diarrhea
	Diarrhea[b]	Other illness[c]	Well[d]	
63	82.6 (5)[e]	60.3 (3)	80.1 (12)	2.5
54	82.4 (12)	—[f]	80.3 (8)	2.1
46	97.5 (2)	103.3 (7)	96.8 (9)	0.7
23	88.3 (4)	85.7 (3)	90.3 (9)	−2.0
35	74.3 (9)	84.5 (6)	78.0 (2)	−3.7
79	102.0 (6)	98.5 (2)	107.6 (8)	−5.6
15	68.5 (2)	72.0 (2)	75.3 (12)	−6.8
80	72.8 (4)	75.0 (8)	82.0 (5)	−9.2
76	83.7 (3)	94.4 (8)	95.7 (9)	−12.0
49	70.0 (3)	64.0 (2)	83.7 (9)	−13.7
24	85.5 (2)	61.8 (5)	101.9 (17)	−16.4
82	65.0 (3)	61.9 (7)	82.2 (5)	−17.2
34	71.2 (11)	69.8 (5)	93.4 (13)	−22.2
91	70.0 (1)	112.0 (1)	99.4 (5)	−29.4
37	69.3 (3)	86.7 (3)	101.1 (11)	−31.8
88	106.6 (5)	—	143.0 (4)	−36.4
69	65.8 (15)	86.8 (14)	122.5 (2)	−56.7

[a]Source: reference 2.
[b]Diarrhea or diarrhea associated with other illnesses.
[c]Respiratory, exanthemic, febrile, skin, eye, ear.
[d]Includes convalescence except 2 weeks following illnesses.
[e]Mean % recommended calories (number of weekly measurements).
[f]No episodes or measurement recorded in period.
Mean % recommended calories for diarrhea = 79.7
Mean % recommended calories for disease-free = 95.9
difference = $\overline{16.2\%}$
Thus, 1- to 2-year-old children consume 12,000 calories (50.209 kJ) less per child per year because of diarrhea.

tant role in the reduction of calorie and protein intake during the acute diarrheas. It is important to note that with rotavirus, anorexia persisted for at least 2 weeks after recovery.

Cultural and Therapeutic Practices. Reduction of food intake during diarrhea is also a result of maternal food-withholding behavior and of various cultural practices in different communities of the world. While the withholding practice might be in part a response to the presence of child anorexia during diarrhea, it extends all the way to starvation during the acute stage. Alterations in dietary composition, such as feeding barley water or addition of herbal infusions to the diet, and cultural beliefs against the feeding of milk and solid foods are likely to contribute to decreased food intake during diarrhea.

ABSORPTION

In Acute Diarrhea of Short Duration. Acute diarrhea has been associated with short-term disturbances of the absorption of almost every nutrient studied. This malabsorption is caused by a number of mechanisms operating singly or in combination: mucosal damage; alterations in motility; dilution; changes in chemical structure of molecules through degradation, fermentation, etc.; competition for uptake of nutrients on the part of the causative agent; effect of bacterial catabolites; etc. In evaluating nutrient losses caused by acute diarrhea, increased baseline excretion secondary to preexisting subclinical environmental ("tropical") enteropathy should be taken into consideration.

Mild to moderate diarrheal disease was reported to reduce nutrient intake by approximately 20% in Guatemalan preschool children (chapter 8), while the more severe toxigenic diarrheas studied in similar children in Bangladesh caused decreased intakes of from 30 to 50%. In addition, absorption of ingested protein was decreased by nearly 20% in Indian preschool children with mild to moderate diarrhea (see chapter 14), and by over 30% in diarrhea caused by rotavirus or *Shigella* in Bangladeshi children of this age.

Nitrogen malabsorption during and following episodes of acute diarrhea has been documented by a number of other studies. Losses may be as high as 200 to 400 mg/kg/day (chapter 11) and may decrease rapidly during recovery. Although the coefficient of nitrogen absorption is low during the acute episode, it is possible to increase the absolute amounts absorbed by increasing the quantities provided by the diet. Some pathogens have greater impact than others (see Ayesha Molla *et al.*, chapter 9, Table VI), probably depending on the mechanisms through which they damage mucosal function. *Shigella* infection, which affects the mucosa of the colon, is associated with decreased coefficient of nitrogen absorption, probably by increasing endogenous losses of plasma, leukocytes, erythrocytes, and intestinal epithelial cells. Some of the protein loss may be a consequence of exudative enteropthy. Increased fecal amino acid losses in acute diarrhea have also been documented by Ghadimi and Tejani.[4] The magnitude of fat malabsorption may depend on the etiology of the diarrhea. Rotavirus infection, which damages the epithelium of the proximal intestine, is associated with greater losses than, for example, *Shigella* infection (see Ayesha Molla *et al.*, chapter 9, Table VII).

Mild diarrhea increases fat excretion from 6 to 14% to about 28%, and in severe diarrhea to over 40%. As with nitrogen malabsorption, the speed of recovery is quite variable. Carbohydrate absorption is decreased in diarrhea caused by rotavirus or *Shigella*, but apparently not in that due to toxigenic *Escherichia coli* or *Vibrio cholerae*. Thus, the effect depends on the invasiveness of the responsible organism.

Invasive infections that cause fever and considerable alterations in systemic metabolism as well as diarrhea produce the greatest metabolic alterations, especially a protein deficit. In adults, the protein losses may reach 0.9 g/kg/day during illness. If there is a loss of serum proteins into the feces as in shigellosis, the protein loss may range from 1.0 to 1.4 g per kg/day.

Considering these consequential losses and the fact that there may be residual defects in nutrient absorption for some weeks after the acute phase of the illness, it should be readily apparent why it takes so long to make up the deficits induced by such infections. It would also seem reasonable that the protein-to-energy ratio would have to increase during repletion. A 30% increase in calories and a 100% increase in protein has been recommended by Whitehead to optimize repletion in young children depleted by infection.[5] Whitehead's estimate of caloric requirements for catch-up growth (approximately 143 kcal/kg) is at the upper range of energy needs specified in the RDA for children in the 6- to 7-kg weight range[6] and found to be required by MacLean and Graham in their treatment of malnourished infants.[7] While Whitehead's estimate of protein requirements (approximately 4 g/kg) is high by present standards (about 2 g/kg), it coincides with the observed intake of recovering children reported by Holt and Fales.[8]

Carbohydrate malabsorption in acute diarrhea has been documented by Lugo-de-Rivera and co-workers.[9] Lifshitz *et al.*[10] have shown that as the severity of diarrhea increases, and as bacterial counts in the upper intestine rise, children develop disaccharide intolerance, the most common being to lactose.

Giardia lamblia infection is usually asymptomatic in individuals over 2 years of age. In children below that age it may be found in the stools in association with diarrheal episodes (Brunser *et al.*, unpublished data, 1981). Acute episodes and chronic, symptomatic *Giardia* infections are associated with increased fecal fat and nitrogen losses.

Total energy losses, resulting from the combination of all of the preceding causes, may reach nutritionally important levels. Schneider has reported fecal losses of about 150 cals/24 hours, or 5% of the intake of 2800 calories in Guatemalan adults.[11]

In Acute, Prolonged Diarrhea. In a few infants, what started as an episode of acute diarrhea will not respond to dietetic or antibiotic therapy. When the duration of the episode exceeds 3 weeks, the name "prolonged diarrhea" is applied. This condition is characterized by nutritional deterioration, severe diarrhea with food intake, and a tendency to dehydration. The intestinal mucosa is thin, with moderate to severe damage. There is a decrease in its digestive and transport capacity. Mortality is very high unless patients are carefully treated. Total parenteral nutrition helps to maintain hydration and to restore nutritional status. At the same time, it probably allows the small intestine lesion to heal. Oral feeding is then carried out with small, frequent feedings of an elemental diet. Volume as well as complexity of the diet are increased, depending on the tolerance of the patient. At the same time, parenteral nutrition is reduced. It may take many months before these patients are able to tolerate a normal diet. While prolonged diarrhea is not common, it is disastrous for the individual in whom it develops.

Subclinical, Chronic Environmental Enteropathy. Chronic ingestion of bacteria originating from a contaminated environment results in morphologic and functional changes in the intestinal mucosa. The former are characterized by blunting of the villi and increases in epithelial and lamina propria lymphoid cells. The functional changes are characterized by malabsorption that may result in important losses of nutrients. Provided that the dietary intake is adequate, some of these intestinal losses may be compensated by other processes. Schneider and co-workers[11] showed that, with protein intakes of about 1.5 g/kg per day, Guatemalan villagers with large fecal volumes absorbed less dietary nitrogen than soldiers who lived in a better sanitary environment and whose fecal volumes were smaller (apparent nitrogen absorptions of 77 and 86%, respectively). Nevertheless, nitrogen balance was similar as a result of compensating differences in urinary nitrogen excretion.

Inadequately compensated losses may result in specific nutrient deficiencies. The adaptive mechanism for inadequate dietary energy absorption is primarily a reduction in physical activity, and if this is not sufficient to compensate, weight loss ensues. This is especially true when repeated episodes of clinical diarrhea are accompanied by inadequate dietary intakes, as this may result in cumulative negative balances for one or more nutrients. Unless these losses are compensated by increased intake and absorption, the result will be deranged nutritional status.

Brunser and co-workers (unpublished data) have shown that apparently healthy adult individuals from the medium and low socioeconomic strata have some blunting of villi and crypt elongation, greater basophilia of the cytoplasm of apical cells, and increased numbers of lymphoid cells in the interepithelial cells and the lamina propria. The microvilli of the brush border have somewhat irregular implantation. These morphological changes of the mucosa are known to be associated with subclinical environmental enteropathy wherever it has been studied. It appears with variable degrees of severity in almost every person living in an unsanitary environment, beginning at a very early age.[12] They also have colonization of the upper intestine by aerobic and anaerobic bacteria.

Metabolic (Urinary) Losses of Nitrogen

Information on urinary losses of nutrients as a direct consequence of diarrheal disease is fragmentary and usually inadequately controlled. As in other systemic infections, it may be assumed that invasive, enteric infections will produce metabolic nitrogen losses, especially when accompanied by fever.[13] Nevertheless, the relationship between urinary nitrogen excretion and dietary nitrogen intake and the tendency to compensate for excessive fecal losses by urinary nitrogen retention make it difficult to interpret data on urinary nitrogen losses during acute diarrheal episodes, such as those presented by Ayesha Molla *et al.* and D. Mahalanabis elsewhere in this volume. The urinary N losses related to fever and other stress conditions in diarrheal disease will be particularly important in children, more so in those under 2 years of age, since diarrheal episodes are often accompanied by a decrease in protein intake because of anorexia and/or maternal behavior in relation to feeding practices.

Diarrheal episodes in the course of metabolic studies are not uncommon, but unfortunately the studies are usually terminated or the data discarded unreported. Moreover, studies based on individuals under diverse experimental conditions do not permit generalization. Negative nitrogen balance during diarrhea is generally observed, but much of it is because of decreased food intake and intestinal malabsorption. Available information on urinary losses is summarized in chapter 11.

Data from Schneider's studies presented by Torún (chapter 15) in this volume suggest that adult men with relatively low chronic absorption of nitrogen, total energy, and D-xylose have lower urinary nitrogen losses and similar nitrogen retentions compared with their counterparts who absorbed better.

Loss into Intestinal Lumen

Loss of protein in the intestinal lumen occurs in children suffering from celiac disease, measles, and kwashiorkor, all of which are manifested by severe loss of body mass and malnutrition. The loss of protein is assumed to be due to extensive ulceration of the large bowel and exudation of the serum protein. Recently, Rahaman and Wahed (Chapter 10) devised a methodology to quantify the loss of protein in the feces of patients suffering from acute diarrheas of various etiologies. Results showed that about two-thirds of the patients studied with enteropathogenic *E. coli* (ETEC), 40% of those with rotavirus, and nearly 100% of patients with *Shigella* lost a substantial amount of protein, as indicated by the marker alpha l-antitrypsin in their feces. Patients with shigellosis on admission were losing between 100 and 500 ml of serum in feces each day. This dropped steadily as the diarrhea subsided and was usually normal by the sixth day.

INTERNAL LOSSES

To ensure the proper nutritional status of the young child, nutrient intake must be sufficient for maintenance of tissues, growth, and physical activity. Under conditions of stress, such as infection, nutrients are required for physiological responses with obvious or presumed survival value, for example, tissue repair or fever, or for the increased synthesis of cellular and soluble protein components of the immune response and the acute phase protein reactants. When intake is limited, these stress requirements may necessitate sacrifice in terms of tissue maintenance, growth, and physical activity. This diversion can be conceptualized as an internal loss of nutrients, and an increase in nutrient supply is essential to restore positive balances.

Fever. Homeothermy in the human is a well-regulated function. Resting energy expenditures are at a minimum at the normal core temperature but increase sharply with either increases or decreases in temperature. Elevation above normal temperature imposes a 13% increase in basal metabolic rate per °C of temperature in adults. Measurement of the metabolic expenditure at rest of hospitalized patients under the stress of surgical procedures and/or infection shows an increase of 25 to 40% in resting metabolic expenditures. The cost is even greater in infants in whom the relatively large surface area/unit body weight imposes more stringent requirements for metabolic heat production. The actual cost in additional energy consumption to raise body temperature depends upon the balance between heat loss (which is decreased under elevated ambient temperatures or by the insulating effect of subcutaneous fat, and is increased by peripheral vasodilitation, etc.) and demands for heat production from muscle (shivering) to raise body temperature. Body temperature is physiologically regulated by adjustments in both heat production and heat loss under thermostatic control by the hypothalamus. In adults, a period of intense shivering for only 10 to 15 minutes will increase energy consumption threefold, and this level of energy use extends for at least 50 to 60 minutes in order to pay off the incurred oxygen debt.

Fever appears to be a primitive response, present even in poikilothermic animals, in which behavioral modification, rather than regulated heat production, is used to raise body temperature. The inflammatory stress that incites the fever response causes release of a small polypeptide from monocytes (a monokine, endogenous pyrogen), which acts to reset the hypothalamic thermostatic set point, apparently via regulation of prostaglandin synthesis. Purified endogenous pyrogen also has immunoregulatory effects, as it appears to be biologically identical to leukocyte-activating factor (LAF). There are reports, largely anecdotal, that severely malnourished children do not develop a normal fever response to infection. It is not known how often this is the case, whether endogenous pyrogen is produced in such patients, if the hypothalamus is fully responsive to the monokine, or if inhibitory substances are present.

Endogenous Energy Sources in Infection. During systemic infections, the pattern of energy utilization is altered. The pool size of glucose increases and glucose oxidation and turnover are augmented. Fasting levels of insulin, glucagon, growth hormone, and corticosteroids are elevated, and the normal response of hormone levels to glucose infusion is distorted, resulting in a diabetic type of glucose disappearance curve. The major source of energy is via *de novo* hepatic gluconeogenesis. This occurs largely at the expense of protein stores via deamination of amino acids, principally alanine. The source of amino acids appears to be the contractile proteins of muscle. Catabolism of muscle has been demonstrated by measurement of 3-methyl-histidine metabolism, which is a marker for muscle protein. The rate of conversion of alanine to glucose, assessed with ^{14}C-alanine, is increased beyond the rate of glucose utilization, accounting for the fasting hyperglycemia. The alteration in normal regulatory feedback mechanisms is also observed here, for the increase in gluconeogenesis in the septic patient is not suppressed by glucose infusion as it is in the fasting normal subject.

These metabolic alterations have not been documented in the common diarrheal diseases but would certainly be expected to be present in diarrheas associated with fever. Catabolic events are reflected in the weight loss that occurs during diarrhea, correcting for dehydration. However, weight loss is certainly in part caused by decreased food intake, estimated to be 160 kcal/day in a field study of Guatemalan children.

Since carbohydrate storage pools are limited, and the induced "pseudodiabetic state" and insulin resistance preclude effective use of energy stored as fat, under conditions of preexisting malnutrition or hepatic damage gluconeogenesis may not be adequate to meet demands, either because of reduced supplies of gluconeogenic precursor amino acids or abnormalities in hepatic function *per se.* Under these conditions hypoglycemia may occur, and hypoglycemic convulsions can occur during acute diarrhea, especially in infants and children.

Turnover of Leukoyctes. Granulocytes are present in three pools: in blood, in tissue, and in the bone marrow. Each of these pools may have several subcompartments, as, for example, the circulating and marginated (endothelium adherent) compartments in the blood. There are approximately 10^{10} granulocytes/kg body weight. Over 90% are present in the marrow, 6 to 8% are in the blood, equally divided between circulating and marginated compartments, and a few percent are transiently present in tissues. Production and maturation occurs in the marrow, the cells are released to the blood pool, which has a half-life of about 7 hours, and these cells transiently pass through tissues where they die or exit from the body via mucous membrane surfaces.

Daily turnover can be estimated from the blood pool size and the half-life, and approximates 10^9 cells/kg body weight/day. Under normal circumstances, and estimating the protein content to be 50 mg/10^9 cells, daily protein synthesis in production of granulocytes is 50 mg/kg body weight. If the energy cost of protein synthesis is estimated at 5 kcal/gram, then the energy requirement for normal granulocyte turnover calculates to be 0.25 kcal/kg body weight/day. Demands for increased granulocyte production during various disease states may accelerate up to about 10-fold, representing a maximum energy cost of 2.5 kcal/kg body weight/day. During acute infection, preformed cells are released from the marrow storage compartment, but the biosynthetic costs do not change if one assumes that the storage compartment must eventually be repleted.

Turnover of Plasma Proteins. Increased consumption and turnover of a number of plasma proteins occur during acute infection. These include the complement proteins, immunoglobulins, and the largely liver-derived acute phase proteins (APPs) such as C-reactive protein, serum amyloid A protein, alpha-1-acidglycoprotein and alpha-1-antitrypsin. For some of the APPs, serum levels increase from barely detectable levels to the mg/dl range, a dramatic increase in specific biosynthetic activity, estimated to be equivalent to a turnover of 350 to 700 grams of protein during the course of systemic infections in adults. This figure should be compared to the total turnover of some 300 to 400 grams of protein per day in normal adults.

At the same time, however, priorities for protein synthesis in the liver are altered and production of albumin decreases. The rapid drop in serum albumin levels during sepsis reflects both the decreased production and increased breakdown of this protein. To the extent that the decreased anabolism of albumin compensates for the increased production of APPs, there may be little or no additional nutrient requirements involved. However, net nitrogen balance is severely affected by the other metabolic changes occurring, particularly the catabolism of muscle protein, deamination, and increased excretion of nitrogen (10 to 15 grams/day in septic adults).

Nutritional Repletion in Adults

Nutrients lost due to diarrheal disease must be repleted during or after the diarrheal episode. The amounts of nutrients to be repleted will depend on the nature, intensity, and duration of the diarrhea. Thus, diarrhea caused by rotavirus, *Giardia lamblia*, or other agents of malabsorptive diarrhea may produce larger nitrogen and vitamin losses than secretory diarrheas do (e.g., cholera, enterotoxigenic *E. coli*). Similarly, chronic diarrheas may produce a depletion of some nutrients that would not be significant if confined to acute episodes. An example is the development of vitamin B_{12} deficiency in tropical sprue.

The extent of possible repletion of nutrients during the acute diarrheal episode will be dealt with in chapter 17 of this volume. During convalescence from diarrhea, allowances should be made for additional amounts of the nutrients that were lost, or that were not ingested because of anorexia or dietary restrictions. It is difficult to specify the precise amounts of additional nutrients or food required, not only because of the great variation in the disease itself but also because of possible adaptive changes. These may include changes in the efficiency of utilization of some nutrients (e.g., greater N retentions after protein depletion) and other complex, not well-understood regulatory mechanisms (e.g., interactions of energy intake, energy expenditure, and weight changes). However, it seems sound to recommend a period of higher energy intake, proportional to the loss of weight, after correcting dehydration, and of more dietary protein, proportional to the duration of anorexia and diarrhea. The need will generally be greater in malabsorptive than in inflammatory or secretory diarrheas. Repletion of vitamins and minerals will depend mainly on the duration of the disease and on the intestinal segment involved (e.g., duodenojejunitis or colitis).

In summary, individuals should be provided with diets with more essential nutrients after a diarrheal disease so that rapid repletion is assured. This can be of critical importance if the patient has had a marginal or inadequate dietary intake and nutritional status before the diarrheal episode.

SIGNIFICANCE OF REPLETION FOR CATCH-UP GROWTH

In children, diarrhea causes both a depletion of lean body mass and a cumulative deficit due to growth failure. While this is true of all infections, the effects of diarrheal infections tend to be greater because absorption is affected as well as intake and metabolic losses. Certainly dietary intake following diarrhea must be significantly higher if rapid repletion is to occur than for individuals who have not been so depleted.

In adults, catch-up growth is not a concern, but repletion is also important and will not occur satisfactorily unless food intake is greater than required for maintenance. The largest effect is on protein needs, but increased dietary calories, vitamins, and minerals are all required for optimum recovery.

PRACTICAL IMPLICATIONS

Table I lists the various kinds of nutrient loss in diarrhea. Individually, some are small, but the cumulative effect is nutrient depletion, weight loss, growth impairment, and sometimes precipitation of clinical nutritional disease. The nitrogen retentions observed during the recovery period from diarrheal and other infectious episodes usually exceed the measured losses. The most likely explanation is that this is due to the considerable nitrogen that is diverted to internal protein synthesis associated with the body's response to infection.

Nevertheless, the effect on *average* requirements of the total population is small and probably negligible in most populations, even those that are underprivileged. This is a misleading way to approach consequences for requirements, however, because they are important primarily during the recovery period and especially so for young children. It is then that the diet may limit repletion and, in children, catch-up growth. Field data indicate that if children do not catch up within a reasonable period, they become stunted. In addition, if the diet is not adequate for prompt repletion and catch-up, the effects of diarrheal and other infections during the weaning period, i.e., in children 6 months to 2 years of age, tend to be additive and lead to the precipitation of clinically evident nutritional disease.

Safe allowances for protein are designed to allow for the needs of nearly all of the population and are now calculated to be 25% above the estimated mean requirement. There is a similar need to specify the additional amount of protein and energy that would be required for the catch-up needs of nearly all children following an episode of diarrheal or other infections. Whether or not the distribution of catch-up is skewed, if an allowance is made for five, seven, or nine times the mean daily growth calculated from annual weight increments, then the diet during the catch-up period must provide 48, 72, and 96 more protein and 8, 12, and 16% more calories, based on the 1981 FAO/WHO/UNU Expert Consultation on Protein-Energy Requirements. In terms of food consumption, children will eat much less than usual during acute episodes of diarrhea and should have available more food than usual during the recovery period when appetite and need are increased.

REFERENCES

1. Mata, L. J. *The Children of Santa María Cauqu^{s}e*. M.I.T. Press, Cambridge, Massachusetts, 1978.
2. Mata, L. J., Kromal, R. A., and Villegas, H. Diarrheal diseases: A leading world health problem. In: *Cholera and Related Diseases*, pp. 1–14. S. Karger, Basel, 1980.
3. Hoyle, B., Yunus, M., and Chen, L. C. Breast-feeding and food intake among children with acute diarrheal disease. *Am. J. Clin. Nutr.* **33**:2365–2371, 1980.
4. Ghadimi, A., and Tejani, A. Protein and amino acid requirements. In: *Total Parenteral Nutrition: Premises and Promises*, A. Ghadimi (Ed.), pp. 213–230. John Wiley, New York, 1975.
5. Whitehead, R. G. Protein and energy requirements of young children living in the developing countries to allow for catch-up growth after infections. *Am. J. Clin. Nutr.* **30**:1545–1547, 1977.
6. Viteri, F. E., Whitehead, R. G., and Young, V. R. (Eds.). *Protein-Energy Requirements under Conditions Prevailing in Developing Countries: Current Knowledge and Research Needs.* The United Nations University World Hunger Programme *Food and Nutrition Bulletin* Supplement No. 3, UNU/WHP, Tokyo, Japan, 1979.
7. MacLean, W. C., Jr., and Graham, G. G. The effect of energy intake on nitrogen content of weight gained by recovering malnourished infants. *Am. J. Clin. Nutr.* **33**:903, 1980.
8. Holt, E., and Fales, H. L. The food requirements of children II. Protein requirements. Am. J. Dis. Child. **22**:371, 1921.
9. Lugo-de-Rivera, C., Rodriguez, H., and Torres-Pinedo, R. Studies on the mechanism of sugar malabsorption in infantile infectious diarrhea. *Am. J. Clin. Nutr.* **25**:1248–1253, 1972.
10. Lifshitz, F., Coelle-Ramirez, P., and Contreras-Gutierrez, M. L. The response of infants to carbohydrate oral loads after recovery from diarrhea. *J. Pediatr.* **79**:612, 1971.
11. Schneider, R. E., Torún, B., Shiffman, M., Anderson, C., and Helms, R. Absorptive capacity of adult Guatemalan rural males living under different conditions of sanita-

tion. In: *Protein-Energy Requirements of Developing Countries: Evaluation of New Data*, B. Torún, V. R. Young, and W. M. Rand (Eds.), pp. 139–149. The United Nations University World Hunger Programme *Food and Nutrition Bulletin* Supplement 5, UNU/ WHP, Tokyo, Japan, 1981.

12. Lindenbaum, J., Harmon, J. W., and Gerson, C. D .Subclinical malabsorption in developing countries. *Am. J. Clin. Nutr.* 25:1056–1061, 1972.

13. Beisel, W. R., Sawyer, W. D., Ryll, E. D., and Crozier, D. Metabolic effects of intracellular infections in man. *Ann. Intern. Med.* 67:744–779, 1967.

17

Therapeutic Interventions in Diarrhea

Jon E. Rohde, Richard A. Cash, Richard L. Guerrant, Dilip Mahalanabis, A. M. Molla, and Aree Valyasevi

Consideration of the formidable array of recent scientific information on the epidemiology, etiology, pathogenesis, and physiologic mechanisms of diarrhea, along with the myriad interrelationships with nutrition, leads, fortunately, to a coherent and relatively concise series of recommendations for the clinical management of these interacting conditions. This summary indicates the practical therapeutic guidelines aimed at the practitioner and community health worker to be derived from the extensive literature. Implementation of these measures will substantially reduce not only the immediate deleterious effects of diarrhea, dehydration, and in some cases death, but also the longer-term, more prevalent, and insidious adverse effects on nutrition.

Fluid and Electrolytes

Extensive reviews have documented the scientific basis as well as the efficacy of oral rehydration therapy (ORT) in acute diarrhea. It is safe,

Jon E. Rohde • Management Sciences for Health, Port-au-Prince, Haiti.   Richard A. Cash • Harvard Institute for International Development, Cambridge, Massachusetts.   Richard L. Guerrant • Division of Geographic Medicine, University of Virginia School of Medicine, Charlottesville, Virginia.   Dilip Mahalanabis • Kothari Centre for Research in Gastroenterology, Calcutta Hospital, Calcutta, India.   A. M. Molla • International Centre for Diarrhoeal Disease Research, Dacca-2, Bangladesh.   Aree Valyasevi • Mahidol University Research Center, Ramathibodi Hospital, Bangkok, Thailand.

more effective, as well as far cheaper than intravenous fluid replacement. While the World Health Organization ORT formula has proved to be effective and safe in the treatment of millions of cases throughout the world, the greatest emphasis should be given to replacement of the fluid and salt losses associated with diarrhea as early as possible in the illness, before the appearance of dehydration. Thus, availability and acceptability of rehydration measures and accessibility of necessary supplies or ingredients are even more critical than precise composition of the resulting formula. Whenever possible, the "complete formula" should be provided, compromising only to ensure acceptance and widespread coverage.

Sodium. The 90-meq/liter solution is effective in all diarrheas, including cholera, but in infants it must be supplemented with low-sodium fluids, preferably breast milk, or, in its absence, dilute feeds, or even plain water. Solutions containing less sodium—50 to 60 mEq/liter—while not effective in the severe secretory diarrheas like cholera, have been used effectively in trials in several countries and may offer a wider margin of safety from electrolyte disorders in the infant age groups.

Bicarbonate. While acidosis invariably accompanies significant fluid loss, the severity is directly related to both volume of diarrhea and degree of dehydration. Thus, early water and salt replacement to avoid dehydration can reduce acidosis even in the absence of base. The acidosis will then resolve through normal renal and respiratory compensatory mechanisms over several days. While the effects of prolonged hypocarbia are not known, it is preferable to provide some base in rehydration solutions. Acetate and citrate are acceptable alternatives to bicarbonate and are easier to incorporate in packaged or tableted ORT production.

Potassium. Although the deficit of total body potassium characterizing malnutrition is invariably exacerbated by acute diarrhea, because of acidosis and extracellular shifts of potassium, this may not be apparent in admission serum measurements. Potassium losses are high, especially in infant diarrheas, and optimal rehydration fluids contain a minimum of 20 meq/liter (WHO formula), with higher concentrations advocated in several studies. As hypokalemia is associated with apathy, decreased appetite, adynamic ileus, and general disturbance of smooth muscle systems, especially in the early rehydrated stage, replacement is an important part of both electrolyte and nutritional therapy. Greater efforts are needed to identify local sources of high-potassium foods and to encourage their use during both home rehydration and convalescence. This specific effect of low body potassium on appetite, however, needs to be defined.

Substrate. An absorbable concentration of 2% glucose (20 gm glucose or 40 gm sucrose/liter) is required for optimal absorption of the salt-water solution. Unfortunately, higher concentrations of sugar are not well tolerated because of high osmotic activity that often exacerbates diarrhea. Thus, ORT provides very few calories (8 kcal/100 cc) at a time when increased energy sources are badly needed. New research in hypoosmotically active substrate sources such as cereal powders, where long-chain molecules (dextrins, starch) provide glucose at virtually no osmotic cost, is extremely promising. Using 30 gm of rice powder/liter, Molla has data indicating less stool output and better urine flow than with the use of standard ORT containing sucrose: this implies better net absorption. Observations of the effectiveness of K mix for the therapy of kwashiorkor showed marked reduction in deaths from diarrhea and hypoglycemia. The easily absorbed, simple carbohydrate (sucrose) combined with casein hydrolysate (a source of small polypeptides) in a liquid mixture contributed to both nutrition and fluid absorption simultaneously. This is supported by earlier work on the synergistic effects of glycine and glucose in an ORT solution. Inclusion of more nutritious substrates absorbed by various noncompeting pathways offers the prospect of a more efficacious and nutrient-dense rehydration solution. Exploitation of multiple absorptive mechanisms affords possible benefits in (1) increased and faster fluid and electrolyte absorption; (2) increased nutrient absorption providing both energy and amino acids (absorbed by at least four independent or quasi-independent intestinal mechanisms); (3) decreased stool volume, thereby overcoming one of the greatest impediments to lay acceptance of oral rehydration solutions; (4) faster recovery due to (a) shorter cell renewal time as a result of readily available basic nutrients for cell metabolism and (b) better absorption of ORT; (5) better digestion of diet in recovery due to continued enzyme induction, offsetting the known effects of starvation in reducing gut enzymes.

Cereals, legumes, and other locally available, simple foods may thus become, in proper quantities, the basis of a combined fluid-protein-energy oral therapy for diarrhea, a single antidote for the FEM-PEM cycle.

Water. The quantity of water used to mix ORT is obviously as critical to final composition as is the measurement of solutes, an obvious but often overlooked fact. Each country should identify the most widely available, reproducible volume measure and adapt packaging or home-made formulas to this standard measure. Larger-size volumes (in the range of 1 liter) have the advantage of cheaper packaging and less percent variation in final volume, while smaller-volume standards are less subject to bacterial growth through standing and reinforce volume-for-volume replacement of losses—one loose motion, one glass of ORT-type messages. Moreover, the small packet may suggest, incorrectly, to the mother that this amount is sufficient to treat diarrhea.

The best quality water available should be used to prepare ORT, but standards of purity that inhibit the use of ORT should be avoided. There is no evidence that ingestion of ORT dissolved in normally consumed water is any more detrimental than the routine daily risk of the water alone.

FEEDING DURING DIARRHEA

The provision of proper and adequate food *during* the course of diarrhea is a critical factor both in avoidance of adverse nutritional effects and in hastening recovery from the illness. Children fed throughout the acute phase of watery diarrhea absorb substantial quantities of nutrients, demonstrate significantly better weight gain over the course of illness, and, in some studies, have a shorter duration of diarrhea than unfed matched controls. The continued presence of food in the intestine may avoid the development of carbohydrate intolerance and other enzyme-deficiency syndromes reported in some studies where introduction of food following fasting is manifested by a recurrence of fluid loss. Patients with chronic diarrhea have been successfully treated with breast milk and, in some studies, elemental diets. The continuation of feeding throughout diarrhea, especially with breast milk, may well avoid these complications.

Breast milk should be continued *ad lib*, even during the rehydration period, alternating with ORT. Important evidence shows that the anorexia of diarrhea, responsible for a considerable part of nutrient deficiency in diarrhea, does not affect breast-milk intake. Taken in normal or increased quantities, associated with more frequent than usual suckling, breast milk contributes both to rehydration and nutrient needs.

Immediately upon rehydration (4 to 6 hours), other foods should be provided, consisting of components of adult diets suitably prepared for babies, and offered five or more times daily. Traditionally used paps, gruels, soups, and "baby foods" should be avoided because of their relatively low calorie density and lack of other nutrients. Fats are absorbed during acute diarrhea, allowing addition of oils to increase caloric density. Food should be offered after breast-feeding to encourage more complete emptying of the breast with consequent stimulus to milk production.

Convalescent Feeding

Immediately following the cessation of diarrhea there is an apparent rise in appetite, often to supranormal levels, as shown by consumption studies in hospitalized patients. Molla has shown appetite recovery in acute rotavirus, enterotoxigenic *Escherichia coli, Shigella,* and cholera diarrheas occurring between the fourth and seventh days of illness, evidenced by spontaneous consumption of RDA quantities or more of usual foods. Supranormal appetite with intake exceeding 130 kcal per kg of body weight has been documented in several hospital studies.

While underlying malnutrition could account for some of the supranormal appetite seen in the hospital studies, limited observations in normally nourished children indicate the same effect.

Field data on episodes of diarrheal illness in Guatemalan children indicate resumption of preillness intake only, without compensatory intake, but limitation of food available within the home and the variable delay in the convalescent intake study may have obscured postillness increases in food intake. The observation of a consistent negative growth associated with diarrhea (average -3.5 g body weight/day of illness) in this group shows that catch-up growth did not, in fact, occur, as one might expect in the absence of extra food intake. Martorell calculated the food supplement required to offset the deficit, using weight gains observed in supplemented children, and expresses this requirement as 66 kcal/day spread over the entire 6-month period of observation. However, expressed per day of illness, his calculations reveal a 600- to 900-kcal deficit per day of diarrheal illness.

Another means of calculation involves estimated calorie requirement for observed deficits in growth. Weight deficit during diarrhea may average as high as 3 gm/kg/day (seen in The Gambia), surely a combination of catabolic and absorptive losses plus lack of normal growth. Given the anorexia and absorptive losses during diarrhea, even with proper dietary management, nutrient balance is below requirements, with perhaps a 25 to 30% shortfall in calories, roughly the requirement above basal needs for normal growth. This expected rate during age 1 to 5 years is roughly ½ gm/kg per day. Body weight deficit can thus be estimated as 3.5 gm/kg times the number of days ill untreated, plus 0.5 g/kg for continued days under proper fluid and dietary treatment. Given a caloric cost of growth of some 12 kcal/g of body mass (it may be as high as 20 kcal/g), this works out to 42 to 70 kcal/kg per day ill to replace lost growth or, in a 10-kg child, 420 to 700 additional kcal for each day ill.

To be comparable with the Martorell data, which use observed growth in response to consumed nutritional supplements, one must make adjustment for absorptive losses, shown to be some 10 to 20% of energy intake some 2 weeks after cessation of diarrhea. Thus, according to this calculation, some 500 to 800 additional kcal are required for each day of diarrheal illness.

Finally, one can simply calculate the catch-up requirement, assuming that unmet RDAs should be fulfilled in the days following illness. Depending upon how much had been consumed during illness (breast-fed children, for instance, may consume normal quantities in spite of illness), the deficit would range from 40 to 100%, or 400 to 900 kcal for a child 12 to 18 months of age. While derived from quite different observations and assumptions, it is evident that all these approaches give comparable estimates that could easily be summarized as (1) feed the child, during the early period after illness, his normal diet *plus* all the food he did not eat during illness; or (2) feed the child 1½ times his normal diet for twice as many days as he was ill; or (3) feed the child extra food daily until he regains or exceeds his preillness weight.

The evidence suggests that food deficits are roughly equal to replacing food not consumed, and that this should be consumed within a period after illness of some two to four times the duration of illness itself. If recovery is prolonged by spreading the nutrient needs over months, stunting will occur and catch-up growth will not be possible after normal weight/height ratios are reached.

Food should be a normal mixed diet with attention to increasing caloric density; the desired additional intake could be achieved by increasing the frequency of feeding by perhaps an extra meal or even two per day. Full-strength milk can form a normal part of the diet by mixing it with other foods and giving it over the day in small increments. Studies in lactase-deficient, malnourished children, postdiarrhea, have demonstrated a high acceptance of total daily lactose if offered in this manner.

While admittedly difficult to achieve in some patients, especially in the home setting, the accomplishment of supranormal food intakes (some 25 to 50% above RDA) for a period two to four times the duration of illness is an effective means to restore growth and obviate the nutritional effects of diarrhea. Nutrition supplement programs highly targeted to this brief but critical period may be the most nutritionally effective intervention point in the diarrhea—malnutrition cycle.

DRUG THERAPY

The effects on nutrition of all pharmacotherapeutic agents must be considered and carefully documented before endorsing their use in treatment of diarrhea. Many time-honored antidiarrheal agents, as well as drugs targeted at newly discovered pathophysiologic mechanisms, have detrimental effects on the digestive and nutrient absorptive function of the gastrointestinal tract. Several groups are considered.

1. *Anti-motility agents* (opiates, Lomotil, Loperamide) increase duration of secretion of fluid, prolong passage of pathogens, increase fever and related catabolism, and may decrease absorption of nutrients through stasis and puddling in the gut. Traditional wisdom notwithstanding, there is no evidence for an inverse relationship of gut transit time and nutrient absorption in acute diarrhea. Antimotility agents should not be used, except for control of severe cramps and tenesmus in children past infancy.

2. *Adsorbents* (Kaolin, charcoal) have no demonstrable effect on either duration or severity of diarrhea. While not apparently harmful, they detract from more important therapy and should be avoided.

3. *Antisecretory agents* (chlorpromazine, indomethacin, aspirin) work pharmacologically on the various cellular mechanisms responsible for secretion in toxin-produced diarrheas. While they can, in certain circumstances, reduce the volume of stool, the effect can be obtained with proper choice of antibiotics (see below), and possible side effects make their use contraindicated.

4. *Membrane-stabilizing agents* (quinicrine, steroids) are potential drugs to prevent the permeability effects of toxins. There are insufficient data to suggest their use, which would also require a thorough review of potential side effects and nutritional effects.

5. *Traditional diarrhea treatment preparations* (astringents, herbal teas, etc.). While useful effects of the myriad agents used to treat diarrhea in traditional cultures around the world are possible, no careful study has been performed demonstrating efficacy. Because diarrhea is so often a brief and self-limited illness, numerous cures have been used and accepted, ranging from exotic concoctions to injected amino glycosides. None are of proven value—many could be harmful.

6. *Antimicrobial agents* (sulfa drugs, antibiotics). Although long viewed as a digestive malady largely related to "improper food ingestion," diarrhea is now clearly recognized as a symptom of infection in a vast majority of cases. This has led to varying use of antimicrobials, waxing to universal treatment of all cases, waning to proscription of the consideration of antibiotics for even the most severe cases of dysentery. It is no surprise that current consensus falls in a middle ground:

- Acute diarrhea of known and documented etiology should be treated with antibiotics proven appropriate for the illness. Guidelines are given by the World Health Organization for the common bacterial pathogens (cholera, *Campylobacter, Shigella, Salmonella*). Note that even among these recognized pathogens there are indications and reasons *not* to treat with antibiotics.

- For the physician faced with a clinical decision, the most useful indicator in favor of antibiotic use is bloody dysentery, especially when accompanied by fever. Unfortunately, the frequent and varying patterns of resistance seen in *Shigella* necessitate an up-to-date knowledge of the sensitivity of organisms prevalent at the time in the affected community. Short, high-dose therapy is not effective; a desired course should last over 5 days.

    Greater degrees of malnutrition, a more ill-appearing child, and longer duration of diarrhea are considered increasing indications for use of antibiotics, but the use of multiple agents or changing of antibiotics in brief succession is harmful and may lead to development of chronic, intractable diarrhea of infancy.

- There is no role for prophylactic antibiotics to prevent diarrhea, with the possible single exception of doxycline, useful for brief visits to tropical areas. Development of resistant strains, overgrowth of unusual microbes or fungi, and even chronic diarrhea can result.

CONCLUSIONS

Management of acute diarrhea involves replacement by mouth of lost fluid, electrolytes, continued breast-milk feeding, and rapid and full reintroduction of the full diet. It should be understood that, while ORT will not necessarily reduce volume of diarrhea (it may and will frequently increase for a brief period as hydration is restored), it will prevent dehydration, restore normal fluid electrolyte balance, and improve appetite. Feeding contributes both to early cessation of diarrhea and to minimizing the detrimental impact of the illness on nutrition.

During convalescence, the days immediately following illness, great attention should be given to increased dietary intake through higher-calorie foods and greater frequency of feeding to achieve an additional food intake roughly equivalent to the food not eaten during illness. Catch-up growth to pre-illness levels should be achieved within three to four times the duration of illness.

While antibiotics are indicated in cases of dysentery and certain other diarrheas with clear bacterial etiologies, their indiscriminate use can be harmful. Indeed, the typical history of a child with intractable diarrhea of infancy, an often fatal chronic disease, includes cessation of breast-feeding, indiscriminate use of multiple antibiotics, and intermittent or prolonged periods of fasting in response to an initial acute diarrheal episode. While chronic diarrhea presents a difficult clinical management problem for which clear therapeutic guidelines are lacking, an effective treatment of acute diarrhea, as outlined in this report, is an important means to avoid the emergence of chronic cases.

18

Prevention and Control of the Diarrheal Diseases

ROBERT E. BLACK, LINCOLN C. CHEN, OSCAR HARKAVY,
M. MUJIBUR RAHAMAN, AND M. G. M. ROWLAND

INTRODUCTION

This chapter deals primarily with those measures that are designed to reduce the incidence of acute diarrheal illness of infectious origin. The two obvious measures are improved environmental sanitation and personal hygiene and better nutrition. However, the outcome of diarrheal disease may be powerfully influenced by management of the acute case, providing an opportunity to prevent some of the sequelae with which this volume is concerned. These consequences include life-threatening dehydration and serious growth impairment. Therapeutic actions, covered in the preceding chapter, are therefore in some sense also essential components of prevention.

Both the incidence of diarrhea and the severity of its consequences decline with increasing age. Children under the age of 5 years bear a major burden of the morbidity, but it is the children under 2 years on whom the impact of diarrhea and associated malnutrition is greatest. The preventive strategies outlined here will therefore be strongly oriented toward reducing morbidity, and hence mortality, in this young age group.

ROBERT E. BLACK • University of Maryland School of Medicine, Center for Vaccine Development, Baltimore, Maryland. LINCOLN C. CHEN • Ford Foundation, New Delhi Field Office, New Delhi, India. OSCAR HARKAVY • Population Office, The Ford Foundation, New York, New York. MUJIBUR RAHAMAN • International Centre for Diarrhoeal Disease Research, Dacca-2, Bangladesh. M. G. M. ROWLAND • Medical Research Council Laboratories, Fajara, Banjul, The Gambia, West Africa.

Epidemiologic Considerations

In general, acute diarrhea is the result of the fecal-oral transmission of an infectious dose of one or more enteropathogens to a susceptible subject. Considerable variation is observed in the precise route followed by different organisms in different circumstances, but certain generalizations may be made.

Enterotoxigenic *Escherichia coli* are pathogens of major importance in early childhood. They are commonly found in early weaning foods, introduced by contaminated water supplies, contaminated utensils, and unhygienic food-handling. The problem is aggravated by the rapid multiplication that occurs in food if it is not consumed soon after preparation. Because *E. coli* is such an important pathogen in childhood diarrhea, interrupting its mode of transmission assumes particular importance in diarrhea prevention and control.

Other important pathogens are rotaviruses, *Shigellae*, and *Giardia lamblia*. These organisms do not usually multiply or even survive in the environment, but they are infectious in relatively small doses, and person-to-person spread is important. Their mode of spread underscores the importance of household and personal hygiene. *Campylobacter jejuni* and *Salmonellae*, in contrast, infect many animal species besides man. They thus may be spread directly by contact with animal feces, as well as through contaminated food or water.

Feces Disposal

It is clear from even this superficial overview of diarrheal disease transmission that the safe disposal of human feces (and the exclusion of animal feces from the home environment) should logically lead to major reductions in transmission of many, if not all, of the above agents of diarrheal disease with a corresponding reduction of morbidity and mortality. In practice, few sanitation schemes have met with success, at least in the short term. Recurring shortcomings of such schemes include failure to assess disease perceptions and culturally entrenched behavior patterns of relevance in a community; maladaptation between sanitary technology and the needs of a specific community; education toward optimal use of the facilities; and in general enlisting the active participation of the community in the program. Particular priority should be accorded to the safe disposal of feces from active diarrheal cases, as they contribute the overwhelming proportion of pathogens in the environment. With the exception of infrequent asymptomatic carriers of enteric pathogens, excreta from healthy persons do not transmit disease.

It should be recognized that in many communities, even where basic sanitation facilities exist and adults use them, young children are often permitted to defecate indiscriminately. Because diarrhea attack rates are highest among children, it is the defecation in this age group that deserves most attention.

WATER SUPPLIES

Contaminated water plays an important role in the transmission of enteropathogens, and there are usually strong desires at many levels of society for the provision of readily available, potable water. However, improved water supplies have many objectives (including lessening the work burden of women and children), only one of which is improved health. Many major capital-intensive water improvement schemes have often been singularly ineffective in reducing diarrheal morbidity. As noted elsewhere in this volume, many diarrheal agents are not primarily waterborne; furthermore, it may be the quality and usage pattern of water in the home, not the purity of water at its source, that largely determines the impact of diarrheal morbidity on individual members of the community, particularly the children.

It is specious, therefore, to limit the consideration of water supplies to the provision of plentiful clean water at a common community source. Effective water improvement schemes should be accompanied by a health education component aimed at improving personal hygiene, with special reference to food hygiene and particularly weaning food preparation, as described later. The provision of comprehensive water supplies is often prohibitively expensive in most situations and may consume large resources, compromising possible investments in other equally or more effective interventions.

CHILD-REARING PRACTICES

Irrespective of the quality of the water and sanitary environment, it is the immediate physical environment to which the child is exposed, determined in large measure by personal hygiene, child care, and feeding practices of the mother, that is crucial in influencing transmission of diarrhea among infants and children. These aspects of the immediate environment of the child are strongly influenced by individual behavior. While relatively underinvestigated, personal behavior represents the most creative and potentially effective area for intervention to prevent diarrhea. This kind of intervention does not depend upon major, capital-intensive investments and thus supports the self-sufficiency of poor families. Two such behavior patterns that might be influenced favorably by intervention are breast-feeding and weaning practices.

Breast-Feeding

Any measures to promote breast-feeding in communities where it is not universally practiced, and to support and sustain the lactating mother and her milk output, are likely to reduce both the prevalence and the impact of diarrhea in infants. These measures might include strong efforts at the national level to limit the promotion and inappropriate use of commercial infant formulas. At the community level, health and nutrition interventions during pregnancy may influence birth weight and subsequent milk production, and delay the time at which other foods are required to complement the diet of the breast-fed infant. In this effort to maximize the quantity of breast milk as a safe supply of appropriate nutrients, it should be recognized that it may be possible in the future to boost the antiinfective properties in breast milk through specific interventions.

In terms of protection against diarrhea, breast-feeding probably has an important direct role for up to 6 months, and an indirect effect, by its contribution to the nutrition of young children, into the second year of life. There is, however, little doubt that even breast-fed infants enter the high-risk category, in terms of both the frequency and the impact of diarrhea, as soon as any kind of supplementary food is introduced.

This introduction of foods should therefore not begin unnecessarily early. The common practice of regular administration of drinks of water, juice, etc., to otherwise exclusively breast-fed infants should be critically examined and eliminated if no demonstrable benefits are documented. Advice on the most appropriate time for the introduction of supplementary foods should ideally be given to individuals on the basis of longitudinal monitoring of infant growth, incorporated into primary health care programs. Attempts at blanket recommendations on the timing of supplements are correctly controversial. They will probably be inappropriate for entire communities, let alone individuals, and may be ignored by mothers.

Weaning Food Technology

Contaminated weaning foods of all sorts have been identified as major vehicles for the transmission of fecal pathogens during early infancy. This contamination appears to be worst in the earliest weaning foods, often dilute cereal gruels or cow's milk, or formula. Three aspects of weaning food technology should be examined for possible preventive interventions.

Preparation of "Dry" Ingredients. Bacterial contamination and multiplication can be reduced by developing and using "dry" weaning foods, which are subject to fewer risks of contamination and do not facilitate bacterial growth as readily as wet preparations do in tropical climates. Food preparation utensils, even when ostensibly cleaned, are commonly fecally contaminated in poor communities. Often, the foods themselves are contaminated with infectious organisms. A further input of pathogens results from food-handling, which could presumably be reduced by improved personal hygiene. A major source of contamination may be the quality of domestic water, reflecting water contaminated either at its source or during subsequent collection and storage in the home. Water for food production should be treated with the same care as drinking water. Much of the bacterial input could be reduced by dry storage and preparation of grains.

Cooking. More complete cooking of foods would reduce or eradicate pathogens. Constraints on cooking may be economic (fuel availability), time, and the effect on the final consistency of food (e.g., boiled cereal gruels become too glutinous). Village technology to reduce this gluey quality already exists in some societies (e.g., germination and malting), hence permitting boiling of the gruel, and incidentally increasing bioavailability of nutrients. However, if the stages prior to cooking result in a "cleaner" product that can be stored safely, there may be little additional virtue in complete cooking.

Delays in Consumption. Usually, traditional foods are time-consuming to prepare and a mother's time is hard-pressed by other work demands. Thus, weaning foods are often made in bulk and fed to young children over the course of 1 or 2 days. Under such circumstances, high levels of enteropathogens in food are almost inevitable, because of rapid proliferation under tropical conditions. Every effort should therefore be made to reduce the standing time of already cooked weaning foods. Again, village technologies exist in some areas to ensure good shelf life and reduce the need for cooking, as in the case of traditionally made yogurts.

Nutrient Density and Quality

In addition to the problem of contamination, many early weaning foods are often grossly deficient in energy and nutrient content. As such, they fail to supply the necessary supplements, while exposing the infant to increased risk of diarrhea. Some of these problems can be overcome by the incorporation of calorically dense oils and fats in the weaning food. More frequent feeds also increase overall intake while simultaneously reducing the standing time of already cooked weaning foods.

HOUSEHOLD HYGIENE

Increasingly, epidemiological and microbiological evidence has demonstrated that high levels of household contamination play a critical role in diarrheal disease transmission. Environmental surveillance invariably documents positive cultures for fecal coliforms in utensils, vessels, dishes, fingers, and other household sources. One key to the interruption of disease transmission, therefore, is use of household "technologies" and practices that either reduce the overall level of household fecal contamination or prevent the oral ingestion of fecally contaminated fluids and foods. Excreta disposal is obviously critical in this regard. Other means include simple, low-cost technologies such as "thin-necked" water storage vessels that prevent hand-contamination of drinking water, the use of alkaline limewater to clean child diapers and soiled hands, simple chlorination of water in the home before drinking, and simple gates and fences to segregate animals from living quarters.

Such technologies and practices should be developed to be consistent with specific local circumstances. It is also possible that behavioral changes, such as hand-washing, may reduce disease transmission. These behavioral and technologic changes often can be achieved at low financial cost. Thus, within specific geocultural settings, it may be feasible to develop and promote practices that are consistent with the economic and cultural realities confronting individual families.

ACCESS TO AND USE OF FAMILY RESOURCES

There is presumptive evidence that some of the differences in diarrheal prevalence and malnutrition between families may be related to the varying efficiency and effectiveness of families, particularly the mother, in the use of available family resources. Promotion of breast-feeding and the preparation, cooking, and serving of uncontaminated nutritious weaning foods cited earlier are two such examples. Other illustrations are improved intrafamilial distribution of food to individual members, particularly to mothers and children. There is some indirect evidence that the educational level of parents, especially mothers, is an important ingredient in effective use of family resources.

Prevention of diarrhea and malnutrition may also be improved by access to, and more effective use of, public and private social services by a family. Prompt and proper treatment of infections at a health center, for example, would not only reduce the nutritional impact of disease but would also enhance host defense systems of the child against the next infection. In this regard, the role and status of women in a society, and their access to modern health knowledge, may be critical in more effective use of external resources.

Role of the Physician and Other Health Professionals

The implementation of many of the preventive interventions at the personal, household, and community levels cited in this chapter will require their integration into community-based health programs. Although not a direct intervention, the training and reorientation of health professionals, especially physicians, are seen as critical adjuncts to successful implementation.

Arguably, the physician, as typically trained in modern, high-technology, hospital-based medicine, is singularly unsuited to direct community-based programs of diarrhea prevention and other elements of primary health care among disadvantaged populations. Furthermore, notions of appropriate diarrhea management, as transmitted in the leading medical textbooks, are outmoded for both developing and developed societies in light of recent research findings, as reported in this volume, and have been shown to be detrimental to the rapid recovery of the patient. Efforts to reorient the physician and other health professionals through training courses, seminars, and wider dissemination of current research results should be considered an essential component of fostering the preventive measures proposed in this chapter.

19

Diarrhea and Malnutrition

Research Priorities

Ranjit K. Chandra, William B. Greenough, Richard
L. Guerrant, Reynaldo Martorell, Leonardo J.
Mata, Kenneth S. Warren, and Cheng-chien Wu

There have been many recent advances in our understanding of the
etiology, pathogenesis, mechanisms, and management of acute and
chronic diarrheal disease. Many studies have investigated the role of
diarrhea in producing or worsening malnutrition. However, the working group identified several areas of diarrhea–malnutrition interactions
where current knowledge is incomplete or nonexistent.

A set of general objectives for future research is given in Table I.
First, it is desirable to continue investigation of causative and contributory factors, both microbial and epidemiologic, that are important in the
occurrence of acute and chronic diarrhea. It is imperative that such studies adopt new technologies, including viral and immunologic diagnostic
methods. The investigation of the etiology of diarrheal disease is most
relevant in those parts of the world where malnutrition continues to be
an important public health problem.

Second, studies should be undertaken to link the severity, duration,
and etiology of diarrhea to its nutritional consequences in terms of food

Ranjit K. Chandra • Memorial Univeristy of Newfoundland, St. John's, Newfound-
land.   William B. Greenough • International Centre for Diarrhoeal Disease
Research, Dacca-2, Bangladesh.   Richard L. Guerrant • Division of Geographic
Medicine, University of Virginia School of Medicine, Charlottesville, Vir-
ginia.   Reynaldo Martorell • Food Research Institute, Stanford University, Palo
Alto, California.   Leonardo J. Mata • Instituto de Investigaciones en Salud, Univ-
ersidad de Costa Rica, San Pedro, Costa Rica.   Kenneth S. Warren • The Rockefeller
Foundation, New York.   Cheng-chien Wu • Chinese Academy of Medical Sciences,
Beijing, People's Republic of China.

Table I.   General Objectives for Future Research on Diarrheal Disease

To further investigation of etiologic and epidemiologic factors in the genesis of acute and chronic diarrhea

To study the nutritional consequences of the severity and duration of diarrhea of various etiologies

To examine sociocultural, behavioral, and anthropologic factors affecting the occurrence of diarrhea and its management

To apply present and emerging technology for reducing the impact of diarrheal diseases in the most cost-effective manner

selection and intake, nutrient absorption, loss and diversion of nutrients, and nutritional cost of catabolic-anabolic processes.

Third, the role of socioeconomic and behavioral factors in the production of diarrheal disease is becoming increasingly apparent. The modern tools of anthropologic research should be used to define some of these contributory factors so that one can better define the most practical and effective methods for control and prevention.

Fourth, the most appropriate methods of intervention must be defined. In order to achieve this, there is need for further research into

Table II.   Checklist of Specific Areas of Research in Diarrheal–Malnutrition Interactions

Nutritional impact	Functional implications	Interventions[a]
Reduced intake	Physical activity	Epidemiologic
Anorexia	Growth and development	Breast-feeding, causes of decline
Diet selection	Socioeconomic cost	Water (at point of use, change with
Reduced absorption	Learning	behavioral alterations)
Increased losses		Physiologic
Nutrients in urine,		ORT[b] delivery
stool		Antimicrobial
Metabolic		Pharmacologic
Protein synthesis		Antisecretory
Cell turnover		Antiattachment
Acute phase reactants		Immunologic
Sequestration		Antiviral
		Antitoxic
		Antiattachment
		Dietary
		Child
		Mother

[a]The most important and feasible form of intervention may vary with culture and stage of development of the region.
[b]ORT = oral rehydration therapy.

Table III. Some Specific Topics for Future Research on Diarrheal Disease

1. Etiopathogenesis and epidemiology
Behavioral, sociocultural, and anthropologic determinants of food and water handling and hygiene in the causation of diarrhea.

Synergism between parasites and accepted agents of diarrheal disease, especially with regard to their combined impact on nutritional status.

Age-related changes in susceptibility to infectious diarrhea (e.g., maturation of local intestinal defense, both antigen-specific and nonspecific, receptors on epithelial cells).

The incidence and nutritional cost of mixed viral-bacterial infections of the intestine.

Investigation of the nature and nutritional implications of environmental enteropathy (tropical sprue, etc.).

Assessment of the magnitude and impact of chronic diarrhea.

Determinants of disease severity with regard to nutritional impact (e.g., extent of mucosal damage, amount of toxin produced).

The role of gut microflora in the causation of diarrhea and its nutritional effects.

Microbial contamination of local foods; how does water contamination contribute to food spoilage?

2. Nutritional impact
What is the nutritional cost of apparently asymptomatic, unrecognized infection with enteric organisms?

What are the catabolic effects of noninvasive microorganisms associated with diarrhea?

How does one distinguish the nutritional effects of diarrhea in terms of the impact of the infection *per se*, and of the secondary complications due to disease (e.g., sugar intolerance) and iatrogenic factors (dietary advice, drugs).

3. Outcome
What s the impact of diarrhea-associated nutritional deficits on growth and development?

What are the effects of the diarrhea-malnutrition complex on physical activity and work performance?

To what extent does nutritional deficiency consequent to diarrheal disease influence learning ability?

Table III. (continued)

4. Interventions
The development and evaluation of weaning foods manufactured by village-level and home technology according to regional and cultural patterns.

The promotion and evaluation of the use of colostrum and breast milk in the prevention and management of diarrhea and other infections frequently encountered in infants.

The study of various practical aspects of oral rehydration therapy (e.g., ingredients, including substrates, delivery, local sources of various ingredients such as potassium, evaluation of effectiveness, impact of rehydration on appetite and food intake).

Detailed observational studies of familial attitudes and practices, sociocultural and anthropologic factors, particularly as they may relate to primary prevention and management of secondary spread within households.

Pharmacologic treatment of diarrhea, including indications, dose, and duration of antimicrobial therapy, and side effects of antisymptomatic drugs.

What are the determinants of clinical and physiologic recovery (e.g., mucosal healing, cell turnover)?

Evaluation of traditional folk medicines.

Management of chronic diarrhea.

the most feasible and practical technology that can be used in the most cost-effective manner to apply current scientific knowledge to reduce the impact of diarrheal disease on individuals and society in terms of nutritional status, growth and development, physical activity, work performance, learning, and other consequences.

Based on these broad general objectives, the working group outlined a few specific areas of research that should receive priority. These are shown in Tables II and III. It is obvious that constraints of various kinds—economic, health, sociocultural, political, etc.—will govern the choice of the particular projects to be undertaken in a given region or institution. But the overall aim is to reduce, in the most expeditious manner, the adverse consequences of diarrheal disease on health and quality of life.

Index